The
Sav-on
Health

self-care

Advisor

The Essential Home Health Guide
for You and Your F

Manufactured in the United States of America
Third edition
First printing: April 2000
10 9 8 7 6 5 4 3 2 1

ISBN 0-7370-1620-5

Medical Advisors

If you don't take care of your body, where will you live?

AARON GOODE, AGE 10

SavonHealth.com
Personal Health Manager

I ntroducing the SavonHealth.com Personal Health Manager! The easiest, most convenient way to manage your health and your family's health. SavonHealth offers comprehensive tools, medical information and records that are available wherever and whenever you need them!

Access
- Determine your personal health status by taking the Health Assessment.
- Use SavonHealth's wealth of content which includes extensive medical information and news articles to learn more about a condition.
- Take a Health Quiz to quickly assess and calculate specific health characteristics.

Record
- Keep track of health information and access it anywhere, anytime!
- Track important health measurements such as your blood pressure.
- Keep track of different facets of your health history such as doctor visits and immunizations.

Improve
- Use SavonHealth's interactive, self-paced improvement programs.
- SavonHealth provides self-paced motivation for a healthy outcome.
- Improve your health and enhance the quality of your life.

Connect
- Create your own personal health manager home page.
- Take advantage of email messaging to receive medication and immunization alerts.
- Access your health record via your wireless phone, PDA or pager!

On SavonHealth, you can also:
- Check for drug interactions.
- Receive email reminders for doctor visits and immunizations.
- Use our convenient link to Savon.com for all your healthcare and prescription purchases!

Health Assessment

Have you ever wondered how your current health and lifestyle impact your future well-being? Curious how your family's health history may influence your risk of disease? Would you like to know what steps you can take today to minimize your risks tomorrow? Would you like to see how your health profile compares to others your age and gender? If you 'answered Yes to any of these questions, then it's time to take the Savon Health Health Assessment.

The Health Assessment is a fast and convenient way to start taking charge of your health. It is a risk-profiling tool based on peer reviewed medical research and recommendations by leading health authorities.

Health Assessment launches a sophisticated program which summarizes your health status, presents your most serious health risks, and recommends actions you can take to minimize those risks.

SavonHealth.com

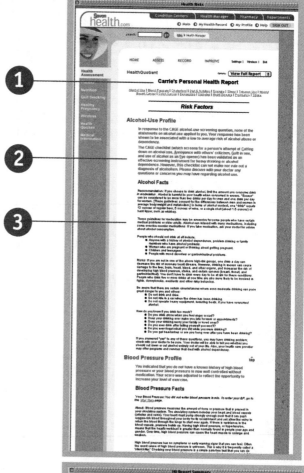

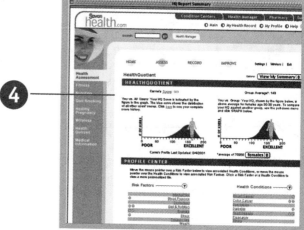

1 ## PERSONAL HEALTH REPORT

Based upon the questions answered during your Health Assessment, a Personal Health Report is compiled based on the following risk factors:

- ➤ Alcohol Use
- ➤ Blood Pressure
- ➤ Cholesterol
- ➤ Diet and Nutrition
- ➤ Exercise
- ➤ Stress
- ➤ Tobacco Use
- ➤ Weight

- ➤ Breast Cancer
- ➤ Colon Cancer
- ➤ Depression
- ➤ Diabetes
- ➤ Heart Disease
- ➤ Pregnancy
- ➤ Stroke
- ➤ Prostate Cancer

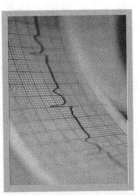

2 ## RISK FACTOR PROFILE

A synopsis of your profile is outlined and categorized. Steps you should take to improve your Health Assessment score are detailed. Your test results are also interpreted in this section.

3 ## RISK FACTOR FACTS

Definitions, risks and treatment options, as well as links for further information and news.

4 ## HEALTH ASSESSMENT SCORE

Scores your overall health and allows you to compare your score to groups of other users. Also access any risk factors or health conditions, be reminded of overdue tests or appointments and recap recommendations.

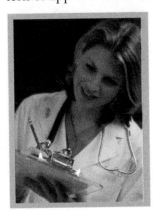

SavonHealth.com

Men's & Women's Health Assessment

GENDER-SPECIFIC, ADVANCED HEALTH ASSESSMENTS

SavonHealth offers two sophisticated Health Assessments that cover topics specific to men's and women's health.

Men's Health Assessment delivers a highly personalized, content-rich report to help men become increasingly proactive about their health. The Men's Assessment covers these vital health issues:

- Stress
- Anger
- Cancer
- Back pain
- Time management
- Sex
- Heart attack risk

Women's Health Assessment is critical for women today as they continue to play the key role in managing their own health and the health of their spouses, children and aging parents. The Women's Assessment covers these vital health issues:

- Birth control
- Stress
- Menstrual Cycles
- Cancer
- Sex
- Hormone replacement
- Heart attack risk

SavonHealth.com

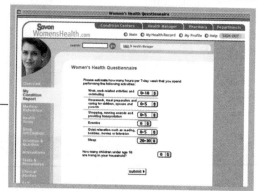

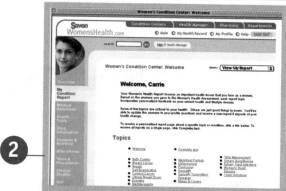

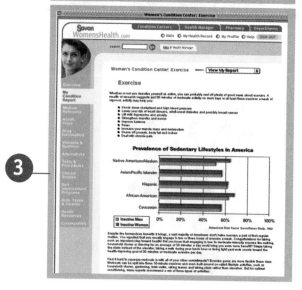

1 GENDER-SPECIFIC HEALTH QUESTIONNAIRE

The Men's and Women's Health program was written by a team of physicians and health educators whose knowledge in this field is based upon over 50 years of practice and research. Find out where you stand on important issues and lifestyle choices facing your gender.

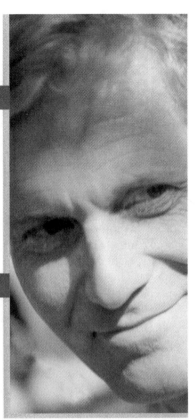

2 GENDER-SPECIFIC CONDITION CENTER

Content is based on recommendations and statistics gleaned from some of the most respected health-related organizations in the country, such as the American Heart Association, the American Cancer Society, and the National Sleep Foundation.

ACCESS

3 PERSONALIZED REPORT PAGE AND CONDITIONS

For selected Risk Factors and Health Conditions, highlights your relative risk and links to clinical feedback personalized to reflect your unique profile.

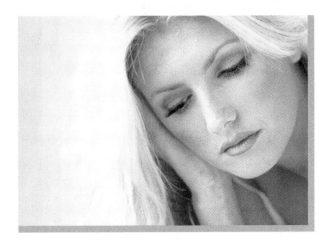

SavonHealth.com

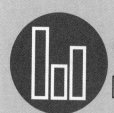

Condition Centers

The SavonHealth condition centers are advanced online assessment tools hat provide educational information, action-oriented next steps and treatment options for specific health conditions. They will help you prepare for doctor visits and also better understand diagnosis of the condition.

The SavonHealth condition centers also provide an integrative approach to prevention and treatment, offering you options in both conventional and alternative medicine.

Condition Center features:
- Immediate, personalized feedback on specific health conditions
- Condition background information
- Lists balanced, unbiased treatment options
- Ranks treatment options according to your preference
- Offers up-to-date, medically valid content

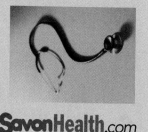

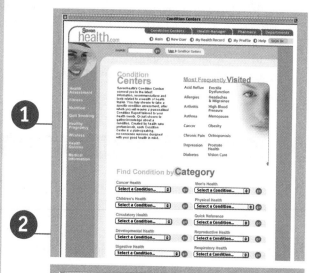

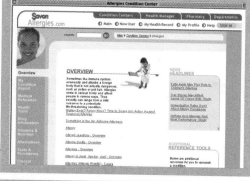

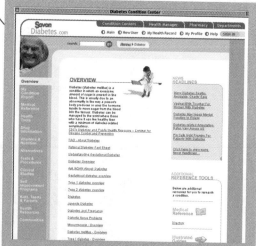

MOST FREQUENTLY VISITED

SavonHealth's Condition Centers connect you to the latest information, recommendations and tools related to a wealth of health topics. You may choose to take a specific condition Health Assessment, after which you will receive a personalized Condition Report tailored to your health needs, or you may choose to gather knowledge about a condition. Created by health care professionals, each Condition Center is a plain-speaking, no-nonsense resource designed with your good health in mind. Here are the most frequently visited Condition Centers:

- Acid Reflux
- Allergies
- Arthritis
- Asthma
- Cancer
- Chronic Pain

- Depression
- Diabetes
- Erectile Dysfunction
- Headaches & Migraines
- High Blood Pressure

- Menopause
- Obesity
- Osteoporosis
- Prostate Health
- Vision Care

2

FIND CONDITION BY CATEGORY

If you are looking for a condition that is not on the Most Frequently Visited list, additional conditions are listed under the following categories:

- Cancer Health
- Circulatory Health
- Children's Health
- Developmental Health
- Digestive Health

- Emotional Health
- General Health
- Infectious Health
- Men's Health
- Physical Health
- Quick Reference

- Reproductive Health
- Respiratory Health
- Skin Health
- Visual Health
- Women's Health

3

CONDITION CENTER OVERVIEW

The Condition Center Overview is the launching point for accessing all the information you need to know about a condition.

From the Overview, you have access to the following condition-specific resources:

- Medical Reference
- Drug Information
- Vitamins & Nutrition
- Alternatives
- Tests & Procedures

- Clinical Studies
- Self-Improvement Programs
- News Headlines
- Illustrated Guides
- Health Tools

SavonHealth.com

ACCESS

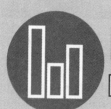

Health Quizzes

Health Quizzes are interactive tools designed to give you a quick risk assessment on a specific health issue.

SavonHealth's Health Quizzes provide:

- Quick assessments with suggestions for follow-up.

- Personalized feedback immediately after submitting your answers

- Suggestions for preventive self-management

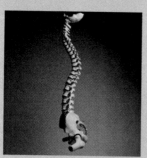

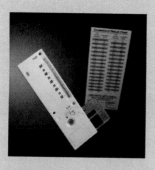

SavonHealth.com

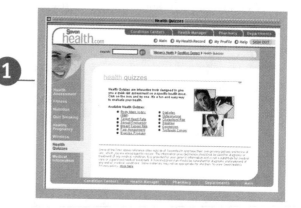

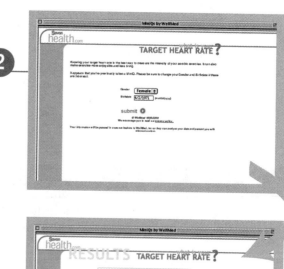

The Health Quiz is a quick way to evaluate your risk assessment. They are easy and instant and cover some of the most frequently asked health issues.

Available Health Quizzes:
- Body Mass Index (BMI)
- Target Heart Rate
- Sexual Frequency
- Breast Cancer Risk
- Pain Assessment
- Exercise Program
- Diabetes
- Osteoporosis
- Cholesterol Risk
- Smoking
- Depression
- Testicular Cancer

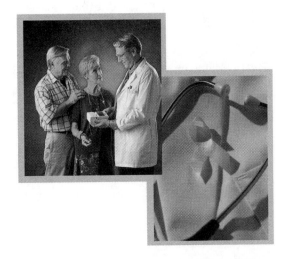

ACCESS

2   HEALTH QUIZ TESTS AND RESULTS

It's a fun and easy way to evaluate your health. Take the quick and easy test for immediate results.

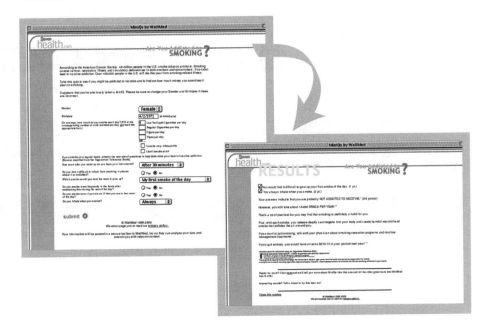

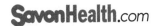
SavonHealth.com

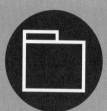

Health Manager

TRACK & STORE FAMILY HEALTH INFO SECURELY & CONFIDENTIALLY

Using the SavonHealth Health Manager, you can:

- Decide what information to store and who will have access to it.
- Add records or data from your doctor, insurance company, hospitals, labs or pharmacies.
- Identify harmful interactions between medications, herbs, vitamins and allergies.
- Use a wireless, internet device to access emergency health information.
- Prepare a pre-visit questionnaire for a doctor or a post-visit report.
- Combine medical information from multiple sources.
- Track lab test or health screening results.
- Learn more about your health status and obtain objective medical information about the conditions, drugs and other items you enter in your Health Manager.
- Receive drug interaction alerts and immunization reminders.
- Fax a summary of information to any health provider.

SavonHealth.com

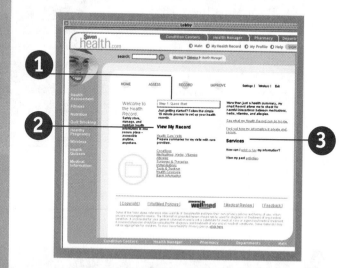

1 QUICK START

Just getting started? Follow this simple 10 minute process to set up your health records.

2 VIEW MY RECORD

More than just a health summary, your smart Record allows you to check for harmful interactions between medications, herbs, vitamins, and allergies; prepare summaries for your visits with care providers and review or amend tests and trackers.

3 SERVICES

Learn how to print or fax your information and view your past activities.

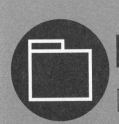

My Trackers

Use SavonHealth's Trackers to help track your progress in matters important to you.

Whether your goal is to lower your blood pressure or to exercise three times per week, trackers are an easy way for you to monitor your activity.

Mini trackers are found within the Health Record. Use these graphical tools to track health measurements over time.

Available Trackers:
- Blood Pressure
- Diet
- Prostate Screen
- Blood Sugar
- Exercise
- Stress
- Cholesterol
- Heart Rate
- Weight
- Height
- Colorectal Screen

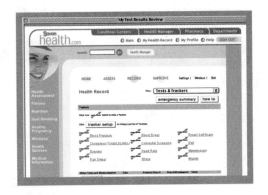

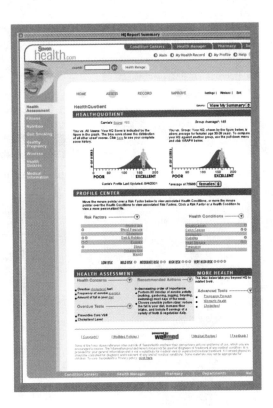

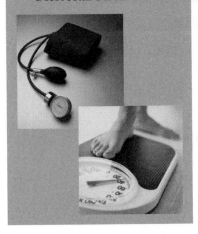

SavonHealth.com

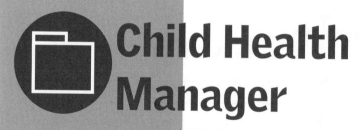

Child Health Manager

TRACKING YOUR CHILD'S HEALTH

SavonHealth's Child Health Manager is an unprecedented tool to track everything about your child's health and development.

Designed to help parents and guardians manage the health and development of children age six and younger, this online program provides a central location to store all the pertinent health information for a child. The Child Health Manager helps parents and guardians keep track of health care visits, immunizations, health conditions, growth and development in language and motor skills and the latest information on child health issues.

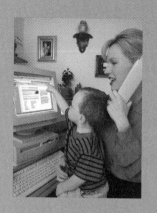

SavonHealth.com

CHILD RECORD

Here you can securely store, manage and maintain your child's health information.

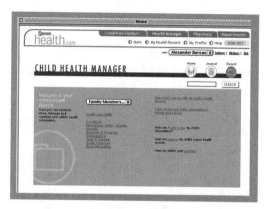

CHILD HEALTH MANAGER HOME PAGE

A "one-stop shop" for all your child's vital information.

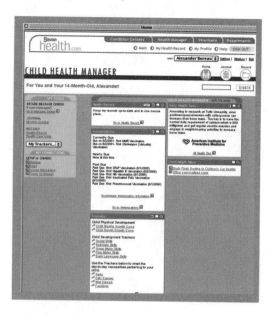

HEALTH CARE VISITS

Questionnaires for before and after doctor visits.

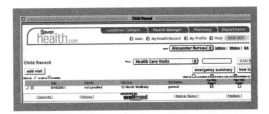

MONTHLY JOURNAL

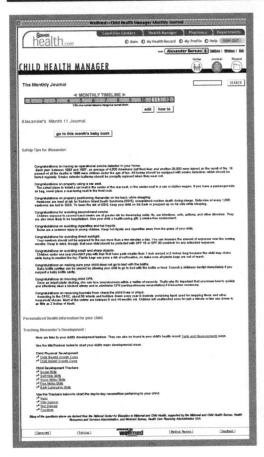

Build a personal chronicle of your infant's growth and development. The Monthly Journal will help parents document all the important information of the first 12 months.

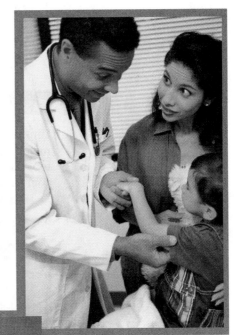

SavonHealth.com

Improvement Programs

These programs can help you through a change, improvement or challenge. SavonHealth offers help for improvement in the following areas:

- Fitness
- Nutrition
- Healthy pregnancy
- Smoking cessation

Improvement Programs motivate you - at your own pace - to achieve healthy outcomes.

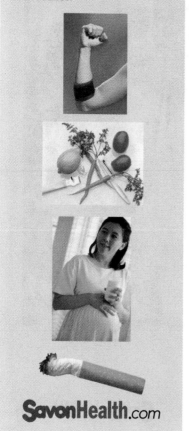

SavonHealth.com

READY, SET STOP! ONLINE SMOKING CESSATION

Find the direction and support you need in this easy-to-follow self-paced program.

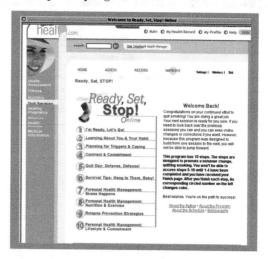

PREGNANCY PLANNER

Your complete resource for the entire 40 weeks of pregnancy. Visit your home page often for information and tools designed to inform and assist you throughout your pregnancy and beyond.

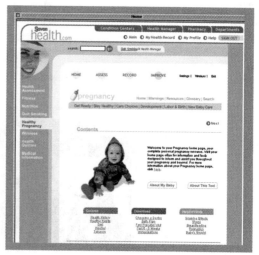

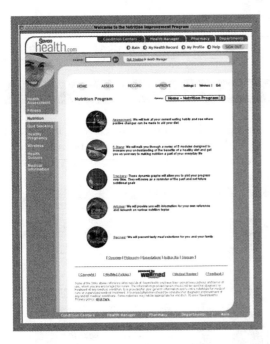

Assess your current eating habits and see where positive changes can be made to aid your diet. Walk through a series of 5 modules designed to increase your understanding of the benefits of a healthy diet. Trackers and dynamic graphs will allow you to plot your progress over time. Read articles and information for your own reference and research on various nutrition topics. Discover tasty meal selections and recipes for you and your family.

IMPROVE

What does being "physically fit" mean to you? SavonHealth has designed this Physical Fitness program to help you answer this question and attempt to achieve your personal desired level of fitness. Whether you want to be able to carry your groceries to your car, reduce stress or run a marathon, this program will provide you with the necessary tools to track, meet and even exceed your goals! Pace yourself and have fun – take it one step at a time – you'll see the positive difference in the long run!

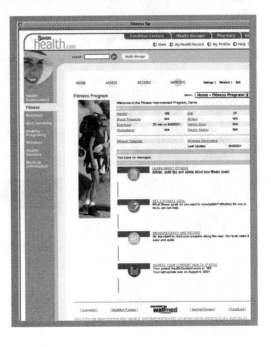

SavonHealth.com

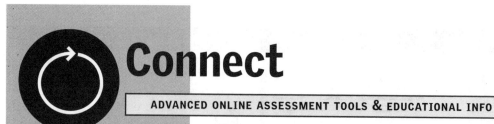

Connect

SavonHealth's proprietary technology and clinical foundation give you instant access to the most accurate and up-to-date health info available.

PERSONAL HEALTH MANAGER HOME PAGE

Receive an up-to-date and completely personalized Home Page with the information products and services you need to track and improve your health and well-being.

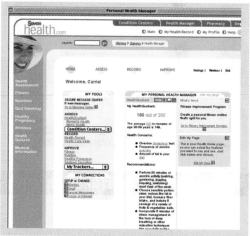

MESSAGING

Be alerted to important and timely information, receive reminders to take your medications and be reminded of important preventive care services.

WIRELESS APPLICATIONS

Access your Health Record via your wireless phone, PDA or pager.

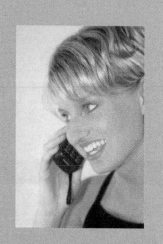

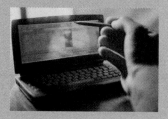

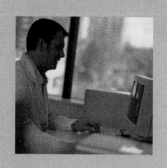

SavonHealth.com

Contents

I PERSONAL HEALTH MANAGER

9 HOW THIS BOOK CAN HELP

11 LIFESAVING SKILLS & FIRST AID

12 LIFESAVING SKILLS

13 Severe Bleeding

14 Rescue Breathing & CPR for Adults & Children Over 8

16 CPR for Infants up to Age 1

17 CPR for Children Ages 1 to 8

18 Choking: Adults & Children

20 Choking: Infants

22 Shock

22 Shock From Allergy

24 FIRST AID

24 Animal Bites

24 Appendicitis

25 Bee & Wasp Stings

25 Blow to the Abdomen

26 Burns

27 Chest Pain

27 Childbirth

28 Cuts, Scrapes & Wounds

30 Drowning

30 Ear Emergencies

31 Electric Shock

32 Eye Injuries

33 Fainting & Loss of Consciousness

34 Food Poisoning

35 Fractures & Dislocations

36 Head, Neck & Back Injuries

37 Heart Attack

38 Heatstroke & Heat Exhaustion

39 Hypothermia & Frostbite

40 Nose Problems

40 Poisoning

41 Seizures

42 Shortness of Breath

42 Snakebites

43 Spider Bites & Scorpion Stings

44 Sprains & Strains

44 Stroke

45 Tick Bites

45 Tooth Knocked Out

47 PROBLEMS & SOLUTIONS

48 HEAD & NERVOUS SYSTEM

48 Alzheimer's Disease

49 Dizziness Chart

52 Headaches

53 Headaches Chart

55 Meningitis & Encephalitis

57 Parkinson's Disease

58 Seizures & Epilepsy

If you don't find what you're looking for here, turn to the index, which begins on page 326.

60 EYES

60 Cataracts

61 Eye & Vision Problems Chart

63 Conjunctivitis

65 Glaucoma

67 Styes

68 EARS

68 Airplane Ear

69 Ear & Hearing Problems Chart

71 Ear Infections

72 Earwax

73 Swimmer's Ear

74 Tinnitus

76 MOUTH

76 Bad Breath

77 Tooth & Mouth Problems Chart

78 Canker Sores

79 Cold Sores

80 Toothache

83 Tooth Grinding

84 NOSE, THROAT, LUNGS & CHEST

84 Allergies

85 Breathing Problems & Coughs Chart

88 Asthma

90 Bronchitis, Acute

91 Chronic Bronchitis & Emphysema

93 Colds

95 Flu

97 Pneumonia

98 Sinusitis

100 Sore Throat

101 Swallowing Difficulty

102 Tonsillitis

104 HEART & CIRCULATION

104 Artery Disease

105 Chest Pain Chart

109 Congestive Heart Failure

111 High Blood Pressure

112 Palpitations

113 Stroke

115 Varicose Veins

116 STOMACH, ABDOMEN & DIGESTIVE SYSTEM

116 Constipation

117 Abdominal Pain Chart

119 Diarrhea

121 Diverticulitis

122 Gallstones

123 Gas & Gas Pain

124 Heartburn

126 Hemorrhoids

127 Hernia

128 Inflammatory Bowel Disease

130 Irritable Bowel Syndrome

131 Rectal Bleeding & Itching Chart

133 Nausea & Vomiting

134 Ulcers & Gastritis

136 URINARY SYSTEM

136 Kidney Stones

137 Urinary Problems Chart

138 Painful Urination

140 Urinary Incontinence

142 SKIN, SCALP & NAILS

142 Acne

143 Rashes Chart

145 Blisters

146 Boils

If you don't find what you're looking for here, turn to the index, which begins on page 326.

147 Bruises
148 Corns & Calluses
149 Dermatitis
151 Poison Oak & Ivy
152 Eczema
153 Fungal Infections
155 Hives
156 Ingrown Toenails
157 Lice & Scabies
159 Psoriasis
160 Shingles
178 Sunburn
179 Skin Cancer
181 Warts

161 THE BODY ILLUSTRATED

161 A New Lens for Cataracts
162 Vision Problems
163 Upper Respiratory
164 Asthma
165 Osteoarthritis
166 Low Back Pain
167 Osteoporosis
168 The Heart
169 Atherosclerosis
170 Bones
171 Muscles
172 Skin Cancer
174 Internal Organs
175 Reproduction
176 Referred Pain

182 MUSCLES, BONES & JOINTS

182 Arthritis
183 Neck Pain Chart
185 Bunions & Hammertoes
186 Shoulder Pain Chart
187 Bursitis
188 Carpal Tunnel Syndrome
190 Low Back Pain
192 Back Pain Chart
194 Leg Pain Chart
195 Muscle Cramps
196 Osteoporosis
198 Overuse Injuries
199 Foot & Ankle Pain Chart
200 Knee Pain Chart
201 Temporomandibular Disorder
202 Tendinitis

204 BEHAVIOR & EMOTIONS

204 Alcohol Abuse & Alcoholism
205 Confusion Chart
208 Anxiety & Phobias
210 Attention Deficit Disorder
211 Depression
213 Drug Abuse
214 Some Street Drugs: Signs & Risks Chart
216 Eating Disorders
217 Grief
218 Stress

220 SEXUAL HEALTH

220 Birth Control
221 Sexually Transmitted Diseases Chart
224 Loss of Sexual Desire

226 MEN'S HEALTH

226 Erection Problems

227 Testicle Problems Chart

228 Prostate Problems

232 WOMEN'S HEALTH

232 Menopause

233 Menstrual Irregularities Chart

236 Pelvic Inflammatory Disease

237 Breast Pain or Lumps Chart

238 Pregnancy

239 How to Do a Breast Self-Exam

241 Premenstrual Syndrome

243 Toxic Shock Syndrome

244 Vaginal Problems

246 CHILDREN'S HEALTH

246 Bed-Wetting

247 Children's Rashes Chart

249 Chicken Pox

250 Childhood Immunization Schedule

251 Colic

252 Croup

253 Diaper Rash

254 Diarrhea in Children

254 Ear Infections in Children

255 Fever in Children

255 How to Take a Temperature

257 Fifth Disease

257 German Measles (Rubella)

258 Hand, Foot & Mouth Disease

259 Impetigo

260 Lead Poisoning

262 Measles

263 Meningitis in Children

264 Mumps

265 Rheumatic Fever

265 Roseola

266 Scarlet Fever

267 Strep Throat

268 Teething

269 Vomiting in Children

269 Whooping Cough

272 GENERAL PROBLEMS

272 Anemia

273 Fever Chart

275 Chronic Fatigue Syndrome

277 Diabetes

279 Hepatitis

281 Infections

282 Sudden Weight Gain or Loss Chart

284 Lupus

285 Lyme Disease

286 Sleep Disorders

288 Thyroid Problems

291 STAYING HEALTHY

292 Eight Ways to Feel Your Best

306 Know Your Health Plan

308 How to Choose a Physician

310 How to Choose a Natural Healer

312 Helping Your Doctor Help You

315 Pain Relief: The Big Four

316 Your Personal Health Record

322 Medicines: Playing It Safe

323 Drug Combinations to Avoid Chart

326 INDEX

If you don't find what you're looking for here, turn to the index, which begins on page 326.

How This Book Can Help

The most useful rule for taking care of your health may be one you seldom hear: Remember who's in charge. The important day-to-day decisions about your own health and vitality are made by one person—you.

Many people go to the doctor when they don't need to. Many do the reverse and don't go when they *do* need to. *The Sav-on Health Self-Care Advisor* steers you clear of both extremes, showing what you can do to take care of yourself and your family and advising you when it's time to call your doctor.

This book covers more than 300 of the most common health concerns in the United States. It is arranged much the way a human body is: If you know where you hurt, you can turn to that section in the table of contents. If you miss what you're looking for there, you'll find it in the comprehensive index that starts on page 326. You'll also find basic emergency and first-aid techniques at the front of the book, and a step-by-step guide to healthy living on pages 291 to 325.

Most sections include quick-reference charts. A chart may provide a ready answer to your question about a symptom; it may direct you to an entry elsewhere in the book; or it may suggest calling your doctor.

If the book directs you to a doctor, you may need to call for advice only, or for both advice and an appointment. If you need to see the doctor right away, the book will say so: "Call for a prompt appointment."

When you need emergency help, you may see "Call 911 or go to an emergency room **right away.**" When the problem could be fatal, the advice is simply "Call 911," because it's safer to wait for paramedics to arrive than to try driving to a hospital; the medics have training and equipment that most of us don't possess.

Some areas of the country don't have 911 service. If yours doesn't, you should find your local emergency number in the front of the phone book. Post it on your telephones and in the **critical information** box on the inside front cover of this book. Use 911 only when you're fairly certain you need it; your health insurance might not cover an ambulance trip for a nonemergency. Use the same guideline to decide whether to go to an emergency room; in some, you may face a longer wait than you would in a doctor's office.

THANKS TO our board of medical advisors and to the many other doctors who helped with *The Sav-on Health Self-Care Advisor*, you can trust the information it contains. Of course, if your doctor's advice conflicts with advice you find in the book, listen to your doctor; he or she should know your medical history and specific needs. In the end, though, it is your health. There's nothing like being a full, informed partner in the choices that you and your family will be making. We hope this book will become a trusted friend along the way and that it helps you enjoy a long and healthy life.

Lifesaving Skills & First Aid

THIS SECTION explains what to do in situations that can be life-threatening and will call for fast action. Read it before you need it, so that you'll be prepared to act without panic. Make a special point of reading "Lifesaving Skills" on pages 12 through 23. This is a guide to the basic life-support techniques you would need for many accidents and injuries—the ABCs, CPR, the recovery position, and handling severe bleeding, choking, and shock. You don't have to memorize the details. If you're familiar with the methods, at least, you may be able to keep someone alive.

First-aid instructions begin on page 24. Common injuries and problems appear in alphabetical order.

Emergency and first-aid advice is sometimes updated. Check with your local chapter of the American Red Cross or American Heart Association every year or so to learn of any changes. Better yet, take one of the CPR or first-aid courses offered by the American Red Cross, the American Heart Association, or your local fire or rescue department.

It's easy to set yourself up with the basic tools for a first-aid kit. They're listed on page 21.

About calling for help: You'll be advised at times to call 911. If your area doesn't have 911 service, you should find your local emergency number in the front of the telephone book. Take time now to write that local emergency number on this page, and also to post it on your telephones.

> **LOCAL EMERGENCY NUMBER**
>
> _____

Lifesaving Skills

When something happens that's a matter of life and death, you will need to know some basic emergency techniques. Don't waste time worrying about doing every step perfectly. Just do the best you can.

SIGNS OF A LIFE IN DANGER

- **Severe bleeding.**
- **No breathing.**
- **No heartbeat or pulse.**
- **Choking:** The person can't get air.
- **Shock:** Irregular pulse and breathing, cold skin. The person may be unconscious.

WHAT TO DO

The American Red Cross suggests 3 basic steps for any emergency:

Check the scene and the person.
Call 911 or your local emergency number.
Care for the person.

- ➤ Check the scene for things that could be a danger to the person or to you—fire, flood, traffic, spilled chemicals, or other threats. Don't be a dead hero. If danger is extreme, wait for professionals—police, firefighters, paramedics—to deal with it.
- ➤ Check the person. Try to find out what's wrong. Is it a life-threatening emergency? Don't move a badly injured person unless he or she is about to be hurt even worse by something on the scene. In that case, move the person and yourself out of harm's way before starting treatment.
- ➤ Call for help. Shout if you're alone with the person. If the person isn't breathing or has no heartbeat, phone 911 or send someone to do it. Don't start emergency treatment until you have called 911.
- ➤ Call on bystanders. See if anyone nearby has had more first-aid or CPR training than you have. Ask them to help.
- ➤ Care for the person. Treat the most serious problem first. Look for a medical alert tag on the person. If you find one, do what it says.
- ➤ Care for yourself. Protect yourself from a stranger's blood and other body fluids. Wear gloves if you have them. Put cloth or plastic between the person's body fluids and yourself, especially if you have open cuts or scrapes. While giving care, don't touch your mouth, nose, or eyes, or eat or drink anything. Wash your hands, or use alcohol wipes, right after giving first aid.

CHECKING THE **ABC**s

Airway. Open it. Gently tilt the person's head back and lift the chin. This will get air to the lungs through the nose and mouth. **Caution:** If you suspect a head, neck, or back injury, do not tilt the head. Moving it could cause further injury (see page 36).

Breathing. Look, listen, and feel for it. Look to see if the person's chest is rising and falling. Listen and feel for exhaled breath by putting your ear to the person's mouth.

Circulation. Check for a pulse. Using 2 fingers, feel for a pulse on either side of the neck slightly under the jaw, between the front of the throat and the long muscle on the side of the neck. For an infant (under 1 year), use 2 fingers to feel for a pulse on the inside of the arm between the armpit and the elbow. Put your ear to the person's chest to listen for a heartbeat.

Severe Bleeding
www.SavonFirstAid.com

SIGNS AND SYMPTOMS

- Spurting or gushing blood.
- Bleeding that won't stop.

Heavy bleeding that spurts or won't stop can quickly threaten a person's life.

WHAT TO DO

➤ Call 911 or go to an emergency room **right away.**

➤ Press right on the wound with a sterile dressing or the cleanest cloth you have—or your hand if you have no cloth. If a cloth becomes soaked with blood, don't remove it. Put a new cloth on top of it, and keep pressing. **Caution:** If an object is stuck in the wound, press around the object, not on top of it. Don't press on an **eye injury** (see page 32) or an open **fracture** (see page 35).

➤ Make the person as comfortable as possible. Raise the place that's bleeding higher than the heart, if you can, to reduce blood flow. **Caution:** If you suspect a **head, neck, or back injury** (see page 36), don't move the person. You might cause further injury.

➤ If the person is bleeding around a broken bone, don't wash or probe the wound. Just stop the bleeding with a clean cloth (see **fractures and dislocations,** page 35). **Caution:** Do not try to remove anything stuck in the wound, especially in a chest or back wound.

➤ If the bleeding spurts or gushes—or if slower bleeding does not stop after 5 minutes—find a pressure point where an artery can be squeezed shut (see box at right).

➤ When the bleeding stops, don't remove the cloths you've been using. Wrap the wound in a bandage or more cloths. If something is stuck in the wound, wrap around it, not over it.

➤ If the person is unconscious, check the **ABCs** (see box on facing page): Lift the chin to open the airway, then check for breathing and pulse. Watch for signs of **shock** (see page 22): weak and rapid pulse, shallow breathing, cold skin, confusion, loss of consciousness.

➤ If the person is not breathing or has no pulse, start **CPR** (see page 14).

When Bleeding Won't Stop

When nothing else works, pressing on an artery may stop the bleeding. Pressure points are places where an artery can be squeezed shut. Use a pressure point between the wound and the heart.

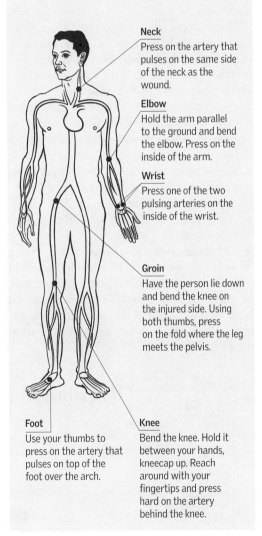

Neck
Press on the artery that pulses on the same side of the neck as the wound.

Elbow
Hold the arm parallel to the ground and bend the elbow. Press on the inside of the arm.

Wrist
Press one of the two pulsing arteries on the inside of the wrist.

Groin
Have the person lie down and bend the knee on the injured side. Using both thumbs, press on the fold where the leg meets the pelvis.

Foot
Use your thumbs to press on the artery that pulses on top of the foot over the arch.

Knee
Bend the knee. Hold it between your hands, kneecap up. Reach around with your fingertips and press hard on the artery behind the knee.

Rescue Breathing & CPR

www.SavonFirstAid.com

Cardiopulmonary resuscitation for adults and children over 8

Cautions:

CPR can cause serious injury, including broken ribs and damage to the liver, lungs, or heart. The information here is meant as a reminder for people with CPR training, not as a replacement for that training.

➤ If you haven't been trained in CPR, ask if anyone else at the scene has.

➤ Don't do chest compressions unless both breathing and heartbeat have stopped. If the person still has a pulse, chest compressions can cause an irregular heartbeat. Use rescue breathing only.

➤ Never practice CPR on a healthy person.

When the heart and lungs stop working, brain damage or death follows within minutes. Rescue breathing and CPR (a mix of rescue breathing and chest compressions) keep feeding blood and oxygen to the brain until the person can breathe alone, or until medical help arrives.

The American Red Cross and a number of other rescue organizations train people in CPR. Think about taking a course.

WHAT TO DO

If you are in a public place such as a mall or a stadium, ask if there's an automated external defibrillator and someone trained to use it. This device sends electrical shocks to jump-start a heart that has stopped beating. While you wait for help to arrive, start rescue breathing and CPR.

For an adult or a child over 8 (for an **infant,** see page 16; for a **child 1 to 8,** see page 17):

➤ Check the **ABCs** (see box on page 12): Lift the chin to open the airway, then check for breathing and pulse. See if the person's chest rises. Put your ear to his or her mouth to listen and feel for breathing for about 5 seconds.

➤ If the person is not breathing, call 911 **right away.**

➤ Lay the person down, face up. Kneel alongside, halfway between the head and chest. **Caution:** If you suspect **choking,** see page 18. If you suspect a **head, neck, or back injury,** see page 36. Moving the person may cause further injury.

➤ Tilt the head back and lift the chin to open the airway.

➤ If the person is still not breathing, start rescue breathing.

Rescue breathing

➤ Pinch the person's nose shut. Put your mouth over his or her mouth and seal your lips tightly against the skin.

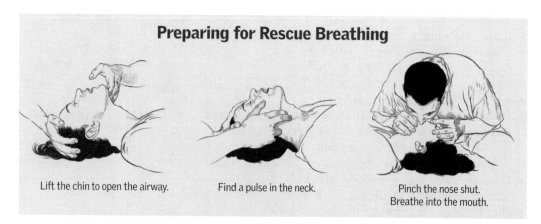

Preparing for Rescue Breathing

Lift the chin to open the airway.   Find a pulse in the neck.   Pinch the nose shut. Breathe into the mouth.

➤ Breathe slowly and gently into the mouth for 1½ to 2 seconds, watching for the person's chest to rise.

➤ Remove your mouth and let the chest fall. Repeat with a second breath. **Caution:** Breathe just hard enough and long enough to make the chest rise. If you breathe too hard, air can be forced into the stomach, and that can cause vomiting.

➤ If the chest does not rise, tilt the head farther back. Give 2 breaths again.

➤ Check for a heartbeat. Using 2 fingers, feel for a pulse on either side of the neck slightly under the jaw, between the front of the throat and the long muscle on the side of the neck.

➤ If you feel a pulse, continue rescue breathing at the rate of 1 breath every 5 seconds. Check the pulse every 12 breaths. Time breaths like this: Count slowly, "A thousand one, a thousand two, a thousand three"; on "a thousand four" take a breath; breathe into the person on "a thousand five," and so on.

➤ Continue until the person can breathe alone, or until medical help arrives.

➤ If you feel no pulse or heartbeat, get ready to do chest compressions.

Chest compressions

Caution: Before you start, be sure you feel no heartbeat. If the person has a pulse, chest compressions are not needed, and they can cause an irregular heartbeat, so you should use rescue breathing only.

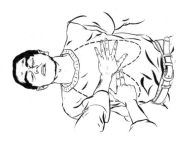

Find the spot for chest compressions.

➤ Kneel beside the person. Put your hands on the person's breastbone, keeping your shoulders right above your hands.

➤ Use the index and middle finger of one hand to touch the notch where the ribs meet the breastbone.

➤ Put the heel of your other hand above this notch, on the midline of the breastbone on the side closer to the person's head.

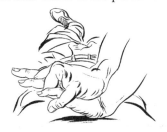

Push with the heel of your bottom hand.

➤ Now lift your first hand and put it on top of the second. Interlace the fingers of both hands and tilt them up so that only the heel of your bottom hand remains on the person's chest. Keep your arms straight and your elbows locked.

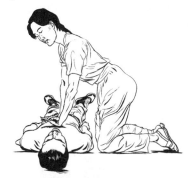

Kneel so you can push straight down with your elbows locked.

➤ Push straight down, depressing the breastbone 1½ to 2 inches.

➤ Release the pressure so the chest rises, but don't take your hands off the chest.

➤ Give 15 compressions, pushing straight down on the count of "*one* and *two* and *three* and *four*. . . ." Use short thrusts.

➤ Alternate with rescue breathing—give 2 breaths, then 15 chest compressions, then 2 more breaths, 15 more chest compressions, and so on. Repeat the series 4 times. Then check for a pulse.

➤ Continue the cycle until the person regains a pulse and can breathe on his or her own, or until medical help arrives. **If you feel a pulse, stop chest compressions and do rescue breathing only, until the person can breathe alone.**

CPR for Infants
www.SavonFirstAid.com

Up to age 1

Caution: CPR can cause serious injury. Babies are small and tender, so be gentle.

WHAT TO DO

➤ Check the **ABCs** (see box on page 12): Open the airway, look at the chest for breathing, check for circulation (a pulse).

➤ Lay the infant face up on a firm surface. Gently tilt the head back to open the airway. Don't tilt a baby's head back very far.

Caution: If you suspect choking, turn to **choking infants,** page 20.

➤ If the infant is not breathing, call 911 **right away.** Then start rescue breathing.

Rescue breathing

➤ Lift the chin with one hand and seal your lips over the baby's mouth and nose.

➤ Breathe slowly and gently into the infant for 1 to 1½ seconds, just hard enough to make the chest rise. An infant's lungs are small and don't need much air.

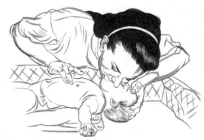

Breathe into the baby's nose and mouth.

➤ Remove your mouth and turn your head to watch the chest fall. Repeat with a second soft breath.

➤ Check for a pulse. Using 2 fingers, feel on the inside of the upper arm, halfway between the armpit and the elbow, for 5 to 10 seconds. Also, put your ear to the chest to listen for a heartbeat.

➤ If the infant has a pulse but still is not breathing, keep giving rescue breathing.

➤ Give 1 breath about every 3 seconds. Time them like this: Breathe into the baby as you count "a thousand one," pause and take a breath at "a thousand two," then breathe into the baby at "a thousand three," and so on.

➤ If breath doesn't go in, see **choking infants** (page 20).

➤ Check for a pulse every 20 breaths, which is about 1 minute.

➤ If the infant has no pulse after you've felt for it for 5 to 10 seconds, start chest compressions.

Chest compressions

Caution: Before you start, be sure you feel no heartbeat. If the baby has a pulse, chest compressions are not needed, and they can cause an irregular heartbeat. Use rescue breathing only.

➤ Place the infant on his or her back on a firm surface.

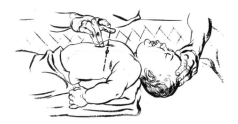

Press in the middle of the baby's breastbone.

➤ Put 2 fingers on the breastbone just below an imaginary line between the nipples. Use your free hand to tilt the head back gently.

➤ Pressing straight down, give 5 chest compressions on the count of "one, two, three," and so on. The infant's breastbone should depress just one-half to 1 inch.

➤ Release the pressure between thrusts, but don't take your fingers off the chest.

➤ After 5 compressions, give 1 rescue breath. Then do 5 more compressions and another rescue breath. Repeat the cycle 20 times. Then check for a pulse. Continue until the infant regains a pulse and begins to breathe on his or her own. **As soon as you know the infant has a pulse, stop chest compressions.**

CPR for Children
www.SavonFirstAid.com

Ages 1 to 8

CPR for children uses less force and faster rescue breathing and compressions than adult CPR. For children over 8, see page 14.

WHAT TO DO

➤ Lay the child face up on a firm surface. Check the **ABCs** (see box on page 12): Gently tilt the head back and lift the chin to open the airway, and check for breathing and pulse. **Caution:** If you suspect choking, turn to **choking,** page 18.

➤ If the child is not breathing, call 911 **right away.** Then begin rescue breathing.

Rescue breathing

➤ Pinch the child's nose shut. Seal your lips over his or her mouth. Breathe slowly and gently into the mouth for 1 to 1½ seconds, with just enough force to make the chest rise.

➤ Remove your mouth and let the chest fall. Repeat with a second breath.

➤ If the child is still not breathing, give 1 breath every 3 seconds. Time them like this: Breathe into the child as you count "a thousand one," take a breath on "a thousand two," breathe into the child on "a thousand three," and so on.

➤ Check for a pulse every 20 breaths, which is about 1 minute: Using 2 fingers, gently feel for a pulse on the side of the neck just under the jaw. Put your ear to the chest to listen for a heartbeat.

➤ If the child has a pulse but still is not breathing, keep giving rescue breaths.

➤ If you are sure the child has no pulse after you've felt for it for 5 to 10 seconds, get ready for chest compressions.

Chest compressions

Caution: Before you start, be sure you feel no heartbeat. If the child has a pulse, chest compressions are not needed, and they can cause an irregular heartbeat. Use rescue breathing only.

➤ Kneel next to the child so your shoulders are directly over the chest. Tilt the child's head back with one hand. With your other hand, find the notch where the ribs meet the bottom of the breastbone (the midline).

➤ Put the heel of that hand on the midline of the child's breastbone. Keep your arm straight and elbow locked.

➤ Push straight down with the heel of your hand just hard enough to depress the breastbone 1½ to 2 inches. Compressions take about 3 seconds.

➤ Release the pressure so the chest rises, but don't take your hand off the chest.

➤ Give 5 chest compressions on the count of *"one* and *two* and *three* and *four* and *five."*

➤ After giving 5 compressions, give 1 rescue breath. Repeat the cycle of 5 compressions and 1 breath 20 times, which is about 1 minute. Then check for a pulse. Continue until the child regains a pulse and can breathe alone or until medical help arrives. **As soon as you know the child has a pulse, stop chest compressions.**

Keep Children Safe

Some safeguards can limit the chances that you'll need to perform CPR for a child. Take these steps:

➤ Put safety covers or tape over electrical outlets.

➤ Store electrical appliances away from the sink, tub, and toilet.

➤ Never leave a child alone in the bathtub, at a pool, or near any body of water. Keep toilet seat lids down. Cover kiddie pools.

➤ Prevent choking: Keep buttons, coins, and other small objects out of reach. Don't give children toys that have small loose pieces.

➤ Prevent strangling: Keep shade and drapery pulls and plastic bags out of children's reach.

LIFESAVING SKILLS

Choking:
Adults & Children
www.SavonFirstAid.com

SIGNS AND SYMPTOMS

- High-pitched wheezing.
- Clutching at the neck, bulging eyes.
- Inability to speak, cough forcefully, or breathe.
- Bluish face.
- Seizure or loss of consciousness.

WHAT TO DO

➤ Watch carefully. Encourage the person to cough. Let him or her try to cough up the object. It's possible to breathe with a partly blocked airway: If a person can cough forcefully or talk, he or she is getting enough air.

➤ Call 911 **right away** if the person can't speak, cough forcefully, or breathe, or if he or she is making a high-pitched wheezing sound.

➤ If the person can't get any air at all, give abdominal thrusts (the **Heimlich maneuver**—see box below).

If the person loses consciousness:

➤ Lay the person face up on a firm surface.

➤ Check and sweep the mouth: Hold the tongue and lift the chin. Looking into the mouth, slip a finger along the inside of the cheek and across the back of the mouth and out to remove objects and fluids. **Caution:** Do not try to remove anything unless you can see and grasp it.

➤ Tilt the head back and lift the chin to open the airway.

➤ Put your ear to the person's mouth to listen and feel for breathing.

➤ If the person is unconscious and not able to breathe, it is more important to get air in than to get the object out. Begin rescue breathing.

➤ Pinch the person's nose shut with one hand. Seal your mouth tightly over his or her mouth. Breathe long enough and hard enough to make the chest rise. Remove your mouth and watch for the chest to fall. Repeat the breath.

➤ If the chest does not move: Tilt the head farther back and give 2 more breaths.

➤ If chest still does not rise, give 5 abdominal thrusts: Straddle the person. Put the heel of one of your hands in the middle of the abdomen just below the ribs and

The Heimlich Maneuver

➤ Stand behind the person. Wrap your arms around his or her waist.

➤ Make a fist with one hand, and put the thumb side against the middle of the abdomen—just below the ribs but above the navel. Grab the fist with your other hand.

➤ Give up to 5 quick, forceful thrusts inward and upward into the abdomen. Pause, then repeat until the blockage comes out or medical help arrives. See the instructions above for what to do if the person loses consciousness.

Caution: If the person is pregnant or obese, give thrusts higher on the chest, against the center of the breastbone.

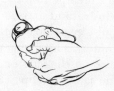

Grab your fist with your other hand.

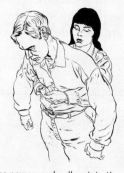

Hug the person and pull up into the abdomen.

How to Avoid Choking

Thousands of people die from choking every year. Most of them are babies and older people. To limit chances of choking:

➤ Cut food into small pieces.

➤ Chew food until it is soft before you swallow it.

➤ If you wear dentures, take small bites, chew slowly, and try to eat soft foods—dentures make it harder to sense when food is soft enough to be swallowed easily.

➤ Don't give babies or little children small, firm, or hard-to-chew pieces of food—such as hot dogs, carrot chunks, or peanuts—that can get stuck in the throat.

➤ Don't eat on the run—haste can make you bolt chunks of food. Sit down and take time to enjoy your meal.

➤ Don't laugh or talk excitedly while you're eating—talk between bites, after you've swallowed.

➤ Don't drink a lot of alcohol and eat—it dims your ability to tell when food is chewed and dulls the nerves that signal your body to swallow.

---

above the navel. Put the other hand on top. Give up to 5 quick thrusts upward and into the abdomen, aiming toward the person's head.

➤ Check the mouth again. Tilt the head and give 2 breaths.

➤ If the chest still does not rise, repeat the 5 thrusts, mouth sweep, and 2 breaths. Continue until the blockage comes out, the person begins breathing, or medical help arrives.

If you are choking and alone:

➤ Give yourself abdominal thrusts with your fist: Put a fist in the middle of your abdomen below the ribs and above your navel. Use your other hand to thrust the fist up and into your abdomen until the object pops out.

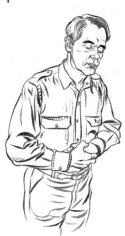

Pull your fist up hard into your abdomen or . . .

➤ Or use a chair back, railing, or other firm object: Bend forward over it, and press your abdomen against it firmly until the object comes out. **Caution:** Don't lean on a sharp edge that could hurt you.

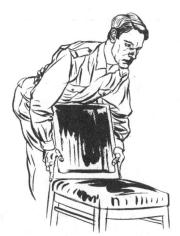

. . . use a chair back to give yourself abdominal thrusts.

➤ If you can see and grasp the object stuck in your throat, try to pull it out. **Caution:** Don't try to grab an object you can't see. You might force it farther down your windpipe.

➤ Even if you get the object unstuck, call your doctor for advice or go to an emergency room. You could have problems from the choking or the first aid.

Choking: Infants
www.SavonFirstAid.com

Up to age 1

SIGNS AND SYMPTOMS

- Gagging or coughing that doesn't stop, or gets weak.
- High-pitched wheezing cough.
- Unable to cry, cough, or breathe.
- Loss of consciousness.

Choking is a serious threat to babies. They can choke on foods or fluids, or on small objects they put in their mouths. Don't give infants small, hard food that can stick in the airway. Don't leave small objects and coins where an infant can find them. Check with your fingers if you suspect an infant has something in his or her mouth.

WHAT TO DO

➤ If the infant can cough or cry, watch him or her carefully.
➤ Call 911 **right away** if the infant can't stop coughing, can't cry or cough forcefully, makes a high-pitched wheezing sound, or stops breathing. **Then:**
➤ Give 5 soft back blows: Lay the infant face down on your forearm so that the head is lower than the chest. Support the head with your hand. With the heel of the other hand, strike the back 5 times between the shoulder blades. **Caution:** Babies are small and tender, so take extra care to be gentle.

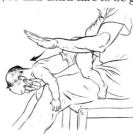

Give back blows with the heel of your hand.

➤ If the object doesn't pop out, give chest thrusts: Turn the infant face up, keeping the head lower than the rest of the body.

Put 2 or 3 fingers in the center of the breastbone. Give 5 thrusts about 1 inch deep. Remember: Do it firmly but gently.

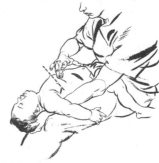

If back blows don't work, give thrusts in the center of the breastbone.

➤ Alternate 5 blows and 5 thrusts until the object comes out, or the infant starts to breathe or cough. Stop as soon as the baby can breathe, cough, or cry.
➤ If the infant is unconscious and not breathing, begin rescue breathing. The goal now is to get air in, not to get the object out.

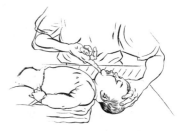

Lift the baby's chin to open the airway.

➤ Put the baby on his or her back. Look into the mouth and sweep the inside with your little finger to remove any visible objects or fluids. **Caution:** Don't try to remove anything you can't see.
➤ Tilt the head back and seal your lips tightly over the baby's nose and mouth. Give 2 breaths. Breathe just long enough and hard enough to make the chest rise.
➤ If the air will not go in, tilt the head farther back and try 2 more breaths. Give 5 back blows and 5 chest thrusts, and check the airway.
➤ If the chest still does not rise, keep repeating 5 back blows, 5 chest thrusts, a check for objects in the mouth, and 2 breaths until help arrives or the object pops out.

Your Home Pharmacy

A well-stocked home medicine chest has what you need for most minor ailments and injuries, when you need it. It can save you the stress of trying to find an open drugstore at 2 AM. The following list covers ills from sprained ankles to the flu. Remember that all medicines should be stored in a cool, dry spot, out of the reach of children.

For headaches, colds, and coughs:
Acetaminophen (adult and children's strength)—for pain and fever
Aspirin—not for children or teenagers (see box on **Reye's syndrome,** page 95)
Ibuprofen—for swelling and cramps
Antihistamine—for allergies
Decongestant—for clogged nose and sinuses
Cough suppressant
For poisoning:
Activated charcoal—to absorb poison
Ipecac—to make someone vomit
For digestion problems:
Antacid—for indigestion, heartburn
Antidiarrhea medicine
Disposable enema
Laxative (bulk-forming)
For skin:
Calamine lotion—for skin irritations
Foot powder—for athlete's foot
Petroleum jelly—for dry lips and skin
Sunscreen (SPF 15 or above)
Witch hazel—for itching
Basic supplies:
Adhesive tape, 1 inch wide
Adhesive bandages, assorted sizes
Elastic bandage (3 inches wide)
Cotton swabs and balls
Antibiotic ointment
Hydrogen peroxide
Rubbing alcohol
Scissors
Thermometer
Tweezers
Eye cup
Eyedrops

A Basic First-Aid Kit

Every household should have at least one well-equipped first-aid kit with an emergency handbook. Every member of the family should know where it is. Keep another kit in your car. You can buy a first-aid kit or make your own. Either way, be sure that it includes these items:
Emergency phone numbers
Gauze pads and rolls, assorted sizes
Adhesive tape, 1 and 2 inches wide
Assorted small adhesive bandages
Triangular bandage
Chemical cold pack
Small and large plastic bags
Disposable gloves
Antiseptic wipes or towelettes
Flashlight and extra batteries
Safety pins
Scissors and tweezers
Thermal blanket
Syrup of ipecac, small bottle
Antiseptic ointment
Activated charcoal

Source: American Red Cross

About Calling 911 . . .

Don't hang up too soon.
When you call, be sure to give the address. Give the phone number you're calling from. Say what's wrong. Tell what happened. Say how many are hurt or sick. Give your name. And don't hang up until the emergency dispatcher does.

Don't cry wolf.
Your local emergency number is for just one thing—emergencies that threaten human life. Use it when you need it, but don't misuse it. About 40 percent of 911 calls are for nonemergencies, and they tie up help that someone else needs.

Shock

www.SavonFirstAid.com

How to spot it, how to treat it

Shock is the body's reaction to a sudden, severe loss of blood from a wound or illness. Blood pressure drops, robbing organs and tissues of vital blood and oxygen. Shock can be caused by **severe bleeding** (see page 13), dehydration, heart disorders, an allergic reaction (**shock from allergy,** see this page), an infection such as **blood poisoning** (see page 29), or **toxic shock syndrome** (see page 243). It can be fatal if not treated right away, so it calls for emergency care as soon as you see it.

SIGNS AND SYMPTOMS

From blood loss, dehydration, heart disorders:
- Weak, rapid, or irregular heartbeat.
- Cold, damp, pale, or bluish skin.
- Shortness of breath or rapid, shallow breathing.
- Dilated (widened) pupils.
- Intense thirst.
- Confusion, dizziness, or feeling faint.
- Loss of consciousness.

From internal bleeding:
Same as blood loss, plus:
- Coughing up or vomiting blood.
- Bleeding from the rectum or vagina.
- Blood in the urine, or abnormally heavy menstrual flow.
- Swelling, hardness, tenderness, or bruising in abdomen or other areas.
- Wounds or other signs of a blow to the head, chest, or abdomen.

WHAT TO DO

For most types of shock:
- Call 911 **right away,** or send someone for help.

Caution: If you suspect a fractured pelvis or a **head, neck, or back injury** (see page 36), do not move the person unless you must. You may do further damage.

- Check the **ABCs** (see page 12): Lift the chin to open the airway, and check for breathing and pulse.
- If the person is not breathing or has no pulse or heartbeat, begin **CPR** (page 14).
- Lay the person on his or her back, with feet propped up 12 inches so blood can flow toward the brain.
- Find the cause of shock. Look for injuries: If you see a bleeding wound, press on it. If you find a **fracture or dislocation,** keep it from moving (see page 35). If the person has been stung by an insect or is having **shock from allergy,** see below.
- Keep the person warm. Loosen tight clothing, and cover him or her with blankets or clothes. If the ground is cold, put blankets or newspapers underneath the person as well.
- Check the **ABCs** often. If the person begins to vomit or to bleed from the mouth or nose, turn the head to the side to keep the airway open.
- Keep the person calm and still.

Cautions:
- Don't give anything to eat or drink.
- Don't put a pillow or padding under the head—it might cause further damage to an injured head or neck, and might bend the neck so that breathing becomes hard.
- Don't use an electric blanket or other form of direct heat.

Shock From Allergy

www.SavonFirstAid.com

Some people get a severe allergic reaction to bee stings, bites from other insects, or certain foods or drugs. This is called anaphylactic shock. The reaction is often immediate. It can be fatal if the throat swells shut, blocking the airway.

If you know you have strong allergic reactions, you may want to keep on hand an emergency kit with some antihistamine pills and a shot of epinephrine. Ask your doctor.

Recovery Position

An unconscious but still breathing person should be put in the recovery position to keep the airway open. **Caution:** Don't put someone in this position if you suspect a **head, neck, or back injury** (see page 36). In that case, moving the person could cause further damage.

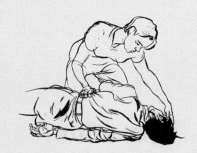

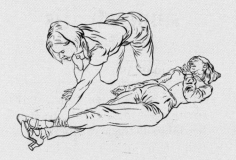

1. Kneel beside the person. Turn the head toward you. Tuck the arm closest to you under the person's body, keeping it straight. Put the other arm across the chest, and cross the far ankle over the one nearest to you.

2. Support the head with one hand. Grip the person's clothes at the far hip with the other hand and pull the person gently over onto his or her side. Support the person's body with your knees as it rolls.

3. Carefully tilt the chin back to open the airway. Then bend the top arm and knee to prop up the body and make breathing easier. Make sure the bottom arm is out from under the body, lying straight beside and behind it.

Check often to see that the person is breathing and has a heartbeat.

It's a good idea to carry the kit to picnics, hikes, and outdoor events.

SIGNS AND SYMPTOMS

- Hot, reddened skin on the face and other places.
- Intense itching, or hives.
- Rapid swelling of face or tongue.
- Speeded-up heart rate.
- Wheezing and trouble breathing.
- Dizziness.
- Abdominal cramps, nausea, and sometimes vomiting.
- Loss of consciousness.

WHAT TO DO

Call 911 **right away,** and treat the person as for other types of shock.

➤ Try to find the source of the reaction. If it's a bee sting and you see a stinger, scrape it off or pluck it out as quickly as you can. Don't waste time looking for a credit card or knife to scrape with. A stinger keeps injecting venom after it's torn off the insect, and even a slight delay means the person will get a bigger dose.

➤ Some people who know they have severe allergic reactions carry an emergency kit. Help the person take the medication, usually a shot of epinephrine. Follow the instructions in the kit. **Caution:** Don't give epinephrine to an older person or one who has heart trouble.

➤ Get the person to an emergency room as soon as possible after giving an epinephrine shot. The shot may have side effects.

➤ If the person stops breathing or does not have a pulse, begin **CPR** (see page 14).

First Aid

Here is basic advice on how to handle the most common injuries and illnesses, in alphabetical order. Many of these problems call for techniques covered in "Lifesaving Skills" on pages 12 through 23.

Animal Bites

WHAT TO DO

➤ Press directly on the wound until the bleeding stops, using a clean cloth (or, if you have to, your hand). Hold the edges of the flesh together (see **cuts, scrapes, and wounds,** page 28).

➤ If the bite is minor, clean it well with soap and water. Then put on antibiotic ointment and a bandage.

➤ If the bite is deep, don't clean the wound after you stop the bleeding. Call your doctor for a prompt appointment. A deep bite may need stitches and could become infected. You may need antibiotics, a tetanus shot, or rabies treatment.

➤ If possible (whether the animal is wild or a pet), have your local animal control center confine the animal and check it for rabies. Unvaccinated pets—along with stray cats and dogs, and wild animals such as raccoons, bats, foxes, and skunks—may carry rabies. Rabies infection is rare but can be fatal if not treated.

➤ Report any wild animal bites to your doctor and local health department or animal control center.

Cautions:

➤ Don't go near an animal that is drooling or foaming at the mouth, acting strangely, or biting for no reason. It may be rabid. Call your doctor and local health department or animal control center.

➤ Watch for signs of infection in a bite wound: redness, pain, swelling, tenderness, pus, hot skin, fever. Call your doctor for advice if you see these signs.

Appendicitis

SIGNS AND SYMPTOMS

■ Pain in the abdomen. It may start in the upper part, then move in a few hours to the lower right. The pain often gets worse until it becomes sharp and severe.

■ Vomiting, nausea, or loss of appetite.

■ Constipation or, less often, diarrhea.

■ Low fever.

An inflamed and infected appendix (appendicitis) can rupture after 24 hours and spread infection to nearby organs. To prevent this, a surgeon removes the appendix before it ruptures.

Pain in the abdomen may also signal **food poisoning** (see page 34), **gallstones** (see page 122), **kidney stones** (see page 136), a urinary tract infection (see **painful urination,** page 138), or an intestinal blockage (see **abdominal pain** chart, page 117).

WHAT TO DO

➤ If abdominal pain lasts for more than 4 hours, call a doctor for emergency advice. If you can't get one, call 911 or go to an emergency room.

➤ Keep the person quiet and as comfortable as possible.

➤ Watch the symptoms for 4 to 12 hours, looking out for severe pain in the lower right abdomen.

Cautions:
- ➤ If the person is constipated, don't give him or her laxatives. They can indirectly cause the appendix to rupture.
- ➤ Don't use an electric blanket or apply direct heat to the abdomen.
- ➤ Painkillers or antibiotics can mask symptoms, so don't give them if you suspect appendicitis.

Bee & Wasp Stings
www.SavonFirstAid.com

SIGNS AND SYMPTOMS

Minor stings:
- ■ Pain that lasts for several hours.
- ■ Redness, swelling, and itching or burning at the sting site.

Allergic reactions to stings:
- ■ Severe itching or hives.
- ■ Dizziness.
- ■ Reddish rash.
- ■ Cramping.
- ■ Trouble breathing.
- ■ Swelling of the eyes, lips, tongue, or throat.
- ■ Fever.
- ■ Drowsiness or loss of consciousness.
- ■ **Shock from allergy** (see page 22).

WHAT TO DO

All stings:
- ➤ If you see a stinger, scrape it off or pluck it out as quickly as you can. Don't waste time looking for a credit card or knife to scrape with. A stinger keeps injecting venom after it's torn off the insect, and even a slight delay means a person will get a bigger dose.
- ➤ Wash the area with soap and water.
- ➤ Apply a cold compress.

Allergic reactions to stings:
- ➤ Call 911 or go to an emergency room **right away.**
- ➤ Watch for the symptoms of **shock from allergy** (see page 22), such as wheezing or severe trouble breathing, rapid heartbeat, nausea, or loss of consciousness.

- ➤ If you have an emergency kit with epinephrine to counter severe allergic reactions, give the drug. **Caution:** Don't give epinephrine to an older person or one who has a heart condition.
- ➤ If needed, begin **CPR** (see page 14).
- ➤ If you know you are allergic to insect bites, wear a medical alert tag and ask your doctor about an emergency kit with a shot of epinephrine. It's a good idea to carry the kit to picnics, hikes, and outdoor events.

Blow to the Abdomen
www.SavonFirstAid.com

SIGNS AND SYMPTOMS

- ■ Hard or tender abdomen.
- ■ Vomiting, nausea, or loss of appetite.
- ■ Bleeding from the rectum or vagina, or blood in the urine.
- ■ Cold, clammy skin.
- ■ Weak, rapid pulse.
- ■ Uneven (rapid or slow) breathing.
- ■ Confusion or memory loss.

Watch for signs of abdominal injuries after any accident. A blow to the abdomen may lead to **shock** from internal bleeding (see page 22), a life-threatening condition.

WHAT TO DO

- ➤ Call 911 or go to an emergency room **right away.**
- ➤ Check the **ABCs** (see box on page 12): Lift the chin to open the airway, then check for breathing and pulse.
- ➤ If you see signs of **shock,** follow the instructions on page 22.
- ➤ If the person is not breathing or has no pulse, begin **CPR** (see page 14).
- ➤ While waiting for medical help, lay the person down, feet higher than heart. Keep him or her warm with a blanket, and loosen any tight clothing. **Caution:** Do not let the person eat or drink.

Burns
www.SavonBurns.com

SIGNS AND SYMPTOMS

- Red marks, dry white marks, or charring.
- Pain.
- Blistering.
- Swelling.

Burns are ranked as first-, second-, third-, or fourth-degree, depending on their depth (not the area they cover or how painful they are). **First-degree burns** sear only the outer layer of the skin, but can be very painful. **Second-degree burns** injure both the outer and inner layers of skin and often produce blisters, swelling, and severe pain. **Third-degree burns**—charred or white skin—are painless because they burn down through all the layers of the skin, including the nerve endings. **Fourth-degree burns** go through all the layers of skin to the tissues and organs below.

WHAT TO DO

➤ Move the person away from the burn source. If his or her clothing is on fire, lay the person on the ground and smother the flames with a blanket, coat, or any other handy cloth. Or tell the person to lie down and roll over slowly. **Caution:** If you suspect a **head, neck, or back injury** (see page 36), don't move the person unless you absolutely have to. Moving may cause further injury.

➤ Call 911 or go to an emergency room **right away** if the burns cover more than one body part; if they involve the face, hands, feet, or genitals; or if they appear to be third- or fourth-degree.

➤ If the person is unconscious, check the **ABCs** (see box on page 12): Lift the chin to open the airway, then check for breathing and pulse. If the person is not breathing or has no pulse, begin **CPR** (see page 14).

➤ Take off clothing or jewelry in the burned area before swelling begins. **Cautions:**

Burns From Chemicals

Signs and Symptoms
- Blisters or burn marks.
- Headache or stomach pain.
- Trouble breathing.
- Seizures or dizziness.
- Loss of consciousness.

What to Do
➤ Move the person away from any contact with the chemical.

➤ Brush off any dry chemicals. Protect your hands with gloves or clothing when doing so.

➤ Run water over the injured area for at least 15 minutes to dilute the chemical. Use plenty of water. If you know what substance caused the burn, read the label on the packaging for the maker's emergency instructions, and call a doctor **right away.**

➤ If the burn is in the eye, pour water over the open eye from the inside corner to the outside (see **eye injuries,** page 32). Go to an emergency room **right away.**

➤ Take off the person's jewelry and any clothing that may have touched the chemical.

➤ Protect the burn with a dry sterile bandage.

➤ Call a doctor for an emergency appointment. If you can't get one, call 911 or go to an emergency room.

➤ If the person is unconscious, check the **ABCs** (see box on page 12): Lift the chin to open the airway, then check for breathing and pulse.

➤ If the person is not breathing or has no pulse or heartbeat, call 911 and begin **CPR** (see page 14).

Don't pull away any clothing stuck to burned skin. Don't blow on burned skin.

➤ If the burned area is smaller than the size of the person's chest, cover it loosely with a cloth that has been soaked in cool water and wrung out, or hold the burned area under cool running water or in a bowl of cool water for about 10 minutes, or until the pain stops or decreases.

➤ If the burn is larger than the size of the person's chest, don't put water on it (this could lead to hypothermia). Cover the burned skin loosely with a clean, dry cloth. If fluid oozes through the cloth, put another cloth over it.

➤ To reduce swelling, raise the burned area higher than the person's heart.

➤ Unless the person is vomiting or unconscious, you may give small sips of water.

➤ If the person is unconscious but still breathing, support the head and roll him or her onto the side, into the **recovery position** (see page 23).

Cautions:

➤ Do not put the person in the recovery position if you suspect a **head, neck, or back injury** (see page 36), or if the burn is on the chest or elsewhere on the front of the body.

➤ Don't put ice, ointments, lotions, butter, or baking soda on the burn.

➤ Don't break any blisters.

➤ Don't use adhesive tape or bandages, or cotton balls. They stick to the skin.

Chest Pain
www.SavonChestPain.com

SIGNS AND SYMPTOMS

■ Dull, sharp, crushing, stabbing, or severe burning pain, or pressure or tightness in the chest. Pain may spread to the jaw, neck, back, or arms, especially the left arm.

See the **chest pain** chart (page 105). Depending on the type of pain and other symptoms, chest pain could signal a number of ailments, including **heart attack** (see page 37), angina, a collapsed lung, pleurisy

(inflammation of the sac around the lungs), an injured rib or a pulled chest muscle, an **ulcer** (see page 134), **heartburn** (see page 124), or **anxiety** (see page 208). Never ignore chest pain that lasts longer than a few minutes.

WHAT TO DO

➤ If you suspect a **heart attack** (see page 37), call 911 **right away.**

Childbirth
www.Childbirth.com
Emergency

SIGNS AND SYMPTOMS

■ Contractions of the uterus 2 to 3 minutes apart.
■ A liquid discharge from the woman's vagina.
■ An overwhelming urge by the woman to push, or to move her bowels.
■ Feeling or seeing the baby's head emerge.

Caution: Childbirth is a natural process, even when it comes unexpectedly at home or on the way to the hospital. If you are in labor or with someone who is about to give birth, don't try to stop the process or delay delivery. Stay calm and call for help.

WHAT TO DO

Before delivery:

➤ Call a doctor for emergency instructions. If you can't get one, call 911 or go to an emergency room **right away.**

➤ If you have no time to get to a hospital and medical help hasn't yet arrived, prepare a place—with a plastic sheet and clean linens and pillows, if possible—for mother and child.

➤ Collect clean towels, sheets, or other cloths. Sterilize scissors or a knife and a few feet of string by plunging them into boiling water.

➤ Keep the woman warm. Make her comfortable. Help her take off her clothes from the waist down.

➤ Remove your jewelry and wristwatch. Wash your hands well with soap and hot water. Scrub under your nails.

➤ Stay calm. Help the woman take slow, deep, calming breaths.

➤ Try to get a medical person—at a fire, police, or rescue department or a hospital—on the phone to talk you through the delivery.

During delivery:

➤ You will see some bloody fluid and other discharge. Watch for the baby's head to appear in the opening to the vagina. Have a clean towel or cloth to wrap the baby in as soon as the baby comes out.

➤ Be ready to support the baby's head as it comes through the vagina. The baby's shoulders and body should follow on the next contractions. **Caution:** Don't pull on the baby's head. Support it gently as the shoulders slide out.

➤ When the head emerges, see if the umbilical cord is wrapped around the baby's neck. If it is, use 2 fingers to gently ease it over the baby's head.

➤ There may be a gush of fluid as the baby's body slides out, and the baby will be very slippery. Have the clean cloth or towel ready to grasp the baby.

➤ If the baby doesn't come out headfirst, don't try to pull the baby out. Support the body as best you can to expose the face so that the baby can breathe, and get medical help **right away.**

After delivery:

➤ The baby may still be wrapped in a bag of fluids (the amniotic sac). If so, rip the sac open with your fingers. Gently clear it away from the baby's mouth and nose.

➤ Hold the newborn with his or her head lower than the body. Turn the head to the side, so that fluids will drain from the baby's mouth and nose.

➤ Place the baby lower than the mother's buttocks to help keep blood flowing to the baby through the umbilical cord.

➤ Wipe the baby's nose and mouth gently with a clean cloth, to remove mucus and other fluids so they won't get into the

baby's lungs. Don't wash the baby. Most babies start to breathe at this point.

➤ If the baby doesn't start breathing within 30 seconds after delivery: Keep the head lower than the body. Tap the soles of the baby's feet. Then rub the baby's back.

➤ If the baby still doesn't start to breathe, begin infant rescue breathing (see page 16). Use only very gentle puffs of air.

➤ When the baby and mother seem okay, make sure that both are warm. Now, you can put the baby on the mother's stomach or chest; this will reduce heat loss.

➤ Encourage the mother to start nursing. The baby's sucking helps release a hormone that makes the uterus contract and prevents further bleeding.

➤ Don't pull on the umbilical cord. It is attached to the placenta, or afterbirth, which will come out 10 to 20 minutes after the baby does.

➤ Don't cut the umbilical cord. Wait for a doctor to do it. Get ready to cut the cord *only* if medical help is far away or if mother and baby are having serious problems: For instance, if the baby can't breathe and needs to be resuscitated, you will probably have to cut the cord to get into position for rescue breathing

If you need to cut the umbilical cord:

➤ Strip the blood in the cord toward the baby several times.

➤ Use the cleanest string you have to tie off the cord at least 7 inches from the baby's navel. Make a second tie about 3 inches beyond that, closer to the mother. Be sure both ties are tight.

➤ Use scissors you have sterilized—or that you have made as clean as you can—to cut between the two knots.

Cuts, Scrapes & Wounds
www.SavonFirstAid.com

Life is full of scrapes, cuts, and punctures. Scrapes can hurt, but they usually bleed only a little. Cuts can bleed heavily. Puncture wounds may not bleed much, unless they rupture major blood vessels or organs, but they can get infected.

WHAT TO DO

➤ Call for emergency medical advice if a wound is deeper than one-quarter inch and longer than 1 inch; if it has jagged edges; or if bleeding doesn't stop after 5 minutes. If you can't get a doctor, go to an emergency room.

Severe bleeding:

➤ Call 911 or go to an emergency room **right away** (see **when bleeding won't stop,** page 13).

Head wound:

➤ If the injury is more than a minor bump or surface cut, call 911 **right away.**

➤ Do not move the person unless you absolutely must; this can cause further injury (see **head, neck, and back injuries,** page 36).

➤ If a head wound is bleeding but not deep, cover the wound with a clean bandage or cloth. Press directly on the wound. If a cloth becomes soaked with blood, don't remove it. Put another cloth on top of it, and keep pressing.

➤ Put a cold compress over the wound to ease pain and swelling.

➤ Keep the person calm and still until medical help arrives.

➤ Watch the person for 24 hours for signs of serious injury—confusion, unusual drowsiness, bleeding from the ears or nose, or loss of movement on one side of the body.

Eye or eyelid cut:

➤ Cover both eyes lightly with bandages. **Caution:** Don't apply direct pressure to a bleeding eye.

➤ Call a doctor for an emergency appointment. If you can't get one, call 911 or go to an emergency room.

Minor bleeding, a puncture wound, or a scrape:

➤ Clean the wound with soap and water.

➤ Cover the wound with a bandage to stop the bleeding and prevent infection. If you are using an elastic bandage, be sure

Blood Poisoning

Blood poisoning (septicemia) is the term for a bacterial infection in the blood. This may spread from a wound, appendicitis, a burn, a urinary tract or lung infection, or dental work, or from injecting street drugs. The bloodstream then carries the infection to other parts of the body.

Signs and Symptoms

- Chills and fever.
- Headache.
- Fatigue or confusion.
- Nausea, diarrhea, or lost appetite.
- Warm, flushed skin.
- Increased heart rate.

What to Do

➤ Call a doctor for emergency advice. If you can't get one, call 911 or go to an emergency room. You may need antibiotics.

➤ Watch for signs of septic shock, a common side effect of blood poisoning with some of the following symptoms: rapid pulse and breathing, temperature below normal, fainting, and possibly confusion or coma. If symptoms appear, call 911 **right away.** If you are waiting for medical help to arrive, see **shock,** page 22.

---

it's not so tight that it cuts off internal blood flow. Make sure you can slip a finger between the bandage and the skin.

➤ For deep puncture wounds, call your doctor for emergency advice.

➤ Watch for signs of infection: redness, pus, swelling, pain, and fever. If the wound becomes infected, call a doctor for advice.

➤ Make sure the person has a current vaccination against tetanus.

Drowning
www.SavonFirstAid.com

SIGNS AND SYMPTOMS

- Pale or bluish skin, especially the lips.
- Cold body.
- Loss of consciousness.
- No breathing.

Drowning occurs when water blocks the air supply to the lungs. Big bodies of water aren't the only places it happens. People also drown at home—in bathtubs, pools, and whirlpool baths. Toddlers can drown in pails and toilets. Knowledge of rescue breathing and CPR can save a life.

WHAT TO DO

In the water:
- If you are a very strong swimmer and see a person floating face down in the water or having trouble swimming, wade out into the water and retrieve the victim face up. Otherwise, tell any nearby lifeguard or emergency worker and call 911 **right away.**
- If you are in the water with a drowning person who has stopped breathing, begin the rescue breathing phase of **CPR** (see page 14), if possible. Tilt the head back, pinch the nostrils closed, and breathe into the mouth. As you pause between breaths, move toward land. **Caution:** Don't try rescue breathing in the water unless you can safely stand up in it, or unless you are a very strong swimmer.

Out of the water:
- If a person has been pulled from the water unconscious, check the **ABCs** (see box on page 12): Lift the chin to open the airway, then check for breathing and pulse. If the person is not breathing or does not have a pulse or heartbeat, begin **CPR** (see page 14). If the person is a young child or an infant, see page 17 or 16.
- People who have almost drowned often cough up water and food during rescue breathing. Turn the head to the side from time to time to allow water and vomit to

drain from the mouth, and sweep out the mouth with your finger.
- If the person is on land and unconscious but breathing, support the head and roll him or her onto the side into the **recovery position** (see box on page 23) to keep the airway open. **Caution:** Don't move the person into the recovery position if you suspect a **head, neck, or back injury** (see page 36)—such as from a diving accident.
- Remove wet clothing, and cover the person with a coat, blanket, or dry clothes.
- Help the person rest quietly until medical help arrives.

Caution: In cold water or icy conditions, watch for symptoms of **hypothermia** (shivering, uncoordinated movements, drowsiness, loss of consciousness). See page 39.

Ear Emergencies
www.SavonFirstAid.com

SIGNS AND SYMPTOMS

- Earache.
- Muffled or lost hearing; ringing in the ear.
- Swelling or redness.
- Blood or other fluids draining from the ear.
- Dizziness, nausea, or vomiting.

While an earache may signal an ear emergency, it is also a sign of less serious problems, ranging from an **ear infection** (see page 71) to a blockage from **earwax** (see page 72). If you have a long-lasting earache, call your doctor for advice.

WHAT TO DO

If blood or fluids are draining from the ear:
- If you suspect a head injury, call 911 or go to an emergency room **right away.**
- Cover the ear loosely with a clean cloth. Tape it in place. Don't try to clean the ear.
- Lay the person face up while waiting for medical help. **Caution:** If you suspect a **head, neck, or back injury** (see page 36),

don't move the person; this could cause permanent injury.

If an eardrum has burst:

➤ If a person suddenly has pain, ringing, or buzzing in the ear; trouble hearing; or discharge (including pus or blood), an eardrum may be ruptured. Call a doctor for a prompt appointment.

➤ To prevent infection, cover the ear with a dry sterile pad.

➤ Give an over-the-counter pain reliever such as acetaminophen or aspirin. Never give aspirin, however, to a child or teenager who has chicken pox, the flu, a cold, or any other illness you suspect of being caused by a virus (see box on **Reye's syndrome,** page 95).

If a foreign object is in the ear:

➤ Shake it out: Have the person tilt his or her head so that the sore ear faces down. Straighten the ear canal by gently pulling the top part of the ear up and back, then shake the head. **Caution:** Don't shake an infant or a young child.

➤ If nothing comes out, look for the object in the ear. If you can see it, use a pair of tweezers carefully to try to remove it. Don't try to remove a live insect or hard object.

➤ If you can't see it, don't try to take it out. Go to a doctor or an emergency room.

If a live insect is in the ear:

➤ Try floating the insect out by pouring a small amount of warm (not hot) oil— baby, mineral, or olive—into the ear. This may also ease pain.

➤ To apply oil: Have the person tilt the head so the sore ear is up. Gently open the ear by pulling it upward and back. Slowly pour in the warm oil and watch for the insect to float out.

Cautions:

➤ Don't push on anything in the ear or push anything into the ear.

➤ Don't try to remove a hard, smooth object such as a BB or bead.

➤ Don't work on the ear if the person (especially a child) won't hold still.

➤ Never strike anyone on the head to try to clear an ear.

Electric Shock
www.SavonFirstAid.com

SIGNS AND SYMPTOMS

■ Deep, charred, or small burns on the mouth or other parts of the body.
■ Tingling sensation.
■ Sudden dizziness or headache.
■ Muscle pains.
■ Loss of consciousness, which may include no breath or heartbeat.

WHAT TO DO

➤ Remove the source of electricity as quickly and safely as possible. **Caution:** Don't touch the person until the current is off or gone. Don't use appliance switches— they may not work. Unplug the appliance or turn off main power switches.

➤ If you can't turn the current off, get the person away from it. **Caution:** Don't use your hands or anything metal or wet. Insulate yourself by standing on a rubber mat, newspapers or books, something wooden, or a pile of clothing or linens. Use a dry, nonconducting object to separate the person from the current: a stick, a wooden chair or small table, or a rope.

➤ When you can touch the person safely, check the **ABCs** (see box on page 12): Lift the chin to open the airway, then check for breathing and pulse.

➤ Look for injuries, especially burns. If you see any, call 911 **right away. Caution:** Electrical burns are often deeper and more serious than they appear.

➤ Give first aid for **burns** (see page 26).

➤ Cover the person and make him or her as comfortable as possible.

➤ If the person might have been struck by lightning, call 911 **right away.** It's all right to touch a lightning victim and begin first aid—the electricity is gone.

➤ For other electric shocks, call a doctor for emergency advice. If you can't get one, call 911 or go to an emergency room, even if the person seems unharmed.

If someone has been shocked by a downed electrical wire:
➤ Stay at least 20 feet away from high-voltage current.
➤ Call 911, then call the power company to have the current turned off.
➤ If the person is inside a car or truck and is conscious, tell him or her to stay there unless there is a fire or other immediate danger. If the person must leave the car, tell him or her not to touch the car and the ground at the same time. Have the person jump clear of the vehicle.
➤ As soon as the power is off or the person is clear of the current, begin first aid.

Caution:
➤ Don't touch any electrical wire, car, or person in contact with a live wire.

Eye Injuries
www.SavonFirstAid.com

SIGNS AND SYMPTOMS

■ Bruise or cut on the eye.
■ Pain.
■ Bloodshot eye.
■ Itching, dryness, or tears in the eye.
■ Blinking, or trouble keeping the eye open.
■ Sensitivity to light.
■ Trouble seeing.
■ Headache.
■ Different-size pupils.

WHAT TO DO

Foreign object in the eye:
➤ Call 911 or go to an emergency room **right away.**

Cautions:
➤ If the object is stuck in the eye, don't try to take it out.
➤ Don't touch the object; keep the person's hands away from the eye.
➤ If a large object such as a pencil is in the eye, tape a paper cone or cup over it to support the object. For a long object, punch a hole in the bottom of the cup.

Cover the person's other eye with a clean cloth; this will help keep the injured eye from moving.
➤ For a small object, tie a clean cloth loosely over both eyes for the trip to the emergency room.

Bleeding in the eye:
➤ If the eye is bleeding, cover both eyes with a clean cloth and raise the person's head above the heart. Then call 911 or go to an emergency room **right away. Caution:** Don't try to move the person if you suspect a **head, neck, or back injury** (see page 36). You may cause further injury.

Foreign objects not embedded in the eye:
➤ If the person is wearing contact lenses and can safely remove them, he or she should do so. The object may come out with the contact lens.
➤ If that doesn't work, clean your hands with soap and water, then ask the person to sit in good light and look up as you gently pull down the lower eyelid. Look inside the eye and the lower eyelid. If the object is there, pull the upper lid gently over the lower. The tears that follow may wash out the object.

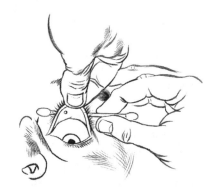

How to fold back the upper eyelid

➤ If tears don't wash the object out, flush the eye with running water—either from a cup or the tap. The person can also try opening his or her eyes underwater in a bowl of fresh tap water.
➤ If you can't see the object in the lower lid or eye, ask the person to look down. Put a cotton swab or wooden matchstick lengthwise against the upper lid. Then pull up gently on the upper lashes and lid and fold the lid over the stick. You may now be able to see the object. Use

running water to wash it out, or take it out using the edge of a clean, soft, damp cloth or cotton swab. **Caution:** If the object is on the colored part of the eye or on the pupil, don't try to remove it with anything but cool running water.

➤ Wash the eye gently with cool water.

➤ If you can't find or remove the object, or you do remove it but the person is still in pain or can't see, tie a clean cloth over both eyes and go to an emergency room.

Caution:

➤ Keep the person's hands away from the eye—rubbing can scratch the surface of the eye.

Scratched eyeball:

➤ Wash your hands. A scratched eyeball can become infected.

➤ Rinse the eye with cool, clean water for 5 to 15 minutes. The water should run from the inside corner of the eye to the outside. Hold the eyelid open to make sure the water gets under it.

➤ Cover both eyes with a clean cloth, and tie it loosely in place.

➤ Go to an emergency room.

Chemicals in the eye:

➤ Ask the person to remove contact lenses, if any. Then flush the eye for 15 to 20 minutes: Hold the eye open under running water from a faucet or cup. Let the water run from the inside to the outside corner of the eye. Make sure water gets under the lids. Keep the injured eye lowest so that chemicals don't run into the other eye.

➤ If both eyes are injured, let water run from the inside to the outside corners of both. Make sure water gets under the lids. **Cautions:** Don't put anything but water in the eye. Keep the person's hands away from the eyes.

➤ Tie a clean cloth over both eyes.

➤ Call 911 or go to an emergency room **right away.** Tell emergency nurses and doctors as much as you can about the chemicals involved.

Fainting & Loss of Consciousness
www.SavonFirstAid.com

SIGNS AND SYMPTOMS

Just before fainting:
- Light-headedness, dizziness, weakness, or yawning.
- Pale, cold, or clammy skin.
- Sweat on the face, neck, or hands.

Prolonged loss of consciousness:
- Lack of awareness or no response for several minutes.

A moment of **fainting**—partial or brief loss of consciousness usually caused by a short-term drop in blood flow to the brain—is seldom harmful. **Loss of consciousness** for more than a minute or two, however, may mean something more serious: concussion, stroke, or other brain damage; abnormal heart rhythm or heart attack; major blood loss; a lack of oxygen in the blood; diabetic coma; epilepsy; or drug reaction. To find out whether someone is unconscious, tap the person on the shoulder and ask, "Are you okay?"

WHAT TO DO

Cautions:

➤ Don't try to revive someone by shaking, slapping, or dousing with cold water.

➤ Don't put a pillow under the person's head—this can bend the neck and block the airway.

➤ Don't give anything to eat or drink (including alcohol) until the person is fully conscious. If you know the person is diabetic, however, try giving sips of juice or soda (not sugarless).

Someone about to faint:

➤ Keep the person from falling, then help him or her lie down.

➤ Raise the legs 8 to 12 inches, so that blood can flow to the brain.

➤ Use a cool, damp cloth to wipe the forehead.

➤ Loosen clothing that seems tight, especially at the neck or waist.

FIRST AID

Someone who has already fainted:

➤ If you find an unconscious person and don't know the cause, look for a medical alert tag or an injury.

➤ Lay the person on his or her back. Raise the legs 8 to 12 inches. **Caution:** Don't move the person if you suspect a **head, neck, or back injury** (see page 36). You may cause further injury.

➤ Check the **ABCs** (see box on page 12): Lift the chin to open the airway, then check for breathing and pulse. If the person is not breathing or has no heartbeat, call 911 and begin **CPR** (see page 14).

➤ Loosen any tight clothing, especially at the neck or waist.

➤ If the person has fallen, check for injuries. Look especially for head wounds. If any, call a doctor for emergency advice. If you can't get one, call 911 or go to an emergency room.

➤ If the person is vomiting, turn the head to the side so that the airway isn't blocked.

Lost consciousness (more than a minute):

➤ If the person is injured, move him or her only to avoid further injury. **Caution:** Don't try to move the person if you suspect a **head, neck, or back injury** (see page 36). You may cause further injury.

➤ Call 911.

➤ Check the **ABCs** (see box on page 12): Lift the chin to open the airway, then check for breathing and pulse. Begin **CPR** (see page 14) if the person isn't breathing or has no heartbeat or pulse.

➤ Keep the airway open: Roll the person onto his or her side while supporting the head. This is the **recovery position** (see box on page 23). **Caution:** Don't place a person in the recovery position if you suspect a head, neck, or back injury.

➤ Keep the person warm.

➤ Use a cool, damp cloth to wipe the forehead.

➤ Check for a medical alert tag that says whether the person has diabetes, epilepsy, or drug allergies. Tell medical people about it. (See page 41 for treatment of epileptic **seizures**; see page 22 for **shock from allergy.**)

Food Poisoning
www.SavonFirstAid.com

SIGNS AND SYMPTOMS

Bacterial:
- Fever.
- Many stools or diarrhea (often severe or explosive), which may be bloody.
- Severe pain and cramping in the abdomen.
- Vomiting.

Botulism:
- Nausea, vomiting, diarrhea.
- Drooping eyelids or blurry vision.
- Dry mouth, trouble swallowing.
- Trouble breathing.
- Muscle weakness or paralysis.

Viral:
- Diarrhea, abdominal cramps, and vomiting.

Chemical:
- Diarrhea and vomiting.
- Sweating.
- Dizziness.
- Confusion.
- Tearing eyes.
- Drooling.
- Stomach pain.

Spoiled or contaminated food can lead to food poisoning. The most common type is **bacterial,** most often passed along by human hands during kitchen work or found in undercooked or unrefrigerated food. **Botulism** is a rare but severe form. It's caused by bacterial poisons that form when foods such as vegetables or fruits are incorrectly preserved or canned at home. **Viruses** that get into food, and **chemical toxins** in certain foods—such as some mushrooms, moldy peanuts, and potato sprouts—can also cause food poisoning.

WHAT TO DO

➤ Call 911 or go to an emergency room **right away** if you see or feel symptoms of botulism (muscle weakness, trouble swallowing and breathing, blurred vision) or chemical food poisoning (vomiting, diarrhea, mental confusion, stomach pain). These can be fatal.

➤ If vomiting and diarrhea are severe, call your doctor for a prompt appointment. You may need treatment for dehydration (see **diarrhea,** page 119, and **nausea and vomiting,** page 133).

➤ Don't take antidiarrhea medicines if you suspect food poisoning. You should allow vomiting and diarrhea to flush the toxins out of your system. Don't eat solid food during periods of vomiting and diarrhea.

➤ As soon as you can keep fluids in your stomach, drink clear liquids such as water, sports drinks, or noncaffeinated tea for about 12 hours to replace fluids you've lost. Liquids should be room temperature, not cold. Sip the drinks; don't gulp. Next, eat bland foods for about 24 hours. Good choices include cooked cereals, rice, bread, and broth.

Fractures & Dislocations

www.SavonFirstAid.com

SIGNS AND SYMPTOMS

- Pain.
- Distorted body part.
- Bruised or discolored skin.
- Swelling.
- A bone showing.
- Numbness.
- Lost function around injury.

Fractures are breaks, cracks, or chips in a bone. When the skin is not broken, it's called a closed fracture. When a bone breaks through the skin, it's called an open fracture. Open fractures are more dangerous, because they may lead to severe bleeding or infection. **Dislocations** happen when bones are moved out of their normal place at a joint, so the joint stops working. Dislocated joints often appear deformed.

WHAT TO DO

Caution:
Don't move the person if you suspect a **head, neck, or back injury** (see page 36). You may cause further injury.

➤ Call 911 or go to an emergency room **right away** if the person shows symptoms of **shock** or **internal bleeding** (see page 22).

➤ Call 911 if he or she is unconscious or can't be moved. Check the **ABCs** (see page 12).

➤ Begin **CPR** (see page 14) if the person is not breathing or has no heartbeat.

➤ Unless you have to, don't move the person if you suspect an injured pelvis—this may also mean an injury to the low back. Keep the person still.

➤ Check for other injuries. If the person has an open fracture, stop the bleeding: Tie a clean cloth over the wound and press on it. Don't wash or probe the injury (see **cuts, scrapes, and wounds,** page 28).

➤ Apply a cold compress for 10 to 30 minutes, leave it off for 30 to 45 minutes, and repeat (see box on **RICE,** page 198).

➤ If the person is mobile and conscious, no matter whether you think a bone is broken or simply dislocated, call a doctor for a prompt appointment. If you can't get one, go to the nearest emergency room.

Cautions:
➤ If you aren't sure whether a bone is broken, treat it as though it is.

➤ Don't try to move a bone or joint that appears distorted.

To immobilize an injured finger or toe:
➤ Put a small piece of cloth or a cotton ball between the injured finger or toe and one that isn't hurt. Tape them together. Raise the finger or toe above the person's heart.

To immobilize a forearm, wrist, or hand:
➤ Supporting the injured area, place the forearm on the person's stomach. Slip a magazine or newspaper padded with towels under the injured arm, wrist, or hand. Then fold the paper and padding around the arm to form a splint. Tie the splint in place on either side of the injury. The splint should go beyond the joints around the injury.

➤ To make a sling, fold a large cloth (a towel or shirt) into a triangle. Ease the wide

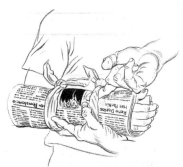

A splint made from newspaper

part under the injured arm, with any extra cloth at the elbow. Tie ends around the neck. Pin the extra cloth around the elbow. **Caution:** A sling should be snug, but not so tight that it cuts off blood flow.

To immobilize the lower leg:

➤ To make a splint using boards: Find 2 boards—broomsticks also work well— one the length of the person's leg from hip to heel, the other from groin to heel. Pad the boards with blankets or pillows, then tie them on either side of the leg at the groin, thigh, knee, and ankle.

➤ To make a splint using a blanket: Roll the blanket and place it lengthwise between the person's legs, then tie the legs together at the groin, thighs, knees, and ankles.

To immobilize the upper leg or hip:

Hip fractures cause bruising, swelling, tenderness, or deformity in the hip, and severe pain when the person tries to walk. **Caution:** Unless you have to move the person, don't splint a broken upper leg or hip.

➤ If you do have to use a splint: Find 2 boards, one long enough to reach from the person's armpit to the heel, the other from the groin to the heel. Pad them and tie them in place at the chest, waist, groin, thigh, knee, and ankle. But don't place a tie directly over the break.

Head, Neck & Back Injuries
www.SavonFirstAid.com

SIGNS AND SYMPTOMS

Head injury:
- Head wound, which may bleed heavily or show up as a lump or bruise.
- Blood or other fluid that drains from the mouth, nose, or ears, even with no direct injury to that area.
- Nausea, vomiting, or headache.
- Bruises around the eyes.
- Slurred speech or trouble breathing.
- Vision changes.
- Dizziness, confusion, seizures, or loss of consciousness.

Neck or back injuries:
- Severe pain.
- Trouble moving.
- Tingling in arms or legs.
- Lost control over bowel or bladder.
- Unusual posture of head, neck, or back.
- Unconsciousness.

Be especially alert for head, neck, and back injuries after vehicle accidents, jumping, falling, or diving accidents, and gunshot wounds to the head or chest. Multiple wounds, a broken helmet, or unconsciousness after physical trauma are other signs. People with head, neck, and back injuries need special care to avoid permanent paralysis. It's important to figure out the kind of injury.

WHAT TO DO

Don't move the injured person unless it's really necessary, as in the case of a fire, an explosion, or other life-and-death situation. Moving someone with a head, neck, or back injury could cause permanent spinal cord damage and even paralysis. If you must move someone, make sure the head, neck, and back are in a line and well supported. Don't turn the head sharply to straighten it.

➤ Call 911 **right away.**

➤ Keep a conscious person still and calm. This can be vital. Talk to him or her, and give emotional support.

➤ If the person is unconscious, check the **ABCs** (see box on page 12). Begin **CPR** (see page 14) if he or she isn't breathing or has no heartbeat or pulse.

Caution: Don't move the neck unless you must to keep the airway open. If you need to place the person face up for CPR, do so very carefully, supporting the head, neck, and back together. Make sure they're in a straight line. Get someone to help.

➤ Treat any injuries such as **cuts, scrapes, or wounds** (see page 28), or **fractures and dislocations** (see page 35).

➤ Keep the person warm and as comfortable as you can until help arrives. Loosen tight clothing and cover him or her with a blanket, coat, or other clothing.

➤ Don't give anything to eat or drink.

➤ To help keep the person's head and spine still, gently place your hands on either side of the head to hold it in line with the body. **Caution:** Don't turn the head or pull on it to straighten it. Don't put a pillow under the head—bending the neck might block the airway.

➤ A person with a head injury may vomit without warning and choke. So watch carefully while waiting for help.

➤ If the person chokes, vomits, or loses consciousness, sweep the airway clear with your fingers. If you have to turn the person on his or her side, do so very carefully, supporting the head, neck, and back together. Make sure they're in a straight line. Get someone to help.

Cautions:

➤ Gently cradle the person's head and neck to keep them in line.

➤ *Don't* place the person in the recovery position described on page 23.

Heart Attack
www.SavonHeartAttack.com

SIGNS AND SYMPTOMS

■ Crushing or squeezing chest pain or tightness that lasts 5 to 10 minutes and doesn't ease with rest. It often starts in the center of the chest, then spreads to the jaw, neck, back, or arms (most often the left arm). Women are less likely than men to have severe chest pain.

■ Shortness of breath.

■ Fear or anxiety.

■ Dizziness.

■ Sweating.

■ Nausea or vomiting.

■ Pale or bluish lips, skin, or fingernails.

■ Uneven heartbeat, or none.

■ Unconsciousness.

WHAT TO DO

➤ Call 911 **right away.**

➤ If the person is unconscious, check the **ABCs** (see box on page 12): Lift the chin to open the airway, then check for breathing and pulse. Begin **CPR** (see page 14) if the person isn't breathing or has no heartbeat or pulse. **Caution:** Don't try to move the person if you suspect a **head, neck, or back injury** (see page 36). You may cause further injury.

➤ Loosen tight clothing.

➤ Keep the person as warm and comfortable as you can until help arrives.

➤ If the person has lost consciousness but is breathing and has a heartbeat, support the head and roll him or her into the **recovery position** (see page 23). **Caution:** Don't try to revive the person by shaking or slapping; don't throw cold water on the person.

➤ If the person is conscious, a sitting or partly sitting position may make breathing easier. Offer comfort. If the person has heart medication, help him or her take it, following label instructions.

➤ Give the person an aspirin to chew. It can help dissolve a blood clot causing the attack. **Cautions:** Don't give aspirin if the person already takes it. If you can, also give the person up to 3 nitroglycerin pills to dissolve under the tongue, 5 minutes apart. Don't give any other medicine, or anything to eat or drink.

➤ Watch the person's breathing and pulse until medical help comes. If breathing or pulse stops, begin CPR.

Heatstroke & Heat Exhaustion

www.SavonFirstAid.com

SIGNS AND SYMPTOMS

Heatstroke:
- Temperature above 104 degrees.
- Hot, dry skin.
- Rapid breathing and pulse.
- Confusion, unconsciousness, or seizures.

Heat exhaustion:
- Rapid pulse.
- Clammy skin.
- Heavy sweating.
- Headache.
- Vomiting, nausea, or both.
- Stomach cramps; cramps in the arms and legs.
- Dizziness.

People get **heatstroke,** which needs emergency treatment, when they have been working or playing in a hot place for a long time. During heatstroke, a person's temperature rises to dangerous levels because the body's normal cooling system becomes overloaded and stops working. Then that person may lose consciousness or have seizures.

Heat exhaustion often happens when people work or exercise in hot weather and don't drink enough fluids. Then the body can't make enough sweat to cool itself. Heat exhaustion is less serious than heatstroke but may lead to it. Both are more common in the very young and the old.

WHAT TO DO

Heatstroke:
➤ Call 911 or go to an emergency room **right away.**
➤ Move the person to a cooler place as quickly as you can.
➤ Remove the person's clothing.
➤ Sponge or splash cool water on the person, or wrap him or her in wet towels or sheets. Also put cool, wet cloths on the forehead.
➤ Fan the person—use your hand, some paper, a fan, or a hair dryer set on cool.

Cautions:
➤ Don't use an alcohol rub.
➤ Don't give food or drink.

Heat exhaustion:
➤ Move the person to a cooler place as quickly as you can.
➤ Have the person sit or lie down if he or she is conscious. Raise the feet and loosen tight clothing. Remove any sweat-soaked clothing.
➤ Sponge or splash cool water on the person, or wrap him or her in wet towels or sheets. Put cool, wet cloths on the forehead.
➤ Fan the person—use your hand, some paper, a fan, or a hair dryer set on cool.
➤ If the person is conscious and can swallow and breathe, give him or her a rehydration drink: Mix 1 quart water with 1 teaspoon table salt, one-half teaspoon baking soda, 4 teaspoons cream of tartar, and 3 to 4 tablespoons sugar. **Caution:** Don't give to children under 12.
➤ If you can't make a rehydration drink, give sports drinks or fruit juices diluted with equal amounts of water.
➤ Be sure to give water or drinks in small sips. The person should drink until his or her urine is clear.
➤ If you take these steps and the person doesn't begin to improve, call 911 or go to an emergency room **right away.**

Cautions:
➤ Don't use an alcohol rub.
➤ Don't force the person to drink. Never give drinks with alcohol or caffeine (many soft drinks are loaded with caffeine).

Hypothermia & Frostbite

www.SavonFirstAid.com

SIGNS AND SYMPTOMS

Hypothermia:
- Shivering.
- Loss of coordination; clumsiness.
- Weakness, sleepiness, or unconsciousness.

Frostbite:
- Cold, numb skin.
- Blue or white skin; blackened, waxy, or hard skin.
- Lost use of the injured part.

Hypothermia occurs when body temperature falls much lower than normal. If not treated, it can lead to loss of consciousness, cardiac arrest, and death. It can occur in mild weather if a person becomes wet and exhausted.

Older people can get hypothermia in cool temperatures, even inside a building. With age, the body becomes less able to maintain an even temperature and to sense cold.

If you suspect someone's temperature has dropped too far, check it with a thermometer. If you don't have one, feel the skin over the abdomen—it's a better gauge than the hands or feet. If it feels cold, the person may be in danger.

Frostbite, caused by long exposure to cold, freezes the skin and damages deeper tissues.

WHAT TO DO

Call 911 or go to an emergency room **right away,** if you can.
- If the person has symptoms of both hypothermia and frostbite, treat the hypothermia first while you wait for medical help.

Hypothermia:
- Check the **ABCs** (see box on page 12): Lift the chin to open the airway, then check for breathing and a pulse. Start rescue breathing if needed, and chest compressions if you can't find a pulse or heartbeat (see **CPR,** page 14). **Note:** People with hypothermia sometimes have slow, weak pulses; take extra time to check for one.
- Guide or carry the person to shelter.
- Change the person's clothing if it is wet.
- Slowly warm the person. Begin by covering his or her head and neck. Use your own body heat, blankets, or aluminum foil. Put warm compresses (cloths soaked in warm water) on the person's chest, neck, and groin. **Caution:** Don't use direct heat such as an electric blanket. Warming should be gradual. Don't rub the hands or feet roughly.
- If the person is conscious, offer sips of a warmed, sweet beverage; don't give any drinks with alcohol.

Frostbite:
- Get the person to shelter.
- Loosen tight clothing; remove any jewelry.
- If the person's hands or feet are frostbitten, soak them for 20 minutes in a bowl of water warmed to no more than 105 degrees (it should feel comfortably warm, not hot, to healthy skin). Stir the water gently; add warm water as it cools. Cover other areas of frostbite for 30 minutes or more with cloths soaked in warm water. As often as needed, resoak the cloths to keep them warm.
- If you don't have warm water, use blankets, newspapers, or your own body to warm the frostbitten skin.
- Dry the damaged area gently when it is soft and warm, and feeling and color have returned. Put clean, dry cloths over the injured area; put dry cloths between frostbitten fingers. Keep the area warm with more dry cloths.

Cautions:
- Don't use direct heat such as electric blankets or a campfire.
- Don't massage frostbitten skin.
- Don't let the person smoke, or drink anything with alcohol.
- Don't thaw frozen skin if it could freeze again before help arrives; refreezing can make the injury worse.

Nose Problems
www.SavonFirstAid.com

SIGNS AND SYMPTOMS

Severe nosebleed:
- Bleeding from the nose or down the back of the throat.
- Gagging or choking.

Objects in the nose:
- Irritation or itching in the nose.
- Trouble breathing through one or both nostrils.
- Bleeding or smelly flow from a nostril.

WHAT TO DO

Severe nosebleed:
- Call a doctor for advice if blood is streaming down the back of the throat; if a nosebleed doesn't stop after 30 minutes; or if you suspect a **head, neck, or back injury** (see page 36). If you can't reach a doctor, call 911 or go to an emergency room.
- Have the person sit down and lean slightly forward.
- Pinch the nostrils shut for 5 to 10 minutes while the person leans forward. This may help keep blood from running down the throat and reduce the risk of vomiting.
- If the nosebleed continues after 10 minutes, have the person gently blow out excess blood. Do this only once.
- Pinch the nostrils shut for another 5 minutes. If the bleeding continues, put a small roll of cloth or tissue just inside the bleeding nostril. (Don't push the packing too far in—it should be easy to pull out.) Pinch the nostrils shut again.
- After the bleeding stops, hold a cold compress (a cloth soaked in cold water and wrung out) over the person's nose and face for about 10 minutes. Keep the person seated.
- After 30 minutes to an hour, take out the packing.
- To prevent drying or more bleeding, dab petroleum jelly inside the nostril.

Cautions:
- For 12 hours after the bleeding stops, the person shouldn't bend over, or blow or pick the nose.
- Watch for signs of a broken nose—it might be misshapen or bent, or you may see pain, swelling, or bruising around the eyes. Hold a cold compress or ice pack on the nose. Go to an emergency room.

Objects in the nose:
- First, ask the person to press a finger against the unblocked nostril and blow—this might help expel the object.
- If that doesn't work, sniffing pepper might help by causing a sneeze. Tell the person to inhale very lightly.
- If nothing works, go to an emergency room. **Caution:** Don't use tweezers or other tools to try to remove the object.

Poisoning
www.SavonFirstAid.com

SIGNS AND SYMPTOMS

- Headache or stomachache.
- Dizziness or seizures.
- Chills and fever.
- Trouble seeing.
- Odd-smelling breath.
- Pale or bluish skin; burn marks.
- Vomiting, nausea, or both.
- Trouble breathing.
- Sleepiness, unconsciousness.

WHAT TO DO

- If the person has inhaled a poison gas such as chlorine, or carbon monoxide from car exhaust or a faulty heater, get him or her to fresh air as fast as you can. **Caution:** Avoid the fumes yourself. Get someone to help you.
- If the person has lost consciousness, call 911 and check the **ABCs** (see box on page 12): Lift the chin to open the airway, then check for breathing and a pulse.
- If the person has lost consciousness but is breathing, roll him or her into the **recovery position** (see box on page 23). **Caution:** Don't try to move the person if you

suspect a **head, neck, or back injury** (see page 36). You may cause further injury.

Caution: A person who has been poisoned may show few symptoms or symptoms that are not listed here, so you should search for clues. Try to find out what the poison is. If the person is conscious, ask what he or she inhaled or swallowed. Sniff for strange odors. Check stoves and heaters. Look around for medicines or chemicals; for detergents, air fresheners, or other household items; and for parts of plants the person may have swallowed.

Poisonous Household Substances

Many household items are poisonous. Among the most common are:

Alcohol	Mothballs
Antifreeze	Oven cleaner
Deodorizers	Paint
Detergents	Paint remover
Disinfectants	Paint thinner
Fuels	Pesticides
Herbicides	Tobacco
Household cleaners	Turpentine

Besides these items, many prescription and over-the-counter drugs are poisonous if you mix them with alcohol or take big doses.

Poisonous Plants

A number of common garden plants and house plants are poisonous. So are many plant parts—seeds, berries, nuts, and bulbs—if swallowed. Call your local poison control center if you have questions about plants around your home. Some common plants to watch out for are:

Castor bean	Philodendron
Foxglove	Poison hemlock
Jimsonweed	Water hemlock
Oleander	

➤ Call your local poison control center. Tell the person at the center what you think may be the cause of the poisoning. Listen to instructions.

Cautions:
➤ Don't try to make the person vomit unless you're told to.
➤ Don't give the person anything to eat or drink unless you're told to.
➤ Don't rely on poison-remedy directions from product labels.

Seizures
www.SavonEpilepsy.com

SIGNS AND SYMPTOMS

- Tingling feelings.
- Muscle spasms, twitching, stiffening, thrashing.
- Drooling.
- Fixed stare, or eyes rolled back.
- Lost bowel or bladder control.
- Sleepiness, confusion, loss of consciousness.

Seizures are seldom fatal, though they can be alarming. Causes include epilepsy, diabetes, heatstroke, fever (in children), electric shock, poisoning, brain injury, drug or alcohol abuse, and abruptly stopping heavy use of alcohol or other drugs.

WHAT TO DO

➤ If someone with you feels a seizure about to start or begins to lose balance, guide him or her to a safe spot. Check for a medical alert tag and any recent injury.
➤ Call 911 if this is the person's first seizure; if another seizure starts within a few minutes; if the seizure lasts more than about 3 minutes; or if the person has diabetes, is pregnant, has been injured, or doesn't regain consciousness after the seizure ends.
➤ If the person stays unconscious for more than a few minutes after the muscles relax, check the **ABCs** (see box on page 12): Lift the chin to open the airway, then check for

breathing and a pulse. If you can't find a heartbeat or pulse, or the person isn't breathing, call 911 **right away** and begin **CPR** (see page 14). **Caution:** Don't try to move the person if you suspect a **head, neck, or back injury** (see page 36). You may cause further injury.

➤ During a seizure, guard the person against self-injury: Take off eyeglasses; push away or pad anything hard nearby, such as furniture. Don't try to restrain the person unless it looks as if he or she is about to be injured.

➤ Lay the person on his or her side to keep vomit from getting into the lungs. Put something soft under the person's head to protect it.

➤ Don't put your hands near or in the person's mouth. Don't try to hold on to the person's tongue or put anything in his or her mouth. Jaws clamping down can inflict a bad bite.

➤ Loosen tight clothing.

➤ When the seizure is over, help the person get comfortable. Offer reassurance. The person may be confused or drowsy, and may fall asleep.

➤ Stay with the person until he or she is completely conscious and safe or until medical help arrives.

Shortness of Breath
www.SavonFirstAid.com

SIGNS AND SYMPTOMS

■ Breathlessness or labored breathing, even with little or no physical activity.

■ Dizziness or light-headedness.

■ See the **breathing problems and coughs** chart, page 85.

WHAT TO DO

➤ Help the person get comfortable. Sitting up can aid breathing.

➤ Offer reassurance. Shortness of breath can lead to panic, which can make breathing even harder.

➤ If the person can answer questions (even with gestures), try to find out the cause of the breathing trouble.

➤ If the person also has chest pain (which may be mild or crushing, burning, or tight, and may spread to the jaw, neck, shoulder, or left arm), nausea, and dizziness, the person may be having a **heart attack** (see page 37). Call 911 **right away.**

➤ If the person is wheezing, coughing, or feels tight through the chest, he or she may be having an **asthma** attack (see page 88). If this is the first attack or if it is more serious than other attacks, call 911 or go to an emergency room **right away.** Help the person take any prescribed asthma medication.

➤ If the person also has a fever over 100 degrees or is coughing, he or she may have **acute bronchitis** (see page 90) or **pneumonia** (see page 97). Call a doctor for advice and an appointment. Give a pain reliever for fever, and a cough medicine. (Never give aspirin to a child or teenager who has chicken pox, the flu, a cold, or any other illness you suspect of being caused by a virus; see box on **Reye's syndrome,** page 95.)

➤ If the person is also wheezing and coughing up mucus, he or she may have **chronic bronchitis** or **emphysema** (see page 91). The person may already be under a doctor's care.

➤ If the person has been worried about something, the symptoms may be related to **stress** (see page 218) or **anxiety** (see page 208).

Snakebites
www.SavonFirstAid.com

SIGNS AND SYMPTOMS

Rattlesnake, cottonmouth, and copperhead bites:

■ Pain that increases at the bitten spot.

■ Rapid changes in skin color and swelling at the bitten spot.

- Twitching skin.
- Sweating, dizziness, nausea.
- Shock; convulsions.

Coral snake bites:
- Pain at the bitten spot.
- Sleepiness.
- Trouble seeing or speaking.
- Tremors, seizures, or delirium.

Four types of poisonous snakes live in the United States: rattlesnakes, coral snakes, cottonmouths (also called water moccasins), and copperheads. It's important to know which type bit you, so the hospital can give the right antivenin.

Rattlesnakes, cottonmouths, and copperheads have triangular heads, rather than the slimmer heads of other snakes. They all have long fangs, and their bites leave marks that are much alike—2 rows of marks, each topped by a fang wound. Copperheads and rattlesnakes shake their tails in warning, but copperheads don't have rattles. Cottonmouths, when angry, open their mouths to show the white lining that gives them their name. Coral snakes have red, black, and white or yellow rings, and black muzzles.

Snakebites seldom kill. The few deaths that occur are mostly from rattlesnakes. Coral snakes are the most poisonous, but they don't bite many people.

WHAT TO DO

If you're not certain a bite was from a poisonous snake, assume it was. Begin first aid:
- ➤ If the person has lost consciousness, check the **ABCs** (see box on page 12): Gently lift the chin to open the airway. Then check for breathing and a pulse. Start rescue breathing if needed, and chest compressions if you can't find a heartbeat or pulse (see **CPR,** page 14). Call 911 or go to an emergency room **right away** if you can. Tell the people there what kind of snake bit the person, if you know.
- ➤ If the person is conscious, keep him or her still and calm. If you can, lay the person down so the bite is below the level of

the heart—blood from the bite, and any venom, will flow more slowly to the heart.
- ➤ Remove any tight clothing or jewelry near the bite.
- ➤ If the bite was on an arm or leg and you know that the snake was poisonous and that it will take more than a half hour to get help, tie a light tourniquet above the bite.
- ➤ If you have to kill the snake, try not to damage the head; it will help with identification. Stay away from the snake.

Cautions:
- ➤ Don't make cuts near the bite. Don't try to suck out venom with a snakebite kit or your mouth—these measures don't help.
- ➤ Don't put a cold compress or ice on the bite.
- ➤ Don't let the person walk. Carry the person if he or she has to be moved.

Spider Bites & Scorpion Stings
www.SavonFirstAid.com

SIGNS AND SYMPTOMS

- Bite mark, sting mark, swelling, or blister at the bitten spot.
- Pain in the bite or sting area, or in the stomach.
- Nausea, vomiting, chills, or fever.
- Trouble breathing or swallowing.
- Severe sweating and excess saliva.

Two types of poisonous spiders live in the United States: the black widow and the brown recluse (fiddleback). Their bites are especially dangerous to children, seniors, and anyone who is ill. The black widow has a red spot on its abdomen and leaves only a faint red bite mark. The brown recluse has a brown, violin-shaped marking on its back; watch for a blister, swelling, and a bull's-eye-shaped bite.

Scorpions have poisonous stingers in their long, upturned "tails," but only a few of the species found in the United States inflict fatal stings.

WHAT TO DO

➤ Wash the wound with soap and water.

➤ Apply an ice pack or cold compress.

➤ Call your doctor for emergency advice. If you can't get one, call 911 or go to an emergency room.

➤ If possible, bring the spider or scorpion to the doctor's office or emergency room.

Caution: Watch for signs of **shock from allergy** (see page 22). If they appear, call 911 **right away.**

heart to reduce fluid buildup and swelling.

➤ Put on an elastic bandage to support the sprained or strained area. Wrap the bandage in an upward spiral, starting several inches below the injured area. You may wrap the bandage over the ice pack temporarily. **Caution:** Don't wrap the bandage too tightly.

➤ If a sling is needed, see **fractures and dislocations,** page 35.

➤ Don't put any weight on the strain or sprain for 1 to 3 days.

Sprains & Strains

www.SavonFirstAid.com

SIGNS AND SYMPTOMS

■ Pain.

■ Swelling.

■ Bruising.

A sprain is a tear or stretch in a ligament, the tough band of tissue that connects the bones of a joint. Sprains are common in the ankles, knees, wrists, and fingers. A **strain** (often called a "pulled muscle") is a tear or stretch in a muscle or tendon, the band of tissue that attaches a muscle to bone. **Strains** often occur in the neck, back, thigh, and calf.

WHAT TO DO

➤ Treat a severe sprain or strain (marked by swelling and intense pain, or a "pop" in a joint when you move it) as though it were a **fracture** (see page 35), and call a doctor for a prompt appointment.

➤ If the sprain or strain seems mild, apply a cold pack—a package of frozen vegetables or a plastic bag filled with ice cubes, wrapped in a damp cloth—several times a day for up to 3 days. Leave it on no more than 10 to 30 minutes at a time. Leave it off 30 to 45 minutes between applications. Use moderate pressure. This should reduce the pain and swelling. (See box on **RICE,** page 198).

➤ Keep the injured area raised above the

Stroke

www.SavonStrokes.com

SIGNS AND SYMPTOMS

■ Abrupt weakness or numbness of the face, arm, or leg (most often on one side of the body).

■ Sudden trouble seeing or loss of vision (often in only one eye).

■ Loss of speech, or trouble speaking or understanding speech.

■ Sudden, severe headache.

■ Dizziness, unsteadiness, or sudden loss of consciousness.

A stroke occurs when blood flow to the brain is cut off, usually because of a blocked artery. Though a stroke can be fatal or disabling, prompt medical help may reduce some of its worst effects.

WHAT TO DO

➤ Call 911 or go to an emergency room **right away.**

➤ If you're waiting for medical help to arrive, check the **ABCs** (see box on page 12): Lift the chin to open the airway, then check for breathing and pulse. If the person is not breathing or has no pulse, begin **CPR** (see page 14).

➤ If the person is unconscious but breathing, support the head and roll him or her onto the side, into the **recovery position** (see box on page 23). **Caution:** Don't place the person in the recovery position if you suspect a **head, neck, or back injury** (see page 36). Moving him or her could cause further injury.

➤ If the person is conscious, offer reassurance. Lay him or her down, with head and shoulders slightly raised by pillows. Loosen any tight clothing.

➤ If vomit or fluid is draining from the person's mouth, or if the person has trouble swallowing, turn him or her onto the side so the airway doesn't become blocked. **Caution:** Don't let the person eat or drink.

Tick Bites
www.SavonFirstAid.com

SIGNS AND SYMPTOMS

Lyme disease:
- A bull's-eye rash, often with a pale center, that may widen to several inches across. The rash begins to show 2 days to a month after the bite, and may last 2 to 4 weeks or longer.
- Flulike symptoms—such as headache, fatigue, fever, chills, and aching muscles and joints—starting within a month of the bite.

Rocky Mountain spotted fever:
- A pink rash that starts near the wrists and ankles 2 to 14 days after a tick bite, then spreads to the face, torso, and other areas of the body. The rash turns deep red, then looks like red pinpricks.
- Fever, chills, and severe headache.

The bite of the tiny deer tick may result in **Lyme disease** (see page 285), which can cause arthritis, heart problems, and vision and hearing problems, among other ailments. Bites of some other ticks can cause **Rocky Mountain spotted fever,** an infection that can be deadly if untreated.

WHAT TO DO

➤ If you can see the tick, remove it as soon as you can to prevent infection. Grasp it with tweezers close to the skin, then pull it out gently and steadily. If you don't have tweezers, use a glove, a piece of paper, or plastic wrap. (If you use your bare fingers, wash your hands right afterward.) Avoid squeezing or twisting the tick; this could spread bacteria into your skin or blood. Don't try to burn a tick off the skin. If you can't get all of the tick out, call a doctor for advice. Save the tick in a jar; rubbing alcohol will help preserve it.

➤ Wash the area of the bite with soap and water.

➤ Apply an antiseptic ointment or alcohol to prevent infection. An ice pack can help relieve pain, and calamine lotion will relieve itching.

➤ Watch for signs of Lyme disease or Rocky Mountain spotted fever.

➤ If you see symptoms, call a doctor for a prompt appointment. Bring the tick with you, if you saved it.

Tooth Knocked Out
www.SavonFirstAid.com

WHAT TO DO

➤ Call a dentist **right away** or go to an emergency room. Teeth replanted within an hour or two can survive. Pick up the tooth by the crown (the part of the tooth that shows when it's in place), not the root. Use sterile gauze. The tooth must be kept as germ-free as possible.

➤ Wash the tooth quickly, either under running water or in saliva, and put it back in the socket at once. Bite down gently on the tooth or hold it in place with a sterile gauze pad for the trip to the dentist.

➤ If the tooth can't be put in the socket, hold it in the side of the mouth, or wrap it in sterile gauze (or paper towels) and put it in a closed container of cool milk for the trip to the dentist.

➤ If the socket is bleeding, cover it with a sterile gauze pad, then bite down to hold the gauze in place until you get to the dentist.

Problems & Solutions

I N THE NORMAL COURSE OF LIFE, the human body needs surprisingly little upkeep beyond some fairly regular feeding, rest, and exercise. But at some times, in some ways, things can go wrong. If that happens, you can do a lot to set your body right again. As a start, you can learn what's really going on and when it's time to call a doctor.

On the following 242 pages, in entries that cover a wide range of health problems, you'll find the facts you need. Each entry guides you through these logical steps: ➤ **Signs and Symptoms** ➤ **What You Can Do Now** ➤ **When to Call the Doctor** ➤ **How to Prevent It** ➤ **For More Help.**

You'll find a concise description of what your symptoms could mean, followed by clear suggestions for your best course of action. Most entries end with a guide to useful organizations, World Wide Web sites, and books.

When you see the name of a condition in bold type—for example, **asthma**—you'll see the number of a page where you can read more about it. You'll also find charts that help you sort out, at a glance, the connections between symptoms that may seem similar, their possible causes, and what you can do.

In addition, the color illustrations on pages 161 to 176 give you a revealing new look at what can happen inside the body.

We trust that you will find helpful advice here on just about any problem your family is likely to encounter or worry about.

Head & Nervous System

Alzheimer's Disease
www.SavonAlzheimers.com

SIGNS AND SYMPTOMS

- Memory problems that get worse over time and disrupt normal life. A person with Alzheimer's often forgets what happened in the last half hour or asks the same question over and over.
- Confusion, faulty judgment and reasoning, loss of ability to complete simple tasks such as shopping or dialing new phone numbers.
- Growing tendency to lose things and to wander and get lost.
- Neglect of personal hygiene.
- Depression, suspicion, and anxiety, either as direct symptoms or as signs of the distress people feel over the baffling loss of basic skills.
- In later stages, failure to recognize places and people.
- Finally, near-total loss of memory, speech, and physical ability; the need for full-time care.

About 4 million Americans have Alzheimer's disease, a breakdown of brain cells that leads to severe memory loss, confused thinking, and personality changes. It gets worse over time, and is always fatal. Still, people with Alzheimer's can live 10 years or more after symptoms first appear.

The cause of the disease is still unknown. It's most likely to appear in people over 65 and seems to run in families. A genetic link has also been found in some cases of early-onset Alzheimer's, a rare form that can strike people in their late 40s or in their 50s.

Alzheimer's has no cure, but new drugs that may slow its progress are being tested.

WHAT YOU CAN DO NOW

If you show signs of Alzheimer's, or a family member does:

➤ See a doctor. Memory loss and confusion don't always mean you have Alzheimer's (see box on **forgetfulness,** page 51, and **confusion** chart, page 205). If someone close to you shows signs of short-term memory loss, have his or her doctor check for other problems. These include depression, hypoglycemia, vitamin shortages, and other conditions in which memory problems may be reversible.
➤ If memory problems get worse over a few months, ask your doctor for the name of a specialist who can do further tests.

If you're taking care of someone who has Alzheimer's disease:

➤ Keep the home calm and neat. In the early stages, routines and aids such as checklists for daily tasks can help a person with Alzheimer's stay self-sufficient.
➤ Be patient. Forgetfulness, sudden mood changes, and rudeness come from the disease, not ill will.
➤ Help him or her remain active and maintain family ties, friendships, and social contacts as long as possible.
➤ If the person with Alzheimer's tends to wander, have him or her wear a medical alert tag that says "Memory Impaired" and shows your phone number.

Dizziness

Dizziness can have many causes. Often it isn't serious. It can be a sign of illness, however, if it comes with other symptoms, is severe, recurs, or lasts a long time.

SYMPTOMS	WHAT IT MIGHT BE	WHAT YOU CAN DO
After blow to head: dizziness and brief loss of consciousness; headache, nausea, and vomiting.	Concussion (see head, neck, and back injuries, page 36).	Call 911 or go to emergency room **right away** after any blow to head that results in these symptoms.
Dizziness and fever over 104; no sweating; rapid pulse; confusion; hot, dry skin; loss of consciousness. Occurs in high heat.	Heatstroke (see page 38).	Call 911 or go to emergency room **right away.** If waiting for medical help to arrive, cool person with cold, wet cloths and fan.
Dizziness, palpitations, shortness of breath, sometimes chest pressure or pain.	Uneven heartbeat (see page 112). ■ Heart attack (see page 37).	Call 911 or go to emergency room **right away.**
Sudden dizziness and headache; weakness or numbness in face, arm, or leg; blurred vision or trouble speaking; confusion.	Stroke (see page 44).	Call 911 or go to emergency room **right away.**
After head injury (often days or weeks later): dizziness and fatigue, weakness or numbness on one side of body.	Subdural hemorrhage and hematoma—bleeding and swelling in brain.	Call 911 or go to emergency room **right away.**
Dizziness; vomiting; sudden high fever; confusion; diarrhea; headache; red rash, often on palms of hands and soles of feet.	Toxic shock syndrome (see page 243). ■ Other bacterial infection in blood.	Call 911 or go to emergency room **right away.**
While working or exercising in hot weather without drinking enough fluids: dizziness, nausea, vomiting, and headache; cramps in arms, legs, or abdomen; cool, clammy skin; excessive sweating; rapid pulse.	Heat exhaustion (see page 38).	Call doctor for emergency advice. Cool person with cold, wet cloths and fan. Give water or rehydration drink (see page 120), or dilute sports or fruit drink with equal amount of water.

(continued)

HEAD & NERVOUS SYSTEM

Dizziness (continued)

SYMPTOMS	WHAT IT MIGHT BE	WHAT YOU CAN DO
Dizziness, frequent head-aches, nausea and vomiting, double vision, seizures, confusion, memory loss.	Brain tumor.	Call doctor for prompt appointment.
Dizziness and headache, intense hunger, shaking, irritability, confusion, anxiety.	Hypoglycemia—low blood sugar, usually in people who take insulin.	People with diabetes should eat or drink something with sugar in it; for others, non-sugared foods. If symptoms persist, call doctor for advice and appointment. If person has seizure or loses con-sciousness, call 911 or go to emergency room **right away.**
Dizziness, weakness and fatigue, pale skin, shortness of breath.	Anemia (see page 272).	Call doctor for prompt appointment.
Earache, fever, chills, stuffy nose, blocked or full feeling in ear, muffled hearing, dis-charge from ear. In infants: tugging at ear, bad temper, restlessness, lack of appetite.	Middle ear infection (see page 71).	Call doctor for prompt appointment.
Sudden, severe dizziness, nausea, and vomiting; loss of balance or hearing.	Ménière's syndrome. ■ Labyrinthitis.	See ear and hearing problems chart, page 69.
Within 24 hours after head or neck injury: pain and stiffness in neck, dizziness, headache, nausea and vomiting, trouble walking (sometimes).	Whiplash, often caused by car collision.	Call doctor for prompt appointment if neck is injured. Apply ice packs and take pain relievers. Sleep with thin pillow under head and thin rolled-up towel un-der neck.
Dizziness, most often when moving head; nausea and vomiting.	Benign paroxysmal posi-tional vertigo—dizziness related to inner ear.	Call doctor for advice and appointment.
Dizziness when sitting up or standing up quickly.	Hypotension—a brief drop in blood pressure.	Don't change positions quickly. Ask your doctor if drugs could be the problem.

➤ Alzheimer's impairs a person's judgment and physical skills. Don't let anyone with the disease drive.

➤ Have someone take over for you now and then to ease some of your stress.

➤ Contact an Alzheimer's support group, which can help both you and the person with Alzheimer's.

HOW TO PREVENT IT

There is no sure way to prevent Alzheimer's disease. But recent studies suggest that daily doses of nonsteroidal anti-inflammatory drugs such as aspirin, ibuprofen, and naproxen sodium may protect some people. Likewise, estrogen replacement therapy appears to decrease the risk for women. Last, there is some evidence that large doses of vitamin E may slow the progression of the disease. Ask your physician for advice.

WHEN TO CALL THE DOCTOR

➤ If someone shows distinct symptoms of Alzheimer's. It can be hard for people to see and accept their own symptoms, so it is often up to others to help.

➤ In the later stages of the disease, at the first sign of illness. Alzheimer's can weaken the immune system.

➤ If the person with Alzheimer's puts himself or herself or others in danger.

➤ If you take care of a person with Alzheimer's and feel you need support.

FOR MORE HELP

Key Websites: *www.SavonHealth.com*. For more information on Alzheimer's disease: *www.SavonAlzheimers.com*.

Organizations: Alzheimer's Association, 919 N. Michigan Ave., #1100, Chicago, IL 60611-1676. 800-272-3900, M–F 8–5 CST; *www.alz.org*. More than 200 chapters nationwide provide literature, referrals, and information on support groups. Website provides facts about current research and links to other Websites.

■ The National Institute on Aging, Alzheimer's Disease Education and Referral Center (ADEAR), P.O. Box 8250, Silver

A Little Forgetful? Don't Fret.

Everyone forgets things once in a while. Most middle-aged and older people find that their memory slows down a bit as they age. They may become more forgetful, and they may take a little longer to remember things than they used to. This does not mean they have Alzheimer's disease.

In people of any age, high fever, poor nutrition, head injuries, and reactions to medication can cause temporary forgetfulness. Older people may sometimes become confused or forgetful because of emotional problems as they deal with major life changes— retirement, the death of a loved one, or other upheavals. That's normal. But if memory problems persist and increase, call your doctor for advice.

Spring, MD 20907-8250. 800-438-4380, M–F 8:30–5 EST; *www.alzheimers.org*. Staff answers questions, provides information, and refers callers to other organizations.

Website: The Alzheimer Page, *www.biostat. wustl.edu/alzheimer*. Created and sponsored by Washington University in St. Louis, this site offers E-mail discussion groups and loads of resources and facts. Supported in part by the National Institute on Aging.

Books: *The 36-Hour Day: A Family Guide to Caring for Persons With Alzheimer's Disease, Related Dementing Illnesses, and Memory Loss in Later Life*, by Nancy L. Mace, M.A., and Peter V. Rabins, M.D., M.P.H. Third edition of a classic. Johns Hopkins University Press, 1999, $13.95.

■ *Alzheimer's (A Caregiver's Day-by-Day Account)*, by Robert V. Rowe. A personal account of caring for a spouse with Alzheimer's. Robert V. Rowe, 1998, $19.95.

■ *Alzheimer's & Dementia: Questions You Have . . . Answers You Need*, by Jennifer Hay. Easy-to-read book in question-and-answer format. People's Medical Society, 1996, $12.95.

HEAD & NERVOUS SYSTEM

Headaches
www.SavonHeadaches.com

Most headaches are mild and harmless, and go away with rest and a dose of an over-the-counter pain reliever. But others are more severe, and some can signal a serious problem such as **stroke** (see pages 44 and 113) or **glaucoma** (see page 65). Some headaches are chronic, meaning they occur almost daily for months or even years. The most common types of headache are tension, migraine, cluster, and sinus.

Ninety percent of headaches are *tension headaches*—a steady, dull pain in the scalp, temples, or back of the head. They are often the result of muscles getting tight because of stress, fatigue, or poor posture.

Migraine pain can be severe, and may come with nausea and vision problems such as light flashes or partial blindness. No one knows exactly what causes a migraine, but the pain is most likely a result of changes in the blood flow to and from the brain. A migraine can be triggered by any number of factors, including stress, certain foods and medications, and hormonal changes. Migraines are more common in women than in men and tend to run in families.

Cluster headaches can be even more agonizing than migraines, with pain that starts around one eye and spreads to that side of the head. Men are more likely than women to suffer from cluster headaches, which strike suddenly 1 to 3 times a day for days or weeks—the "cluster"—before fading, often for months or years. Then they may return.

Sinus headaches are caused by sinus infections or congestion (see **sinusitis,** page 98).

The past few years have brought stunning advances in headache care; for example, a new family of drugs called triptans is proving to be very effective in the treatment of migraines. If you repeatedly get headaches but haven't consulted a doctor lately—or ever—now is the time to do so. An expert who's up on current ways to diagnose and treat headaches can help you keep the pain from ruling your life.

WHAT YOU CAN DO NOW

➤ Try an over-the-counter painkiller such as acetaminophen, ibuprofen, or aspirin. (Never give aspirin to a child or teenager who has chicken pox, flu, a cold, or any other illness you suspect of being caused by a virus; see box on **Reye's syndrome,** page 95.) Be aware that in some people daily use of these pain relievers over the course of several weeks may actually perpetuate headaches.

➤ Rest in a dark room, but don't lie down if you have a cluster headache (see entry in **headaches** chart, page 54, for symptoms). Lying down can make a cluster headache worse. Put an ice pack or a cold, wet cloth on your forehead, or a warm one if that feels better.

➤ Massage your forehead and temples for 10 minutes. Place 2 fingers at the middle of your forehead at the hairline. Using gentle pressure, work them slowly down the sides of the forehead to your temples.

➤ Stretch your neck by rolling your head, gently pressing forward at the base of your skull, and shrugging your shoulders. A self-massage of your neck can also ease the pain for a while. Starting where the neck muscles meet your skull, work your way down, across your shoulders, and up again to the base of the skull.

WHEN TO CALL THE DOCTOR

Call 911 or have someone take you to an emergency room **right away:**
➤ If your headache is sudden and severe, and you have other symptoms such as dizziness, visual changes, numbness, or weakness of a limb.
➤ If you also have a fever and a stiff neck.
➤ If your headache comes on after a head injury.
Call for an appointment right away:

Headaches

Most people have an occasional harmless headache, but many Americans—some 50 million—have intense, chronic head pain. Symptoms vary from person to person; you may have all or only some of them. Headaches can also be a sign of serious illness.

SYMPTOMS	WHAT IT MIGHT BE	WHAT YOU CAN DO
Sudden, severe headache; paralysis, weakness, or numbness on one side of body; nausea, vomiting; delirium; often seizures or loss of consciousness; trouble speaking, moving, or seeing; dizziness and confusion; possibly fever.	Stroke (see page 44).	Call 911 **right away.**
Fever, headache, nausea and vomiting, stiff neck, aversion to light, red rash (sometimes), confusion.	Meningitis (see page 55).	Call 911 or go to emergency room **right away.**
Headache on waking that gets worse when you lie down, nausea and vomiting, double vision, dizziness, loss of memory, personality changes. Head pain comes on slowly but persists and grows worse over time (often months).	Brain tumor.	Call doctor for prompt appointment.
Intense eye pain, headache, nausea and vomiting, vision problems.	Glaucoma (see page 65).	Call doctor for prompt appointment.
Sudden, intense headache; dry mouth; sticky saliva; fatigue; thirst (sometimes).	Dehydration—particularly if headache follows nausea and vomiting (see page 133) or diarrhea (see page 119).	Call doctor for prompt appointment if symptoms are severe. Drink small amounts of liquids often.
Severe, throbbing pain, often on one side of head; vision problems; aversion to light and noise; dizziness; nausea; vomiting.	Migraine headache (see facing page).	Use over-the-counter painkillers. Rest in dark room. Apply ice packs. See doctor about stronger medication or other help if pain persists or recurs.

(continued)

HEAD & NERVOUS SYSTEM

Headaches (continued)

SYMPTOMS	WHAT IT MIGHT BE	WHAT YOU CAN DO
Extreme, nonthrobbing pain, usually around one eye; bloodshot or watery eye; red face; stuffed-up nose.	Cluster headache (see page 52).	Apply ice packs and take hot showers. See doctor after first attack (symptoms could be caused by other, more serious problems). Doctor may prescribe medicine or pure oxygen (to be inhaled).
Lasting pain that can be dull or intense and often feels like a tight band around head; stiffness and tightness in neck, shoulders.	Tension headache (see page 52).	Try over-the-counter pain-killers. Get a deep muscle massage. Learn stress reduction, such as medita-tion. Apply ice packs and take hot showers. See doc-tor if pain persists.
Fever, pain behind fore-head and eyes, with stuffed-up nose and sinus.	Sinus headache (see sinus-itis, page 98).	Call doctor for advice and appointment. Infec-tions can be treated with antibiotics. Use nasal decongestants, but for no more than 2 days.
Pain focused in front of and behind ear, sometimes spreading to face, neck, and shoulders; pain or clicking sound when open-ing mouth.	Temporomandibular disorder (see page 201).	Try over-the-counter painkillers. Try heat and massage. Call doctor for advice and appointment if symptoms persist.
Pounding headache and fatigue in coffee drinkers who skip their morning cup or quit abruptly.	Caffeine withdrawal.	Have cup of coffee for quick relief. Cut back slowly if you're trying to break caffeine habit.

➤ If the headache is more painful or unlike any you've had before.

➤ If your headaches are severe and you have other symptoms such as nausea, flashes of light, runny nose, or a stuffed-up nostril. These are signs of migraines or cluster headaches.

Call for an appointment:

➤ If your headaches occur as often as once a week—or last longer than 24 hours.

➤ If your headaches often seem to be caused by allergies, sinus infection, or de-pression. Treatment for these ailments can ease the pain.

HOW TO PREVENT IT

➤ Keep a headache diary. Note the time and date of each headache and its symp-toms. Write down all you can remember about what you ate and drank and what you did in the 6 to 8 hours before it came on. Look for "triggers" for the headaches, and do what you can to avoid them.

➤ Avoid foods that contain the substance tyramine if they seem to cause your headaches. Such foods include ripe cheeses, nuts, peanut butter, pizza, and red wine.

➤ Practice correct posture. Sit up straight and don't keep your neck bent for long.

➤ Take rest breaks every hour if you're doing hard work such as moving furniture or digging in your garden.

➤ When reading or writing, make sure you have enough light, but not so much that it glares off the page; squinting can tighten muscles. Take 10-minute rest breaks every hour.

➤ If your headaches seem to be caused by allergies, make sure your house is free of dust and mold. Don't go outside when pollen is high (see **allergies,** page 84, for other ways to prevent allergy attacks).

➤ Don't skip meals, sleep too little, or sleep too much on weekends. These can all produce headaches.

➤ Some drugs, such as birth control pills, can provoke migraines. If your headaches seem to be caused by a drug, talk with your doctor.

➤ Don't smoke, and avoid smoky places such as bars. Smoke can cause migraines.

COMPLEMENTARY CHOICES

➤ Some people find that acupuncture and acupressure can relieve the pain of tension and migraine headaches. See page 310 for suggestions on finding a reliable acupuncturist.

➤ Biofeedback, a technique through which you learn to control processes such as heart rate and body temperature, may help ease head pain and relieve the stress that sometimes causes it. Your doctor can recommend a clinic where you can learn the basics.

➤ A massage therapist can help relieve head pain by loosening tight muscles and relieving tension.

➤ Reduce stress (see **relax,** page 303). Try regular exercise, a meditation class, and taking breaks during a hectic day.

➤ Both vitamin B2 (riboflavin) and magnesium have reduced the frequency of migraines in study subjects. Try taking 400 milligrams of vitamin B2 or 20 milli-moles of magnesium every day.

FOR MORE HELP

Key Websites: *www.SavonHealth.com.* For more information on headaches: *www.SavonHeadaches.com.*

Organizations: The American Council for Headache Education, 19 Mantua Rd., Mt. Royal, NJ 08061. 800-255-2243, M–F 9–5 EST; *www.achenet.org.* For a $20 member's fee you get a quarterly newsletter, pamphlets, and a list of doctors.

■ National Headache Foundation, 428 W. St. James Pl., 2nd Floor, Chicago, IL 60614-2750. 888-643-5552, M–F 9–5 CST; *www.headaches.org.* Staff answers questions about headache types, causes, and treatment; also sends free brochures on headaches and a list of doctors who are members. For a $15 member's fee you get a quarterly newsletter, a list of foods to avoid, and handbooks on headaches.

Books: *An Alternative Medicine Definitive Guide to Headaches,* by Burton Goldberg, Robert Milne, M.D., and Blake More. Covers causes and offers drug-free treatments for sufferers of chronic headaches and migraines. Future Medicine, 1998, $18.95.

■ *The Hormone Headache,* by Seymour Diamond, M.D. Describes the link between headaches and hormones, and how to prevent and treat migraines and other headaches. Macmillan, 1995, $11.95.

Meningitis & Encephalitis

www.SavonMeningitis.com

SIGNS AND SYMPTOMS

The following symptoms need prompt treatment. Call your doctor. If a doctor is not available, call 911 or go to an emergency room.

Meningitis or encephalitis in adults:
- Fever, other flulike symptoms, and headache with:
- Sensitivity to light.
- Confusion, drowsiness, lethargy, or bad temper.
- Delirium, seizures, or coma.
- Sometimes, with encephalitis only, paralysis.
- Stiff neck, shoulders, or back. With meningitis only, shooting pain in the neck and back when head is bent forward.
- Rarely, with meningitis only, a bumpy red or purplish rash anywhere on the body.

Meningitis in children:
- Rectal temperature of 100 degrees or higher, with:
- Headache or stiff neck. When child lies down, the head can't be bent toward the chest (except in infants less than 12 months old) because of shooting pain in the neck and back.
- Bad temper or listlessness.
- Loss of appetite.
- Turning away from bright lights.
- Sometimes nausea and vomiting.
- In infants, bulging of the soft spot of the skull.
- Sometimes seizures.
- Rarely, a bumpy red or purple rash anywhere on the body.

Encephalitis in children:
- Same symptoms as in adults.
- In infants, bulging of the soft spot of the skull.

within hours if not treated, but early care most often results in complete recovery. Treatment includes a hospital stay and injected antibiotics.

Viral meningitis is usually a milder form of the illness that goes away on its own. It is treated with bed rest and plenty of liquids.

Encephalitis is an inflammation of the brain that is almost always caused by a virus. In the United States, it is most often caused by herpes simplex, the virus that brings cold sores. The illness can also be brought on by a chicken pox, mumps, or measles virus. Another form is spread by mosquitoes and ticks.

People with mild encephalitis most often recover in 2 to 3 weeks. Severe cases, which are rare, can lead to brain damage or death.

WHAT YOU CAN DO NOW

➤ If a child or an adult has a fever, headache, stiff neck, and any alteration in consciousness (lethargy, confusion, coma), call your doctor for advice. If a doctor is not available, call 911 or go to an emergency room **right away.**

HOW TO PREVENT IT

➤ Get early treatment for any serious infection or high fever.
➤ Shots for meningitis are part of most childhood immunization series—be sure your child gets them.

Meningitis and encephalitis are brain diseases with similar symptoms. Both need prompt medical treatment.

Meningitis is an inflammation of the fragile membranes that cover the spinal cord and brain. Bacteria, viruses, and fungi can cause it. Bacterial meningitis can follow an illness such as pneumonia or a sinus or ear infection. A skull fracture or other head injury also raises the risk. Some forms of viral meningitis can spread through the air.

Bacterial meningitis can lead to death

Red Flag for Children

The bacterial form of meningitis, which strikes infants and young children more than it does adults, can lead to death within hours—or to permanent brain damage—if it isn't treated. Very young children are in particular danger, because they can't describe their symptoms. Call 911 or go to an emergency room **right away** if a child has the symptoms listed. Early treatment usually results in full recovery.

➤ If you have had close contact with a person who has bacterial meningitis, or your child has, call your doctor. You may be advised to take antibiotics (even if you show no symptoms) to prevent infection.

➤ Avoid ticks by wearing long pants and long-sleeved shirts in grassy or wooded areas (see **tick bites,** page 45).

➤ Prevent insect bites by using repellent.

FOR MORE HELP

Key Websites: *www.SavonHealth.com.* For more information on meningitis: *www.SavonMeningitis.com.*

Organizations: Massachusetts Department of Public Health Epidemiology Program, 305 South St., Jamaica Plain, MA, 02130. 617-983-6800, M–F 9–5 EST; *www.magnet.state.ma.us/dph/cdc/epiimm2.htm.*

■ National Institute of Neurological Disorders and Stroke, 31 Center Dr., MSC 2540, Bethesda, MD 20892-2540. 800-352-9424 and 301-496-5751, M–F 8:30–5 EST; *www.ninds.nih.gov.* Ask for the fact sheet on meningitis and encephalitis. At Website, click on *Search* and type in *encephalitis and meningitis.*

Parkinson's Disease
www.SavonParkinsons.com

SIGNS AND SYMPTOMS

Early symptoms:
■ Weakness.
■ Slight tremor of the head or hands.
■ Depression (sometimes).
■ Masklike face, almost no blinking.
■ Muscle stiffness.
■ Slowed movement.

Later symptoms:
■ Loss of balance.
■ Tremors in the hands and/or head when at rest.
■ Confusion and memory loss (in severe cases).

Parkinson's disease most often shows up in people over 60. It occurs when nerve cells begin to die in an area of the brain that controls movement. Genes, brain injury, and environmental poisons may trigger the disease in some people, but in most cases its causes are unknown.

Parkinson's disease has no cure, but many people find that medication—most often levodopa, used with other drugs—controls their symptoms. Some drugs, such as selegiline, may even slow the progress of the disease.

WHAT YOU CAN DO NOW

➤ Some prescription drugs—most often those used to treat mental illness—can cause symptoms like those of Parkinson's. Check with your doctor. Changing the drug may stop your symptoms.

After diagnosis:

➤ Experts agree that it is good for people with Parkinson's to remain active and to exercise. But be careful not to tire yourself out, since stress and fatigue can make symptoms worse.

➤ Physical therapy, deep muscle massage, and yoga may help you move more easily. Talk to your doctor before starting any new program.

➤ Some experts believe it helps to eat significantly more carbohydrate (from vegetables, grains, and pastas) than protein (from meat and dairy). Protein delays the body's production of levodopa, the chemical that people with Parkinson's lack.

➤ Because constipation can be a problem, eat plenty of vegetables and bran, and drink at least 6 glasses of water a day.

➤ Safeguard your home. Tape or tack down small rugs. Stick nonskid decals on the tub or shower floor. Keep the floor clear of shoes and other small objects so that you won't trip over them.

➤ Sit in chairs with armrests and firm seats to make getting up easier. Put a firm pillow on low chair seats.

➤ Use silky sheets and pajamas. They make it easier to move in bed. A cardboard box under the sheets at the foot of the bed will hold bedclothes off your feet.

➤ Join a support group. Many people with Parkinson's find that company eases the depression that can come with the disease.

➤ If you see symptoms of Parkinson's disease in yourself or someone close to you.

➤ If you have any new symptoms during treatment. They may be side effects of the medication you're taking, or they may mean the illness is getting worse.

There is no known way to prevent Parkinson's disease.

Key Websites: *www.SavonHealth.com*. For more information on Parkinsons disease: *www.SavonParkinsons.com*.

Organizations: American Parkinson's Disease Association, 1250 Hylan Blvd., Staten Island, NY 10305. 800-223-2732, M–F 9–5 EST; *www.apdaparkinson.com*. Has 800 support groups and 65 chapters nationwide. Provides education, facts on diet and exercise, counseling, and names of doctors near you.

■ National Parkinson Foundation, 1501 NW Ninth Ave., Miami, FL 33136. 800-327-4545, M–F 8–5 EST; *www.parkinson.org*. Provides free pamphlets about nutrition and general facts about Parkinson's.

Book: *Caring for the Parkinson Patient: A Practical Guide,* 2nd edition, by J. Thomas Hutton, M.D., Ph.D., and Raye Lynne Dippel, Ph.D. A basic guide for patients and their families. Prometheus Books, 1999, $19.95.

Seizures & Epilepsy
www.SavonEpilepsy.com

■ Many people with epilepsy get a warning sign, known as an aura, that lasts a few seconds. It's often marked by nausea, unique smells and tastes, feelings of dread, and warped vision. Auras vary widely, but each person tends to have the same aura before each seizure

Petit mal, or absence, seizure:
■ Person abruptly stops and stares blankly for several seconds, sometimes blinking or making chewing motions.

Grand mal, or tonic-clonic, seizure:
■ Convulsions, jerking motions, and loss of consciousness, often with loss of bladder control and sometimes bowel control. Should stop after 1 to 2 minutes; followed by confusion and sleepiness.

Other epileptic seizures:
■ Seeing or hearing things that aren't there.
■ Incoherent talk or out-of-character actions and speech—sometimes mistaken for drug abuse.

Two and a half million Americans have epilepsy, an illness that results in seizures—brief events in which the brain's electrical system overloads and misfires.

A single seizure probably doesn't mean a person has epilepsy. It's not rare for a very young child with a high fever to have a seizure. This may need medical attention, but does not by itself mean the child has epilepsy (see **fever in children,** page 255). In adults and children, other triggers for nonepileptic seizures include diabetes, meningitis, and encephalitis. Pregnancy, poisoning, heatstroke, and alcohol or drug abuse also can bring them on.

Epilepsy can start at any age, but it usually begins when a person is a child or young adult. Children who have petit mal seizures usually outgrow them. In most cases of epilepsy, the cause is unknown. In the rest, causes include severe head injury, brain tumor, stroke, poisoning, infection, and brain damage. Experts believe genes can also play a role.

Up to 85 percent of people with epilepsy can control it with antiseizure drugs. Brain surgery may help those who can't control their seizures any other way.

WHAT YOU CAN DO NOW

If you have epilepsy, take steps to avoid seizures or to lessen their effects:

➤ Take your medication—missing doses can trigger a seizure. Consult a doctor before switching to a generic brand; your body may absorb different brands in different ways.

➤ If you get a seizure warning sign, or aura, avoid a fall by lying down or moving away from any hazards.

➤ Be aware that stress, fatigue, and alcohol or drug abuse can bring on seizures.

➤ Keep a seizure diary, noting the kind of seizure, the time, and likely triggers. This can help you keep medication to a minimum and gain some control over the illness.

➤ Wear a medical alert tag to help others quickly understand the problem.

➤ Exercise and relaxation techniques can help reduce stress and tension.

➤ Ask your doctor whether it is safe for you to drive.

➤ Ask your doctor about the ketogenic diet, which has been shown to control certain types of seizures in children.

If you are with someone who has a seizure:

➤ See **seizures,** page 41, for first aid.

WHEN TO CALL THE DOCTOR

Call 911 or go to an emergency room **right away:**

➤ If the seizure lasts more than 3 minutes, if a second seizure begins shortly after the first, or if the person does not seem to regain consciousness after the seizure.

➤ If the person is pregnant or diabetic.

Call your doctor for emergency advice, or if your doctor isn't available, call 911 or go to an emergency room:

➤ If your child has a high fever and has a seizure or what you suspect to be one.

Call for advice and an appointment:

➤ If someone you know, especially a child, goes through periods of blank staring, loss of consciousness, confused memory, fainting spells or falls, or odd blinking or chewing motions.

➤ If your doctor has prescribed antiseizure drugs and you have side effects such as drowsiness, hyperactivity, disorientation, or sleep problems.

HOW TO PREVENT IT

There is no known way to prevent most kinds of epilepsy. To guard against it, get good prenatal care, don't abuse alcohol or other drugs, and protect yourself and your children from head injuries by using seat belts, child safety seats, and bicycle helmets.

FOR MORE HELP

Key Websites: *www.SavonHealth.com.* For more information on seizures or epilepsy: *www.SavonEpilepsy.com.*

Organizations: Epilepsy Foundation of America, 4351 Garden City Dr., Landover, MD 20785. 800-332-1000 and 301-459-3700, in English and Spanish, M–Th 9–5 and F 9–3 EST. Staffs sends brochures, answers questions, and refers callers to other resources. Offers recreational and educational programs for children with epilepsy, as well as information on local chapters and support groups.

■ National Institute of Neurological Disorders and Stroke, 31 Center Dr., MSC 2540, Bethesda, MD 20892. 800-352-9424, M–F 8:30–5 EST; *www.ninds.nih.gov.* Call and ask for the information packet on epilepsy.

Books: *A Guide to Understanding and Living With Epilepsy*, by Orrin Devinsky, M.D. Provides in-depth information about epilepsy and how to cope with it. F. A. Davis, 2000, $19.95.

■ *Epilepsy* (The Natural Way series), by Fiona Marshall. Explains treatments and alternative therapies. Approved by the British and American Holistic Medical Associations. Penguin USA, 1998, $5.95.

■ *Your Child and Epilepsy*, by Robert J. Gumnit, M.D. For the parents of an epileptic child. Demos Vermande, 1995, $26.25.

HEAD & NERVOUS SYSTEM

Eyes

Cataracts

www.SavonCataracts.com

SIGNS AND SYMPTOMS

- Hazy or blurry vision.
- Discomfort or trouble seeing in bright light.
- A feeling of film over the eyes or of looking through fog.
- Double vision or triple vision in only one eye.
- "Second sight"—a temporary change in near vision, so that you may find you don't need your reading glasses for a brief time.
- White or opaque area visible in the pupil of the eye (in advanced cataract).

A cataract is a fogging of the eye's clear lens (see color illustration, page 161). It can cloud vision like steam on a window. Cataracts often come on slowly, over years, and many people don't notice them until vision loss begins to interfere with the tasks of daily living, such as driving or reading.

Most cataracts start as the lens breaks down with age. They can also be caused by some diseases, such as diabetes, as well as eye injuries, years of exposure to bright sunlight, and the prolonged use of drugs such as corticosteroids (prescribed for illnesses such as arthritis). Smoking cigarettes or abusing alcohol may also increase the risk. Sometimes a baby is born with cataracts in one or both eyes if the mother had **German measles** (see page 257) during pregnancy.

Surgery is the only treatment for cataracts, but it's not needed unless the cataracts begin to cause problems with work or daily activities. The entire lens of the eye, or the inside of the lens, is removed. It's usually replaced by a clear plastic lens. Less often, instead of putting in a new lens, the doctor prescribes special eyeglasses or contact lenses. You can have the cataract operation in the doctor's office and go home the same day.

WHAT YOU CAN DO NOW

➤ If you think you have cataracts, call your doctor for advice on whether you should see an ophthalmologist (a medical doctor licensed to treat all eye conditions). He or she can tell you if you'll need surgery.

WHEN TO CALL THE DOCTOR

➤ If you have even a few of the symptoms, especially blurred vision or trouble with bright lights.

HOW TO PREVENT IT

➤ Be sure your sunglasses protect your eyes from the sun's ultraviolet A (UVA) and ultraviolet B (UVB) rays. Glasses that block out UVA and UVB light are labeled as "fulfilling the American National Standards Institute requirement." The label should also say they "eliminate 99 percent of UVA and UVB."
➤ If you are a woman and plan to become pregnant, protect your baby by getting vaccinated for German measles if you haven't had the disease already.

Eye & Vision Problems

This chart includes some of the most common eye and vision problems, as well as some of the most serious. If you have any concerns about your vision, call your doctor for advice right away.

SYMPTOMS	WHAT IT MIGHT BE	WHAT YOU CAN DO
Sudden vision changes, such as blindness, double vision, blurring, flashes of light, floating dark shapes, loss of peripheral (side) vision; acute, sustained pain.	Stroke (see page 44). ■ Transient ischemic attack—temporary blockage of artery, with symptoms like stroke. ■ Optic neuritis—inflammation of optic nerve.	Call 911 or go to emergency room **right away** if you have sudden blindness or loss of part of visual field.
Redness, watering, pain, or a feeling of having something in the eye.	Foreign body in eye (see eye injuries, page 32).	Go to emergency room if something is in colored part of eye or if you can't get particle out of white of eye.
Blurred vision; slow loss of peripheral (side) vision; sudden, severe eye pain; halos around lights; teary, aching eyes; headache; nausea; vomiting.	Glaucoma (see page 65).	Call doctor for prompt appointment. Prescription drugs may help.
Blurred vision, sensitivity to light, ache or pain in eye, headache, redness (no discharge).	Iritis/uveitis—inflammation inside eye.	Call doctor for prompt appointment. Prescription drugs may help.
Rapid or gradual vision loss; dim or distorted vision, especially when reading; dark, empty area in center of visual field; straight lines look wavy.	Macular degeneration— the macula, a tiny spot at center of retina, begins to break down or scar. Symptoms usually appear after age 55.	Call doctor for prompt appointment. Some forms can be slowed with laser treatment. **For more help:** Association for Macular Diseases, 428 E. 72nd St., Suite 200, New York, NY 10021. 212-605-3777, M–F 11–3 EST; *www.macula.org*.
Flashes of light, floating dark shapes, loss of peripheral (side) vision.	Retinal detachment—hole in retina. Risk increases with age, with severe myopia, and after cataract surgery.	Call doctor for prompt appointment. In early stages, vision can be restored with surgery.

(continued)

EYES

Eye & Vision Problems (continued)

SYMPTOMS	WHAT IT MIGHT BE	WHAT YOU CAN DO
Small, painful red bump at base of eyelash.	Stye.	See styes, page 67.
Red and itchy eyelids.	Blepharitis—inflammation and scaling of eyelids.	Wash eyelids with warm water containing a few drops of baby shampoo, or with over-the-counter eyelid wash. Call doctor for advice and appointment if ailment doesn't clear up with home treatment.
Hazy vision, blurriness around lights, frequent changes in eyeglass prescriptions, white area visible in pupil.	Cataracts.	See cataracts, page 60, and color illustration, page 161.
White of eye is bloodshot, sticky or watery discharge, itching.	Conjunctivitis.	See conjunctivitis, facing page.
Blurred vision when looking at nearby objects, eyestrain, headaches.	Presbyopia—inability to focus for near vision. Occurs with age as lens loses elasticity.	Call doctor for advice and appointment. Eyeglasses or contact lenses can help.
Blurred vision when looking at distant objects.	Myopia, or nearsightedness. May run in families.	Call doctor for advice and appointment. Eyeglasses or contact lenses can correct it.
Red spot covering all or part of white of eye.	Subconjunctival hemorrhage—bleeding from small blood vessels in membrane over eyeball.	Harmless, though can look alarming. Usually no apparent cause; may follow injury, coughing, or sneezing. Should clear up in 2–3 days. Call doctor for advice if painful or if bleeding recurs.
Dry, hot, or scratchy eyes.	Lack of moisture due to aging, medications, or air pollution.	Moisten eyes with over-the-counter "artificial tears." Apply cold compresses.
Spots or "threads" that float across field of vision.	Floaters—collagen fragments floating in the jelly-like liquid that fills the eye.	Usually harmless. Call doctor for advice the first time you see them.

➤ Wear safety glasses to prevent eye injury during sports, or when using power tools or chemicals such as paint remover.

➤ Eat plenty of green and yellow vegetables. These contain substances (antioxidants) that may help prevent cataracts.

FOR MORE HELP

Key Websites: *www.SavonHealth.com*. For more information on cataracts: *www.SavonCataracts.com*.

Organizations: The Foundation of the American Academy of Ophthalmology Public Service Programs, 800-222-3937, M–F 8–4 PST. Refers low-income senior citizens to ophthalmologists who provide low-cost medical care.

■ National Eye Institute, National Institutes of Health, Bldg. 31, Room 6A32, 31 Center Dr., MSC 2510, Bethesda, MD 20892-2510. 301-496-5248, M–F 8:30–4:30 EST; *www.nei.nih.gov.* Provides brochures, fact sheets, and advice about eye disease.

■ Prevent Blindness America, 500 E. Remington Rd., Schaumburg, IL 60173. 800-331-2020, M–F 8–5 CST; *www.preventblindness.org.* Provides material on eye diseases and has a national network of support groups.

Website: EyeNet, American Academy of Ophthalmology, *www.eyenet.org/public/faqs.* Click on *Cataract.* Covers treatments and resources.

Books: *The Eye Book: A Complete Guide to Eye Disorders and Health,* by Gary H. Cassel, M.D., Michael D. Billing, O.D., and Harry G. Randall, M.D. Discusses cataracts and other eye problems. Johns Hopkins University Press, 1998, $18.95.

■ *The Crystal Clear Guide to Sight for Life: A Complete Manual of Eye Care for Those Over Forty,* by Johnny L. Gayton, M.D., and Jan Roadarmel Ledford. Covers common eye problems, treatments, and how to choose a doctor. Starburst Publishers, 1995, $15.95.

Conjunctivitis
www.SavonConjunctivitis.com

SIGNS AND SYMPTOMS

Redness of the whites of the eyes is common to all types of conjunctivitis. Other signs include:

In bacterial conjunctivitis:
■ Discharge of pus from the eye or crusting on the eyelashes in the morning.

In viral conjunctivitis:
■ Watery discharge, often from one eye only, occasionally with crusting.
■ Sore throat, runny nose, and/or swelling of lymph glands in front of the ears.

In allergic conjunctivitis:
■ Itchy eyes.
■ Burning and watery eyes.
■ Swelling of the tissues around eyes.
■ Runny nose, sneezing.

In conjunctivitis caused by dirty air, fumes, or dust:
■ Burning and watery eyes.
■ A feeling of something in the eye.

Conjunctivitis—often called pinkeye—is an inflammation of the membrane (the conjunctiva) that covers the inside of the eyelid and the white of the eye (see illustration, page 64). It is annoying but rarely serious. Causes include:

➤ Bacterial or viral infections.
➤ Allergies to such things as grass pollen, house dust, mold, or cosmetics.
➤ Smoke and fumes.
➤ In newborns (rarely): infection from the mother's birth canal. This is a serious problem that must be treated at once, because it can cause blindness. Most hospitals treat infants' eyes at birth to prevent conjunctivitis; if the infection breaks through in the first 2 weeks of life despite this early treatment, the baby should be taken to the emergency room.

When caused by bacteria or a virus, conjunctivitis is easy to spread to others through direct contact or through towels, handkerchiefs, or washcloths. Your doctor can give you eyedrops or ointment to make the eye feel better and speed healing. Allergic conjunctivitis

EYES

The Eye

The main layers of the eye are (1) the retina, which translates light into nerve impulses that travel to the brain through the optic nerve; (2) the uvea, rich with blood vessels; (3) the sclera, the tough white outer layer. The conjunctiva is a clear membrane that covers the outer surface of the sclera and the inside of the eyelids.

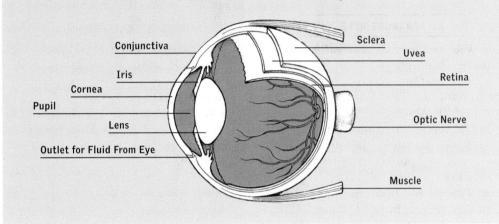

may be chronic—meaning it keeps coming back—or it may be a problem only in allergy season. You can't give it to others.

WHAT YOU CAN DO NOW

General:
➤ Use warm water to gently soak and wipe away any crusted or sticky discharge around the eyes.
➤ Use a clean, wet (warm or cold) washcloth as a compress to relieve discomfort.
➤ If bright light causes pain, wear dark glasses while out in the sun.
➤ Avoid things that irritate your eyes, such as tobacco smoke or the water in swimming pools.
➤ Don't wear eye makeup.
➤ Don't wear contact lenses.

Bacterial or viral conjunctivitis:
➤ To soothe infected eyes, apply a clean, warm, damp cloth. Wash used cloths in hot water with detergent so that you don't spread the infection.
➤ If your child has it, keep him or her at home so it won't spread. The teacher and other parents will thank you.

Allergic conjunctivitis:
➤ Apply a cold, damp washcloth to the eyes to relieve itching.
➤ Try over-the-counter allergy eyedrops or pills to reduce redness and itching. Be aware that the pills can cause drowsiness.

Conjunctivitis caused by dirty air, fumes, or dust:
➤ To soothe sore eyes, use artificial teardrops, available over the counter.

WHEN TO CALL THE DOCTOR

Go to an emergency room **right away:**
➤ If your newborn's eyes redden and produce a discharge; this must be treated quickly to prevent eye damage.

Call for a prompt appointment:
➤ If conjunctivitis affects your vision or causes lots of pain or discharge; you may have a staph or strep infection that requires treatment right away.

Call for advice:
➤ If you injure your eye; it could become infected.
➤ If your conjunctivitis gets worse after a week of home care; you may need treatment for an infection.
➤ If you get conjunctivitis often.

➤ If you have symptoms of conjunctivitis that don't seem to be caused by an infection, a cold, or allergies. A number of eye diseases, including **glaucoma** (see next entry), also can cause redness and tears.

➤ If you notice your vision is blurred, you're bothered by light, or your eyes are red; these may be signs of advanced glaucoma.

HOW TO PREVENT IT

➤ Don't share eye makeup or eyedrops.

➤ Replace eye makeup every 6 months, or after an infection.

➤ Don't share handkerchiefs, washcloths, or towels.

➤ If you wear contact lenses, wash your hands before touching them. Always soak them in fresh, sterile contact lens solution; never reuse solution.

➤ If you have conjunctivitis, don't touch your eye and then touch someone else; you can spread it to others.

➤ Wash your hands often if you have conjunctivitis or someone you live with has it.

➤ If you have allergies, try to avoid the things that cause them, such as pollen, dust, mold, or pets.

➤ During allergy season and periods of high air pollution, filter the air in your car and house by running the air conditioners, if you have them; keep the windows and doors in your home closed.

➤ Wear goggles on the job if you work around chemicals or fumes.

FOR MORE HELP

Key Websites: *www.SavonHealth.com*. For more information on conjunctivitis: *www.SavonConjuntivitis.com*.

Organizations: American Academy of Ophthalmology, Customer Service/ess-conj, P.O. Box 7424, San Francisco, CA 94120-7424. Send a business-size self-addressed stamped envelope and request a fact sheet on conjunctivitis. To order information through fax-on-demand, call 732-935-2761 (24-hour automated line) and request document #1303.

■ The Foundation of the American Academy of Ophthalmology Public Service Programs, 800-222-3937, M–F 8–4 PST. Refers low-income senior citizens to ophthalmologists who provide low-cost medical care.

■ National Eye Institute, National Institutes of Health, 301-496-5248, M–F 8:30– 4:30 EST; *www.nei.nih.gov.* Provides facts about eye diseases.

Book: *Your Eyes . . . An Owner's Guide,* by James Collins, M.D., F.A.C.S. Discusses the care, problems, and treatments of eyes. Prentice Hall, 1995, $12.95.

Glaucoma
www.SavonGlaucoma.com

SIGNS AND SYMPTOMS

Glaucoma often has no symptoms at first. By the time symptoms do appear, some vision may have been lost, so it's vital to spot and treat glaucoma early.

In chronic glaucoma:
■ Blurred vision.
■ Over time, loss of peripheral (side) vision.
■ Teary, aching eyes.
■ Headaches.

In acute glaucoma (an emergency):
■ Severe, sudden eye pain.
■ Blurred vision.
■ Halos around lights.
■ Headaches.
■ Nausea and vomiting.

In secondary glaucoma (after an injury or certain diseases):
■ Blurred vision.
■ Halos around lights.
■ Headaches.

Think of the eye as a sink with a faucet and a drain. The "faucet" consists of a membrane behind the pupil that secretes fluid into the space in front of the lens. The "drain" lets out excess fluid, so the pressure inside remains constant. Glaucoma occurs when the drain becomes clogged; pressure builds, affecting the optic nerve and its small blood vessels. When not treated, glaucoma can cause vision loss and even blindness.

EYES

Glaucoma is one of the most common eye problems in people over 60. It runs in families. African Americans and people with severe myopia (nearsightedness) or diabetes are also at greater risk than others. Some drugs can cause glaucoma. These include certain antidepressants, as well as drugs for asthma or irritable bowel syndrome. People with past eye injuries may be prone to secondary glaucoma.

About 10 percent of glaucoma is acute—it gets worse quickly and requires prompt treatment. Chronic glaucoma accounts for the other 90 percent of cases. It's often called the "sneak thief" of sight because it comes on slowly to steal vision.

Glaucoma can usually be treated with eyedrops, pills, or shots that lower pressure in the eye. Doctors sometimes perform in-office laser surgery to widen clogged drains or to create new ones.

WHAT YOU CAN DO NOW

Glaucoma can be detected only with a test of eye pressure (see **tests,** page 319). Get regular eye checkups, especially if you're in a high-risk group.

WHEN TO CALL THE DOCTOR

➤ If you have symptoms of glaucoma. You'll need treatment right away.
➤ If you are being treated for glaucoma and another doctor prescribes drugs for some other ailment.
➤ If you are taking eyedrops or pills for glaucoma and you learn that you have anemia or you have side effects such as headaches; red eyes; stinging in the eyes; blurred vision; changes in heartbeat, pulse, or breathing; tingling fingers and toes; drowsiness; loss of appetite; bowel problems; kidney stones; or easy bleeding.
➤ If you feel drowsy, tired, or short of breath after taking eyedrops for glaucoma. The drug may be making a heart or lung problem worse.

HOW TO PREVENT IT

➤ Get an eye exam with a glaucoma test every 3 to 5 years after age 39.
➤ Get an eye exam every 1 to 2 years if someone in your family has glaucoma or severe myopia, if you have African ancestors, if you have ever had a serious eye injury, or if you are taking antidepressants or any medications for asthma or irritable bowel syndrome.

FOR MORE HELP

Key Websites: *www.SavonHealth.com.* For more information on glaucoma: *www.SavonGlaucoma.com.*

Organizations: American Foundation for the Blind, 800-232-5463, M–F 10–12 and 2–4 EST; *www.afb.org.* Covers visual impairment, including career advice for people who have trouble seeing.

■ The Foundation of the American Academy of Ophthalmology Public Service Programs, 800-222-3937, M–F 8–4 PST. Refers low-income senior citizens to ophthalmologists who provide low-cost medical care.

■ Glaucoma Research Foundation, 800-826-6693, 24-hour recording. 415-986-3162, M–F 8:30–4:30 PST; *www.glaucoma.org.* Sends free publications and coordinates a national telephone-based support network for glaucoma patients and their families. Website covers glaucoma and current research, and gives links to other organizations.

■ National Eye Institute, National Institutes of Health, Bldg. 31, Room 6A32, 31 Center Dr., MSC 2510, Bethesda, MD 20892-2510. 301-496-5248, M–F 8:30–4:30 EST; *www.nei.nih.gov.* Provides fact sheets and brochures about eye disease.

Website: EyeNet, American Academy of Ophthalmology, *www.eyenet.org/public/faqs.* Click on *Glaucoma.* Covers treatments and resources.

Book: *Coping With Glaucoma,* by Edith Marks. A comprehensive guide to medications and procedures used to diagnose and treat glaucoma. Avery Publishing Group, 1997, $13.95.

Styes

www.SavonStye.com

SIGNS AND SYMPTOMS

- A small, painful red bump on the upper or lower eyelid near the base of an eyelash.
- Burning, itching, or a feeling of having something in the eye.
- A teary eye.

A stye is a bacterial infection of a gland at the base of an eyelash. Styes are often painful, but they're rarely serious.

Styes usually swell, fill with pus, and break open in 3 to 7 days, easing the pain. They may also go away without bursting. You can easily spread them by touching your eyelid, by squeezing the stye, or by using contaminated makeup or towels.

WHAT YOU CAN DO NOW

- ➤ Don't rub the eye and don't squeeze or pick at the stye.
- ➤ Apply a soft, clean washcloth that has been soaked in warm water and wrung out. Hold for 10 to 15 minutes. Repeat 2 to 4 times a day until the stye bursts or goes away. Use a new washcloth each time so you don't spread the infection. Wash used washcloths in hot water with detergent.
- ➤ If the stye comes to a head and bursts, gently and thoroughly wash the pus from the eyelid.

WHEN TO CALL THE DOCTOR

- ➤ If the stye worsens or does not respond to home care within a week. A doctor may prescribe antibiotic drops or ointment, or may lance and drain the stye.
- ➤ If the stye swells but doesn't go away or break open and drain.
- ➤ If styes keep coming back. Rarely, this can be a sign of cancer of the eyelid.
- ➤ If you have any signs of skin infection (redness and roughness) spreading on the eyelid.

HOW TO PREVENT IT

- ➤ Wash your hands often with soap and water.
- ➤ Try not to touch or rub your eyes. Styes can come back if the bacteria spread.
- ➤ Don't share towels or washcloths.
- ➤ Change towels and pillowcases often.
- ➤ Don't share eye makeup or eyedrops, and throw away used cosmetics after 6 months.
- ➤ If styes come back often, clean the outside of your eyelids every day: Dip a cotton swab into a cup of warm water and a few drops of baby shampoo. Wash the lashes of each closed eyelid with this mixture once or twice a day.

FOR MORE HELP

Key Websites: *www.SavonHealth.com.* For more information on styes: *www.SavonStye.com.*

Organizations: American Optometric Association, 243 N. Lindbergh Blvd., St. Louis, MO 63141. 314-991-4100, M–F 8–5 CST; *www.aoanet.org.* Sends free pamphlets on eye and vision problems. For information on styes, send a business-size self-addressed stamped envelope to the Communications Center, or call and ask for Ext. 219.

- National Eye Institute, National Institutes of Health, Bldg. 31, Room 6A32, 31 Center Dr., MSC 2510, Bethesda, MD 20892-2510. 301-496-5248, M–F 8:30–4:30 EST; *www.nei.nih.gov.* Provides brochures and fact sheets about eye problems.

EYES

Ears

Airplane Ear
www.SavonHearing.com

SIGNS AND SYMPTOMS

- Feeling of fullness in the ears.
- Pain in the ears.
- Ringing in the ears.
- Dizziness.

You may get "airplane ear" (barotrauma) when you take a plane trip, especially if you have a **cold** (see page 93), **sinusitis** (see page 98), or **allergies** (see page 84). But any rapid air-pressure change—from an elevator ride in a high-rise, say, or scuba diving—can cause airplane ear.

The problem is in the middle ear. This is the part connected to the back of the nose by the eustachian tube (see illustration, page 73). A cold, sinusitis, or allergies can swell the tube, trapping air. You'll feel pressure in the ears, especially during descents.

WHAT YOU CAN DO NOW

- Yawning or swallowing opens the tube to the middle ear. Just before and during descent, chew gum or suck on candy so that you'll swallow more often.
- When flying, don't sleep during descent. If swallowing and yawning don't work, try this: Take a deep breath; then close your mouth and hold your nose, and try to breathe out through the nose gently and slowly. This can force air through the tubes between your nose and ears. You may have to do this a few times.

If you're flying with an infant:
- Wake your baby before descent.
- Give your baby something to drink or a pacifier during landing. Babies can't "pop" their ears on purpose, but sucking on a bottle or pacifier may do the trick.

WHEN TO CALL THE DOCTOR

- If your ears don't clear, or if pain lasts for several hours after flying.
- If you're planning a plane trip and have just had ear surgery. Ask your doctor how soon you may safely fly.

HOW TO PREVENT IT

If you have a cold, a sinus infection, or an allergy attack—or a child traveling with you does—it's best to postpone a plane trip. If you can't:
- Some air travelers get relief from taking an over-the-counter decongestant pill or nasal spray about an hour before landing.
- People with allergies should also take their medication about an hour before landing.

FOR MORE HELP

Key Websites: *www.SavonHealth.com*. For more information on airplane ear: *www.SavonHearing.com*.
Organization: American Speech-Language-Hearing Association, 10801 Rockville Pike, Rockville, MD 20852. 800-638-8255, M–F 8:30–5 EST; *www.asha.org*. Staff members answer questions and give written advice on airplane ear and other disorders.

Ear & Hearing Problems

Your ears serve two functions—hearing and balance. Some problems affect one or the other function, and some affect both. Try to find the cause of such a problem and treat it early; you can do a lot to prevent or treat most conditions that affect your ears.

SYMPTOMS	WHAT IT MIGHT BE	WHAT YOU CAN DO
Severe pain and swelling behind and in ear, fluid coming from ear, fever, temporary hearing loss.	Mastoiditis—inflamed mastoid bone behind ear.	Call doctor for prompt appointment. Antibiotics or surgical drainage may be required.
Pain, hearing loss, sometimes discharge or bleeding from ear.	Ruptured (perforated) eardrum—often caused by object pushed into ear. ■ Serious middle ear infection (see page 71). ■ Blow to ear or injury while diving or waterskiing.	Call doctor for prompt appointment. Treatment includes medications, patch over eardrum, or surgery. To relieve pain, cover ear with heating pad set on low and take painkillers.
Loss of balance, dizziness, ringing in ears, hearing loss, nausea or vomiting.	Labyrinthitis—infection often caused by a virus, in area of inner ear that controls balance.	Call doctor for advice and appointment. Treatment includes medications and bed rest.
Repeated sudden and severe dizziness, hearing loss, or ringing in ear; loss of balance; headache; nausea or vomiting.	Ménière's syndrome—from fluid buildup in inner ear.	Call doctor for advice and appointment. Treatment includes medications and sometimes surgery. Rest to reduce symptoms. Cut back on fluids and salt. Avoid alcohol, caffeine, tobacco. **For more help:** Ménière's Network, EAR Foundation, 800-545-HEAR, M–F 8–4:30 CST.
Hearing loss over time, dizziness, ringing in ear.	Otosclerosis—overgrowth of bone in middle ear. Often runs in families. More common in women; may get worse during pregnancy.	Call doctor for advice and appointment. Simplest treatment is hearing aid; surgery can help.
Trouble hearing, often at higher frequencies and with background noise; trouble understanding speech.	Presbycusis—hearing loss due to age. Usually begins between 40 and 50. Most common and severe in men.	Call doctor for advice and appointment. Hearing aid is usual treatment.

EARS

(continued)

Ear & Hearing Problems (continued)

SYMPTOMS	WHAT IT MIGHT BE	WHAT YOU CAN DO
Feeling of fullness, discomfort, or pain in ears during or after flying; temporary hearing loss; ringing in ears; dizziness.	Airplane ear.	See airplane ear, page 68.
Throbbing pain and/or tender lump in ear canal; discharge of pus or blood from ear.	Boil (see page 146).	Usually heals by itself. Antibiotic drops or heating pad may help.
Feeling of fullness or blockage in ear, temporary hearing loss, pain or discomfort, ringing in ear.	Earwax (see page 72). ■ Ear infection (see facing page). ■ Early sign of throat cancer (rarely).	If symptoms persist, call doctor for advice.
Earache, fever and chills, stuffy nose, feeling of fullness or blockage in ear, muffled hearing, discharge from ear. In young children: tugging at ear, bad temper, restlessness, lack of appetite.	Middle ear infection.	See ear infections, facing page.
Itchy or blocked ear, pain or tenderness, yellowish discharge, flaky skin around ear, temporary hearing loss.	Swimmer's ear—infection of outer ear canal.	See swimmer's ear, page 73.
Ringing or buzzing in ears—noise that can't be heard by others.	Tinnitus.	See tinnitus, page 74.
Earache with pain in jaw and/or face; headache; clicking noise or locked feeling when opening or closing mouth.	Temporomandibular disorder (TMD).	See temporomandibular disorder, page 201.

Ear Infections

www.SavonEarInfections.com

SIGNS AND SYMPTOMS

In adults:

- Earache (either a sudden, sharp pain or a constant, dull pain).
- Muffled hearing.

Sometimes with:

- Fever of 100 degrees or higher, perhaps with chills.
- Stuffy nose.
- Sore throat.
- Feeling of fullness in the ear.
- Pus or blood from the ear.
- Nausea or diarrhea.

In young children, especially those who aren't yet talking, watch for:

- Tugging at the ear.
- Bad temper.
- Restlessness.
- Lack of appetite.
- Rectal temperature of 100 degrees or higher (101 or higher oral).
- Discharge from the nose or ear.

A middle ear infection (otitis media) is the most common cause of earaches. It's the number one reason children go to the doctor, but it also affects adults.

Ear infections are most often caused by **colds** (see page 93) or **flu** (see page 95). These ailments swell the tissues of the middle ear, trapping fluids and creating an ideal place for bacteria or viruses to thrive. **Allergies** (see page 84) or irritants such as smoke or fumes can have the same effect.

Infections that go on for weeks or happen again and again can cause permanent hearing loss. In young children, any hearing loss is cause for concern, because it may delay speech and language development; prompt treatment is vital.

An ear infection can lead to other problems, including mastoiditis (an inflamed mastoid bone behind the ear), perforated eardrum, **meningitis** (see page 55), and facial nerve paralysis.

WHAT YOU CAN DO NOW

- Hold a warm compress to the ear. Inhaling steam may also help. Or use a vaporizer if you have one.
- Gargle with warm salt water to soothe a sore throat and help open blocked ears.
- Drink plenty of water or other clear liquids.
- Use pillows to raise the head when lying down. This helps drain the middle ear.
- People with allergies may get relief from over-the-counter antihistamines. Some people use decongestant nasal sprays to open the ears. But after a couple of days, sprays can lead to "rebound" congestion that makes the problem worse.
- Over-the-counter drugs such as aspirin, ibuprofen, or acetaminophen may help with pain. (Never give aspirin to a child or teenager who has a cold, chicken pox, flu, or any other illness you suspect of being caused by a virus; see box on **Reye's syndrome,** page 95.)

WHEN TO CALL THE DOCTOR

- If your child has symptoms of an ear infection or trouble hearing.
- If an earache lasts more than 2 days.
- If your temperature or your child's rises above 100 degrees.
- If you have frequent ear infections, or if your child does.

HOW TO PREVENT IT

- Remove irritants and things that cause allergies, such as dust, cleaning fluids, and tobacco smoke, from your home.
- Clean your ears gently with a soft cloth.
- Avoid flying, if you can, when you have a cold. If you must fly, use an over-the-counter nose spray or decongestant 1 to 2 hours before takeoff. While the plane lands, keep clearing your ears by chewing gum and making yourself yawn a lot. And don't scuba dive or dive into a swimming pool if you have a cold. Changes in air pressure when your ears and nose are clogged up can damage the eardrum and make it more susceptible to infection.

EARS

➤ If you have food allergies, or your child does, cut back on the foods that you know cause allergic reactions.

➤ If you're not breast-feeding your baby, hold him or her upright during bottle-feeding to keep milk from getting into the tube that connects the back of the nose and the ear.

FOR MORE HELP

Key Websites: *www.SavonHealth.com*. For more information on ear infections: *www.SavonEarInfections.com*.

Organizations: American Academy of Otolaryngology–Head and Neck Surgery, 1 Prince St., Alexandria, VA 22314-3357. 705-836-4444, M–F 8:30–5 EST; *www.entnet.org*. Send a self-addressed stamped envelope to receive the brochure on earaches and otitis media.

■ American Speech-Language-Hearing Association, 10801 Rockville Pike, Rockville, MD 20852. 800-638-8255, M–F 8:30–5 EST; *www.asha.org*. Staff answers questions on hearing loss; ask for the pamphlet on otitis media.

■ National Institute on Deafness and Other Communication Disorders Information Clearinghouse, 800-241-1044, M–F 8:30–5 EST; *www.nih.gov/nidcd*. Ask for ear infections packet and for fact sheet on otitis media.

Earwax
www.SavonHearing.com

SIGNS AND SYMPTOMS

■ Blocked or plugged feeling in ear.
■ Trouble hearing.
■ Ear pain or discomfort.
■ Ringing in the ear.

Earwax coats and protects the outer ear canal that leads to the eardrum (see illustration, facing page). Usually earwax is soft, drains easily, and doesn't cause trouble.

But sometimes the wax builds up and becomes hard and dry. Then it's one of the most common causes of hearing problems, especially when it mixes with dust, dirt, or water in the ear.

WHAT YOU CAN DO NOW

Infants and young children with built-up earwax should be taken to a doctor; do not attempt to remove the wax yourself. Adults can try the following, but don't do this if you have an earache, fever, discharge from your ear, or a punctured eardrum (see **ear and hearing problems** chart, page 69), or if you've just had ear surgery:

➤ Mix 1 tablespoon hydrogen peroxide, mineral oil, or baby oil with 1 tablespoon warm water. (Make sure it's warm—cold water in the ear can make you dizzy.)

■ Tilt your head, and put a few drops of the warmed liquid into your blocked ear. Leave it there for 3 minutes, keeping your head tilted.

■ Let the liquid run out onto a towel or tissue. The wax should be soft enough to be wiped away from the outer ear with a cotton ball. Repeat if needed.

➤ Over-the-counter liquid earwax softeners can help loosen earwax. But don't use wax softeners if you suspect you have an ear infection or ruptured eardrum (see **ear and hearing problems** chart, page 69), or have had recent ear surgery.

➤ Never attempt to remove earwax with a cotton-tipped stick or swab. You can damage your eardrum or cause an infection.

WHEN TO CALL THE DOCTOR

Call for a prompt appointment:
➤ If you have sudden or total hearing loss in one or both ears.
➤ If pus, fluid, or blood drains from your ear. This can mean an ear infection or a punctured eardrum.

Call for advice and an appointment:
➤ If wax becomes so firmly lodged that home care doesn't work. Your doctor may need to clean the ear.

HOW TO PREVENT IT

➤ Wear earplugs if you work around a lot of dust, which can trigger wax buildup.
➤ Each week, put 1 or 2 drops of mineral oil in each ear to keep wax soft.

The Ear

The outer ear canal carries sound waves to the eardrum. From there, vibrations travel to the middle and inner ear. One part of the inner ear translates vibrations into signals that your brain "hears"; another part keeps you balanced. A second canal, the eustachian tube, connects the middle ear to the back of the nose and throat.

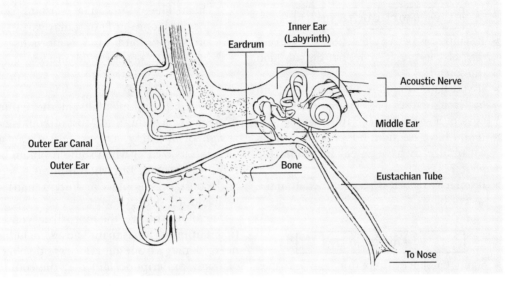

Swimmer's Ear

www.SavonHearing.com

SIGNS AND SYMPTOMS

- Itching or blocked feeling in the ear.
- Ear pain and tenderness that is worse when you move your head or pull on your earlobe.
- Foul-smelling, watery, or yellow discharge from the ear.
- Patches of broken, flaky skin around the opening of the ear.
- Muffled hearing.

You don't have to be a swimmer to get "swimmer's ear" (otitis externa), an inflamed outer ear canal. It's often caused by moisture in the ear, perhaps from frequent showers or shampoos, or from swimming, particularly in polluted water.

The dampness can make the skin inside the ear canal crack or flake, letting bacteria or fungi invade. Some skin problems, such as **dermatitis**

(see page 149) and **psoriasis** (see page 159), can also cause swimmer's ear. Another common cause is having too little earwax to protect the ear canal from moisture. Swimmer's ear is seldom serious.

WHAT YOU CAN DO NOW

Swimmer's ear often clears up on its own. If not, it responds quickly to treatment. Here's what you can do to speed recovery:

➤ Keep the infected ear dry. Wear earplugs or big, loose-fitting cotton balls coated with Vaseline when showering or washing your hair. Stay out of swimming pools.

➤ Use over-the-counter antiseptic eardrops. Or make your own, using equal parts rubbing alcohol and white vinegar. Warm the drops first. Leave them in your ear for a couple of minutes, then tilt your head to let them drain out.

➤ Hold a warm compress over the ear to relieve pain. Over-the-counter painkillers may help. (Never give aspirin to a child or teenager who has a cold, chicken pox, flu, or any other illness you suspect of being caused by a virus; see box on **Reye's syndrome,** page 95.)

➤ To keep the problem from coming back, don't let any water get in the ear canal for 3 weeks after symptoms disappear.

WHEN TO CALL THE DOCTOR

➤ If symptoms persist after more than 4 or 5 days of self-care. It's rare, but the infection can spread.

➤ If you have symptoms and your eardrum has ever ruptured or been injured in other ways, or if you've had ear surgery.

➤ If you have frequent bouts of swimmer's ear or already have an **ear infection** (see page 71).

➤ If you have diabetes or a weakened immune system.

HOW TO PREVENT IT

➤ Squirt lanolin eardrops (or baby oil) into your ears before you swim to protect them from the water. Tilt your head so the drops get to the bottom of the ear canal, then let the liquid drain out.

➤ Try to keep your ears dry. Wear earplugs while swimming (remove them right after), and pull a shower cap over your ears before showering.

➤ Dry the outer parts of your ears after swimming or showering, and use rubbing alcohol eardrops to help evaporate water inside.

➤ Use antiseptic eardrops if you get water in your ears and you tend to get swimmer's ear.

➤ Be careful when cleaning **earwax** (see page 72) from your ears. Don't use any object that could scratch the ear canal.

FOR MORE HELP

Key Websites: *www.SavonHealth.com.* For more information on swimmer's ear: *www.SavonHearing.com.*

Organization: American Academy of Otolaryngology–Head and Neck Surgery, 1 Prince St., Alexandria, VA 22314. 703-836-4444, M–F 8:30–5 EST; *www.entnet. org.* Ask for the swimmer's ear brochure and names of doctors near you.

Tinnitus
www.SavonTinnitus.com

SIGNS AND SYMPTOMS

■ Ringing, whistling, buzzing, humming, or roaring that only you can hear. The sound can be constant or may come and go. It may vary in pitch or loudness; it is more distinct when other sounds are low.

About 50 million adults in the United States have tinnitus. Most often it is not a sign of anything serious, and it can go away on its own or when some problem behind it is treated. But when tinnitus is loud and constant, people can find it hard to concentrate, sleep, or work.

The older you are, the more likely you are to get tinnitus. It has many causes, including nerve damage from loud noises, side effects of many prescription and over-the-counter medications, and chronic stress (see **stress,** page 218). Tinnitus can also be a symptom of other health problems, such as **high blood pressure** (see page 111).

If you have tinnitus along with dizziness, you might have fluid buildup in your inner ear or damage to the small bones in your middle ear (see Ménière's syndrome, otosclerosis, and labyrinthitis in the **ear and hearing problems** chart, page 69).

WHAT YOU CAN DO NOW

Tinnitus can't always be cured, but you can take steps to get relief:

➤ If you have trouble sleeping, cover the tinnitus with a recording of soothing sounds or music.

➤ Try a tinnitus masker, a small device worn like a hearing aid; it makes a pleasant sound to compete with the tinnitus.

➤ Avoid caffeine, alcohol, tobacco, and aspirin, which can make tinnitus worse.

➤ Exercise often. This may provide relief by bringing more blood to the head.

➤ If allergies cause your tinnitus, stay away from things that bring them on. Try a decongestant to relieve stuffiness (but don't use it for more than 2 days at a time, to avoid "rebound" congestion).

WHEN TO CALL THE DOCTOR

Call for a prompt appointment:
- If you have sudden or total hearing loss.
- If you have tinnitus and feel dizzy.
- If you have tinnitus and pus or pain in your ear.

How to Save Your Ears

At least 28 million Americans have some form of hearing loss. In about a third of these cases, excessive noise is likely to blame. Just how dangerous a sound is depends on how loud it is and how long it lasts. A single blast—such as the crack of a shotgun at close range—can instantly kill many of the sensitive hair cells in the inner ear that translate sound waves into nerve impulses. More common, though, is injury from frequent exposure to milder levels of loud noise. Most such exposure takes place on the job, but the culprits are all around us. Among the sounds that can do damage are the buzz of a leaf blower, the roar of a motorcycle, and the wail of a personal stereo turned up too high. It all adds up.

What can you do? First, get out of places that are too loud, just as you would get out of the sun when you start to burn. When a screaming fire truck heads your way, stick your fingers in your ears until it's gone. Monitor your personal stereo: If someone else can hear the music coming from your headset, it's loud enough to do harm—turn down the volume. If you work in a noisy setting, give your ears regular rests. Last, take advantage of a simple device humans have relied on for at least a century: earplugs. Inexpensive foam plugs give plenty of protection if you get at least half of the cylinder into your ear canal. For a proper fit, roll the plug into a skinny log, then pull your earlobe forward as you insert it.

Call for advice and an appointment:
- If you think your tinnitus is caused by another health problem.

- If self-care doesn't work and tinnitus interferes with your concentration, daily activities, or sleep.

HOW TO PREVENT IT

- Wear earplugs or earmuffs when exposed to loud noise. (Cotton balls don't block enough sound.)
- Keep the volume down when listening to music through earphones.
- Cut down on salt. It can cause fluid to build up in your middle ear, and that raises your chances of having tinnitus.
- Get enough rest, avoid stress, and practice relaxation techniques.
- Don't let wax build up in your ears (see **earwax,** page 72).
- If you're taking any medications, ask your doctor if they could be causing your tinnitus. Are there alternatives?
- Keep a diary listing what you eat each day and when you're around dust, chemicals, or other irritants. Note when your tinnitus comes on. This may help you find the cause, so you'll know what to avoid.
- Allergy-proof your home—keep it free of dust, mold, pet hair, and other common causes of allergies. Change filters in your heater or air conditioner often.

FOR MORE HELP

Key Websites: *www.SavonHealth.com*. For more information on Tinnitus: *www.SavonTinnitus.com*.

Organizations: American Speech-Language-Hearing Association, 10801 Rockville Pike, Rockville, MD 20852. 800-638-8255, M–F 8:30–5 EST; *www.asha.org*. Staff answers questions and sends out brochures on tinnitus and other ear disorders.

■ American Tinnitus Association, 1618 SW First Ave., Suite 417, Portland, OR 97201. 503-248-9985, M–F 8:30–5 PST; *www.ata.org*. Ask about membership, publications, and support groups near you.

■ National Institute on Deafness and Other Communication Disorders Information Clearinghouse, 800-241-1044, M–F 8:30–5 EST; *www.nih.gov/nidcd*. Ask for the tinnitus packet.

EARS

Mouth

Bad Breath

www.SavonOralConditions.com

SIGNS AND SYMPTOMS

- Foul odor from the mouth.
- Bad taste in the mouth.
- Inflamed and bleeding gums.

Many people have bouts of bad breath (halitosis) not explained by the effects of strong-smelling food and drink. Most of the time, bad breath is no cause for alarm. But it can be a sign of a health problem, such as gum disease, tooth decay (see **toothache,** page 80), **sinusitis** (see page 98), **tonsillitis** (see page 102), **strep throat** (see page 267), or **diabetes** (see page 277).

Bad breath is mostly caused by bacteria mixed with food bits and saliva that form a smelly film on the teeth called plaque. Smoking is a major culprit, too. A dry mouth adds to the problem, causing "morning breath." Simply not drinking enough water can make it worse. So can some drugs, such as diuretics, tranquilizers, and antihistamines.

WHAT YOU CAN DO NOW

- ➤ Brush your teeth at least twice a day, and floss once daily.
- ➤ Gently clean the top of your tongue with the toothbrush. Be sure to reach in back.
- ➤ Postnasal drip—from a cold, allergies, or sinusitis—can cause bad breath. To flush away mucus and bacteria, try gargling with a saltwater mix: Dissolve a half teaspoon of salt in 8 ounces of warm water. Use the same mix to flush out your nose: Squirt it in with a dropper or a bulb syringe, or put the mix in the palm of your hand and sniff it in, 1 nostril at a time. Wait a few minutes and then blow your nose gently.
- ➤ For a quick cover-up, eat fresh parsley or mint, an orange, an apple, or celery. Or use a mouthwash.

WHEN TO CALL THE DOCTOR OR DENTIST

- ➤ If your bad breath persists for no clear reason after you've flossed and cleaned your teeth, gums, and tongue extra well for a week.
- ➤ If you have a toothache with bad breath. You may have a cavity or an abscess.
- ➤ If your gums are inflamed and bleeding. This could be a sign of gum disease.
- ➤ If you also have a fever or cough and mucus. This could be a symptom of a lung abscess.

HOW TO PREVENT IT

- ➤ Brush at least twice a day and floss daily.
- ➤ Brush your tongue every morning, especially the back.
- ➤ Use mouthwash daily to kill bacteria that brushing might miss.
- ➤ Have your teeth cleaned every 6 months, and see a dentist once a year.
- ➤ Don't smoke.
- ➤ Go light on coffee and alcohol; spicy foods such as garlic, hot peppers, and salami; and strong-smelling foods such as anchovies and tuna.

Tooth & Mouth Problems

Even minor tooth and mouth problems can hurt. You can prevent many of them by brushing your teeth and flossing daily; seeing a dentist every year can help you take early action if a problem does come up.

SYMPTOMS	WHAT IT MIGHT BE	WHAT YOU CAN DO
White or red patch on gums; lump or discoloration anywhere in mouth; sore in mouth that bleeds and/or doesn't heal in 3–4 weeks; trouble swallowing; swelling in jaw or neck.	Oral cancer—tumors can occur anywhere in or around mouth or in upper throat.	Call doctor for prompt appointment. Most oral cancers can be treated if found early. **For more help:** Cancer Information and Counseling Hotline, 800-525-3777, M–F 8:30–5 MST.
Toothache and red, swollen, or bleeding gums; sometimes earache; often fever; facial swelling; bad taste in mouth.	Tooth abscess. See toothache, page 80.	Call dentist for prompt appointment.
Red, swollen gums that sometimes bleed; bad breath; loose teeth; pus discharge in mouth.	Periodontitis—advanced inflamed gums: end result of gingivitis (see below).	Call dentist for advice and appointment. Prompt treatment is needed to save teeth. **For more help:** American Academy of Periodontology, 737 N. Michigan Ave., Suite 800, Chicago, IL 60611-2690. Write for fact sheets and brochures on periodontitis.
Reddish, shiny, swollen gums that bleed easily; bad breath.	Gingivitis—also called gum disease. Most often caused by plaque buildup on teeth.	Call dentist for advice and appointment. Treatment includes removing plaque. Brush teeth after meals at least twice a day. Floss daily.
Red, swollen, painful gums; sore jaw; headache; bad taste in mouth; bad breath.	Impacted teeth—caused by lack of space in mouth.	Call dentist for advice and appointment. Treatment may include pulling a tooth.
Lump or sore in mouth or on tongue.	Noncancerous mouth or tongue tumors. Cause is unknown.	Call doctor for advice and appointment if lump or sore doesn't clear up in 3 weeks.

(continued)

MOUTH

Tooth & Mouth Problems (continued)

SYMPTOMS	WHAT IT MIGHT BE	WHAT YOU CAN DO
Creamy yellow patches in mouth and throat that leave raw, red spots when rubbed.	Thrush—a fungal infection (see page 153) common in people with HIV and in infants. Caused by some antibiotics and steroid inhalers.	Call doctor for advice and appointment.
Painful, swollen glands under tongue, behind ear, or in neck; bad taste in mouth; dry mouth; fever.	Salivary gland disorders. Causes include mumps (see page 264) and bacterial infection.	Call doctor for advice and appointment. Treatment may include antibiotics. Avoid spicy foods and citrus fruits.
Jaw, mouth, and facial pain; headache; clicking noise when opening or closing mouth; locked jaw.	Temporomandibular disorder (see page 201).	Call doctor or dentist for advice and appointment.
Pain and/or tightness in face and jaw muscles; toothache; worn teeth.	Tooth grinding (see page 83).	Call dentist for advice and appointment.
Gray film on gums; red, painful, bleeding gums; bad breath; bad taste in mouth.	Trench mouth—bacterial infection of gums; appears suddenly, often returns.	Call dentist for advice and appointment. Left untreated, can cause permanent gum damage, loss of teeth.

➤ Chew sugarless gum after meals when you can't brush, or rinse your mouth out with water.

➤ Drink at least 8 glasses of water every day.

FOR MORE HELP

Key Websites: *www.SavonHealth.com*. For more information on tooth and mouth problems: *www.SavonOralConditions.com*.

Organizations: American Dental Association, 211 E. Chicago Ave., Chicago, IL 60611. 312-440-2500, M–F 8:30–5 CST; *www.ada.org*. Offers advice on brushing and flossing, and lists dentists by state. At Website, select *Patients & Consumers*, then click on *Bad Breath, Cleaning Your Teeth and Gums,* or *Your Diet and Dental Health*.

■ Richter Center for the Treatment of Breath Disorders, 800-210-2110, M–F 8–8 EST; *www.profresh.com*. Treats and gives information on chronic bad breath.

Canker Sores
www.SavonCankerSores.com

SIGNS AND SYMPTOMS

■ Painful sores on the gums and tongue and inside lips. They can be white, gray, or yellowish, with a red rim.

■ A tingling feeling just before a sore appears.

■ Pain that may increase when eating or talking.

■ Fever and swollen glands (sometimes).

A tear or break in the flesh inside the mouth can lead to canker sores. They're a common ailment; teenagers and women are the most likely to get them. Most often, they heal themselves in 7 to 10 days. They are not contagious. The causes aren't clear, but some triggers include:

➤ Injury to the mouth's lining from chipped or jagged teeth, dental work, or dentures.
➤ Damage from rough toothbrushing.
➤ Burns from hot foods or liquids.
➤ Soreness from sour foods (such as lemons) or acidic foods (tomatoes or oranges).
➤ Food allergies.
➤ Vitamin and mineral shortages.

WHAT YOU CAN DO NOW

Home treatments can help ease the pain of canker sores. Try these:

➤ Rinse your mouth about 4 times a day with 8 ounces of warm water mixed with a half teaspoon of salt. Don't swallow.
➤ Rub an ice cube or Popsicle on the sore.
➤ Apply a paste of baking soda and water.
➤ Avoid spicy, sour, or acidic foods, which may make the sore worse.
➤ Put a wet tea bag on the sore area.
➤ Use an over-the-counter salve or an antiseptic mouthwash made for canker sores.

WHEN TO CALL THE DOCTOR OR DENTIST

➤ If you get sores and a fever of 100 degrees or higher, or swollen glands.
➤ If the sores last longer than 3 weeks; this may indicate a serious problem, such as oral cancer.
➤ If you have severe pain. Your doctor may prescribe painkillers or antibiotics.
➤ If you suspect that tooth or denture problems are causing your canker sores. Talk to your dentist; the sores are not likely to heal until the cause is fixed.

HOW TO PREVENT IT

➤ Clean your teeth gently with a soft brush, and floss daily. Buy toothpaste that's free of the detergent sodium lauryl sulfate, which may dry out the lining of the mouth, leaving the insides of the cheeks and the gums easy to irritate.

➤ Don't eat foods that appear to trigger the sores.
➤ Take a multivitamin/mineral supplement.

FOR MORE HELP

Key Websites: *www.SavonHealth.com*. For more information on canker sores: *www.SavonCankerSores.com*.

Organizations: The American Academy of Otolaryngology–Head and Neck Surgery, 1 Prince St., Alexandria, VA 22314-3357. 703-836-4444, M–F 8:30–5 EST. Ask for the brochure on canker sores.

■ American Dental Association, 211 E. Chicago Ave., Chicago, IL 60611. 312-440-2500, M–F 8:30–5 CST; *www.ada.org*. At Website, click on *Search* and type *canker sores*.

Website: Healthtouch, *www.healthtouch.com/level1/leaflets/NIDR/NIDR003.htm*. Offers information on canker sores and what causes them.

Cold Sores
www.SavonColdSores.com

SIGNS AND SYMPTOMS

■ Painful blisters on or around the lips or mouth.
■ Tingling, prickling, or itching on the lips or mouth (often just before cold sores appear).
■ Fever and swollen neck glands with the first outbreak only.

Cold sores are caused by the herpes simplex virus. After a first outbreak, often during childhood, the virus may lie dormant for years, but it can become active at any time. Triggers include fever (the sores are sometimes called fever blisters), infection, stress, sun or windy weather, and certain foods such as chocolate, nuts, or seeds.

Like **canker sores** (see facing page), cold sores are common and aren't a major health concern unless your immune system is weak-

MOUTH

ened by another illness, such as AIDS.

But they are contagious, so take care not to spread the virus by contact. Don't touch a cold sore and then touch your eyes: You could cause a serious eye infection. Also, herpes cold sores on the mouth can be spread to the genitals (see **sexually transmitted diseases** chart, page 221). When you have a cold sore or are with someone who does, don't kiss or have oral sex.

WHAT YOU CAN DO NOW

Cold sores most often clear up on their own in 7 to 10 days. You can't cure them, but to relieve pain:

➤ Apply an ice cube to the sore spot for a few minutes at a time.
➤ Don't eat sour, spicy, or acidic foods. They may make the sores worse.
➤ Use a lip salve—plain petroleum jelly works well—to ease dryness and prevent cracked lips.
➤ If you get cold sores often, ask a doctor to prescribe medicine you can use when you feel the first signs of an outbreak.

WHEN TO CALL THE DOCTOR

Call for a prompt appointment:

➤ If you have a cold sore and feel any eye pain, or if your vision is affected. You may have a herpes infection in your eye.

Call for advice:

➤ If you get sores and a fever of 100 degrees or higher and/or chills.
➤ If your cold sores last longer than 2 weeks or come back often.

HOW TO PREVENT IT

➤ Get a new toothbrush after you've had cold sores.
➤ Wear a hat and use sunblock on your lips if sun appears to trigger cold sores.
➤ Take 500 to 1,000 milligrams of the amino acid lysine daily. Or eat foods (such as kidney beans, split peas, and corn) that are high in lysine.
➤ If stress seems to bring on cold sores, find ways to relax: Exercise and practice yoga or meditation (see **relax,** page 303).

These sores are contagious. To keep from spreading them:

➤ Wash your hands often, and don't share tableware, towels, or razors.
➤ Don't share lip products or kiss anyone during an outbreak.
➤ Don't touch the infected area.
➤ Don't touch a cold sore and then touch your eye. This can cause a serious eye problem.

FOR MORE HELP

Key Websites: *www.SavonHealth.com.* For more information on cold sores: *www.SavonColdSores.com.*

Organization: The American Academy of Otolaryngology–Head and Neck Surgery, 1 Prince St., Alexandria, VA 22314-3357. 703-836-4444, M–F 8:30–5 EST. Ask for the brochure on fever blisters.

Website: Healthtouch, *www.healthtouch.com/ level1/leaflets/NIDR/NIDR001.htm.* Offers information on fever blisters.

Toothache
www.SavonToothache.com

SIGNS AND SYMPTOMS

Tooth decay:
■ Sharp pain in a tooth, often when you bite or chew.
■ Ache or soreness in teeth, gums, or jaw.
■ Bad breath or bad taste in your mouth—a sign of severe decay or an abscess (infection).

Tooth abscess:
■ Severe pain in the tooth or jaw.
■ A loose tooth.
■ Red, swollen, or bleeding gums.
■ Fever.
■ Earache.
■ Swollen glands in the neck.

Cavities are the most common reason for toothache. They are caused by dental plaque, a sticky substance made up of food

Sensitive Teeth

If heat or cold makes a tooth hurt, you could have an ailment known as dentinal hypersensitivity. This occurs when enamel, the outer covering of the tooth, thins, cracks, or wears away. It is brought on by age, receding gums, dental surgery, or repeated brushing with hard-bristled toothbrushes or "whitening" toothpastes with abrasives.

You can help relieve it and prevent further damage by using a toothpaste made for sensitive teeth and a brush with soft bristles. If pain persists, see your dentist.

bits, saliva, and bacteria. Plaque makes acids that eat away the enamel on teeth. A toothache can also be caused by a bit of food stuck between the gum and a tooth, a broken filling, or something as serious as:

➤ Impacted teeth (teeth that don't grow out fully or that come in at a bad angle) pressing on other teeth or trapping food.
➤ **Tooth grinding** (see page 83), which can crack teeth.
➤ Gum disease.
➤ Pressure from infected or stuffed-up sinuses (see **sinusitis,** page 98).
➤ Jaws that don't line up right (see **temporomandibular disorder,** page 201).

WHAT YOU CAN DO NOW

You'll need to see the dentist, especially if you have signs of an abscess. Until then, these home treatments can relieve some of the pain:

➤ Use dental floss to remove trapped food bits. Rinse with warm salt water. (See **tips on tooth and gum care,** page 82.)
➤ Suck on an ice cube to numb your gums, or put a cold pack on your jaw.
➤ If cold doesn't work, try heat. Put a hot compress on your jaw, and rinse your mouth with warm salt water.
➤ Put a wet tea bag (black tea) on a sore gum for 30 minutes to ease soreness or to stop bleeding.

➤ Put oil of cloves on an aching tooth with a cotton swab every 20 minutes for pain.
➤ Make a temporary filling for a broken or lost filling from an over-the-counter product sold in many drugstores.
➤ Take an over-the-counter pain reliever. Don't take aspirin if you think you might be about to have dental work—it can increase bleeding. (Never give aspirin to a child under 12 who has chicken pox, flu, a cold, or any other illness you suspect of being caused by a virus; see box on **Reye's syndrome,** page 95.)
➤ Don't put aspirin directly on the gums—it can burn the tissues.

WHEN TO CALL THE DENTIST

Call for a prompt appointment:
➤ If you have any symptoms of an abscess. You may need emergency care.
Call for advice:
➤ If your toothache lasts longer than a day or two; if you have throbbing pain in a tooth that doesn't go away; or if heat, cold, or pressure makes the tooth hurt. You may have a cavity.
➤ If you have swollen, red, and painful gums. You may have gum disease or an impacted tooth.

HOW TO PREVENT IT

➤ Brush at least twice a day using a toothpaste with fluoride and a soft-bristled toothbrush. Floss every day. Replace your toothbrush every few months.
➤ Don't eat sweet and sticky foods, which damage tooth enamel.
➤ Get a cleaning every 6 months, and see a dentist every year.

FOR MORE HELP

Key Websites: *www.SavonHealth.com*. For more information on tootaches: *www.SavonToothache.com*.
Organizations: American Academy of Periodontology, 737 N. Michigan Ave., Suite 800, Chicago, IL 60611-2690; *www. perio.org*. Write to request brochures on dental care. Include a business-size

MOUTH

Tips on Tooth & Gum Care

Safeguard your smile by cleaning your teeth and gums at least twice a day. Before you buy a toothbrush, toothpaste, or floss, look for the American Dental Association's seal of approval.

➤ Get a good toothbrush. Soft, "end-rounded" bristles are best. Make sure the brush fits your mouth—you should be able to reach every tooth easily. Be sure your child's toothbrush isn't too big or too hard.

➤ Replace your toothbrush monthly, or sooner if the bristles become bent or splayed. Worn brushes don't clean well and can hurt your gums. Many brushes have colored markers that change when it's time for you to buy a new one.

➤ Keep your brush clean, and don't let others use it.

➤ An electric toothbrush works well if you use it right. And it may get a child to brush more often. Ask your dentist for advice.

➤ Devices that use a jet of water to remove food particles from teeth are helpful for people who wear braces, bridges, or partial dentures. But they don't take the place of regular flossing and brushing.

➤ Use a toothpaste or gel with fluoride, which helps protect teeth from decay.

➤ Some products that claim to whiten teeth may not be safe. They can harm the enamel. Ask your dentist before you use these or other tooth products that make special claims.

➤ Start dental care with your baby's first teeth. Don't let your child fall asleep with a bottle of milk or juice—sweet liquids cling to baby teeth and invite decay that can cause tooth loss.

➤ Take your child to the dentist before his or her first birthday—sooner if you think there is a problem.

Cleaning tips

➤ Don't rush. Take 2 to 3 minutes to reach all the surfaces of all of your teeth.

➤ Hold the brush at a 45-degree angle to your gums so that the tips of the bristles point into the gumline. Move it gently back and forth in very short strokes, brushing about half a tooth at a time.

➤ Be sure to brush the inner surfaces of your teeth. Get the inside of your front teeth as well.

➤ Don't forget to brush your tongue, but be gentle.

How to floss

Floss once a day to clean places that your toothbrush can't reach.

➤ Floss comes in many types: Choose one that feels comfortable and that doesn't cut your gums.

➤ To floss: Break off about 18 inches of dental floss and wind it around the middle finger of each hand. Pinch it between your thumbs and forefingers, leaving about an inch of floss. Use a gentle sawing motion to slip it between your teeth. Do not jerk or snap the floss into the gums.

➤ When the floss reaches the gumline, curve it into a C shape against one tooth. Slide it gently under the gum. Don't press hard; you don't want to cut the gum.

➤ Hold the floss against the tooth. Scrape the side of the tooth gently, moving the floss away from the gum. Repeat with clean floss for each tooth. Don't skip the back of your last tooth.

➤ Your gums may bleed a bit the first 5 or 6 days after you begin flossing. But if they bleed after that, call your dentist. You may be hurting your gums.

➤ You can buy other products besides floss for cleaning between the teeth—picks, sticks, and small brushes.

self-addressed stamped envelope.

■ American Dental Association, Department of Public Education and Information, 211 E. Chicago Ave., Chicago, IL 60611. 312-440-2593, M–F 8:30–5 CST; *www.ada.org*. Write for pamphlets on caring for teeth and gums.

Books: *Tooth Fitness: Your Guide to Healthy Teeth,* by Thomas McGuire, D.D.S. A reader-friendly guide to tooth care. Diane Publishing, 1998, $17.

■ *The Columbia University School of Dental and Oral Surgery's Guide to Family Dental Care,* by Rebecca W. Smith. W. W. Norton, 1997, $29.95.

Tooth Grinding
www.SavonOralConditions.com

SIGNS AND SYMPTOMS

■ Tension, tightness, or pain in the face and jaw muscles.
■ Toothache.
■ Mild to severe headache or migraine.
■ Looseness or aching in the teeth, often upon waking.
■ Worn or broken teeth.

Tooth grinding (bruxism) is a common problem, mostly among women. It is thought to be caused by many factors, such as an abnormal bite, crooked or missing teeth, high levels of stress, or a **sleep disorder** (see page 286).

Until you have symptoms, you may not know you're grinding or clenching your teeth, especially if you do it in your sleep. But you may be wearing down your teeth and cracking them.

WHAT YOU CAN DO NOW

➤ During the day, practice letting your jaw relax while keeping your teeth slightly apart.
➤ Don't chew gum, tobacco, pencils, or any other nonfood object.
➤ Hold a warm washcloth to the side of your

face. This may help to relax your jaw.
➤ If you suspect that stress is the problem, try to reduce it with exercise and relaxation techniques such as meditation, deep breathing, or yoga (see **stress,** page 218, and **relax**, page 303).

WHEN TO CALL THE DENTIST

➤ If you still have symptoms after a month of home treatment, or if you think a bad bite or a missing tooth is causing the problem. You may need to have your dentist fit you with a mouth guard or bite plate.
➤ If you have tooth pain or a jaw ache for more than a day or two. These symptoms could be the result of tooth decay (see **toothache,** page 80) or a sign of **temporomandibular disorder** (see page 201).
➤ If you think stress is still causing problems. You may want to seek counseling or ask your dentist to prescribe a muscle relaxant for your jaw.

HOW TO PREVENT IT

➤ Learn how to ease your stress and stay as relaxed as you can, especially around bedtime. Take a warm bath or shower before bed, listen to soothing music, and practice meditation, deep breathing, or yoga.
➤ Cut down on food and drinks with caffeine, such as chocolate, coffee, tea, and many colas.
➤ Be aware of your posture. Slouching or hunching can trigger teeth clenching.

FOR MORE HELP

Key Websites: *www.SavonHealth.com*. For more information on tooth grinding: *www.SavonOralConditions.com*.

Organization: American Dental Association, Department of Public Education and Information, 211 E. Chicago Ave., Chicago, IL 60611. 312-440-2593, M–F 8:30–5 CST; *www.ada.org*. Write for the pamphlet "Do You Grind Your Teeth?"

MOUTH

Nose, Throat, Lungs & Chest

Allergies

www.SavonAllergies.com

> ### SIGNS AND SYMPTOMS

Hay fever (allergic rhinitis):
- Frequent sneezing.
- Itchy or teary eyes.
- Runny or stuffy nose.
- Itching in back of throat or on roof of mouth.

Allergic asthma:
- Sneezing, wheezing, and coughing.
- In some cases, trouble breathing.

Food allergies:
- Outbreaks of itchy, red, or bumpy skin.
- Upset stomach.

Drug allergies:
- Outbreaks of itchy, red, or bumpy skin, sometimes with flulike symptoms such as headache, low fever, and joint pain.

You have an allergy when your body overreacts to things that don't bother other people. To fight what it mistakes as a threat, your immune system unleashes a compound called histamine that can provoke the sneezing, itching, and other symptoms of allergies.

Hay fever is one of the most common allergies—nearly 1 in 5 Americans has it. Pollen, bits of animal skin called dander, household dust, dust mites, and molds can set it off.

Food allergies—which are rare—occur more often in children than adults; children tend to outgrow them by the age of 3. The foods that most often cause allergies include nuts, eggs, and milk. Seafood and peanuts tend to produce the strongest reactions, even shock or death in rare cases; the treatment is a shot of epinephrine. People seldom outgrow seafood and peanut allergies. Reactions to drugs such as penicillin or to insect stings can be just as deadly (see **bee and wasp stings,** page 25, and **shock from allergy,** page 22).

Many allergies can be handled with minor changes at home. If yours are severe, though, your doctor might prescribe antihistamines, steroid nasal sprays, or shots to relieve your symptoms. Some people with allergies find a measure of relief in complementary treatments such as homeopathy, acupuncture, or herbs.

> ### WHAT YOU CAN DO NOW

➤ If you're allergic to pollen, try to stay indoors with the windows closed when pollen levels are likely to be high, especially if it's windy. To keep cool, use your air conditioner if you have one, or open a window and put a clean ordinary furnace filter across it.

➤ To relieve hay fever symptoms, try an over-the-counter antihistamine or decongestant. Antihistamines block the action of histamine, so they help relieve itchy eyes, sneezing, and runny nose; they can also cause drowsiness, though some prescription versions don't. Decongestants reduce stuffiness. They aren't always as effective as antihistamines, but they can bring relief without the sleepiness. Check with your

Breathing Problems & Coughs

The causes of most breathing problems and coughs—flu, colds, and allergies—clear up with time. If your problem doesn't go away, it could signal an illness that needs treatment.

SYMPTOMS	WHAT IT MIGHT BE	WHAT YOU CAN DO
Wheezing; tight chest or throat; itching and hives; swollen eyes, lips, and tongue; panic; stomach cramps or vomiting; bluish skin (sometimes).	Shock from allergy (see page 22).	Call 911 **right away.**
Shortness of breath; crushing chest pain, pressure, or squeezed feeling (perhaps spreading to jaw, neck, back, or arms); sweating; nausea.	Heart attack (see page 37).	Call 911 **right away.**
Shortness of breath, sharp chest pain, dry cough; symptoms of shock—cold hands and feet, rapid pulse, confusion, moist skin.	Collapsed lung.	Call 911 or go to emergency room **right away.**
Wheezing and shortness of breath; lasting wet (mucus-making) or dry cough.	Chronic bronchitis or emphysema (see page 91). ■ Croup (see page 252).	If skin turns blue or purple, call 911 or go to emergency room **right away.** If not, call doctor for prompt appointment.
Sudden shortness of breath and sharp chest pain, cough (sometimes with bloody phlegm), anxiety, loss of consciousness (sometimes).	Blood clot that travels through body to block artery in lungs.	Call 911 or go to emergency room **right away.**
Wheezing; quick, shallow breathing; coughing (sometimes with thick mucus); tightness in chest; gasping for breath.	Asthma (see page 88).	If skin turns blue or person becomes confused, call 911 or go to emergency room **right away.** If not, call doctor for prompt appointment.

(continued)

NOSE, THROAT, LUNGS & CHEST

Breathing Problems & Coughs (continued)

SYMPTOMS	WHAT IT MIGHT BE	WHAT YOU CAN DO
"Smoker's cough" (sometimes with bloody mucus), wheezing and shortness of breath, chest pain, fatigue, weight loss, lack of appetite.	Lung cancer. ■ Pneumonia (see page 97). ■ Tuberculosis—a chronic infection in the lungs.	Call doctor for prompt appointment.
Cough; fever; runny nose; sore throat; muscle aches; red, itchy bumps all over body.	Measles (see page 262).	If bumps start to bleed or seizures occur (very rare), call 911 or go to emergency room **right away.** If they don't, treat at home with rest and fluids. Call doctor for advice if symptoms last longer than a week.
In children: first symptoms like a cold; after 2 weeks, cough becomes almost constant and is followed by whooping sound, vomiting, choking.	Whooping cough (see page 269).	If child turns blue or stops breathing, call 911 and start CPR (see page 14). Call doctor for advice if symptoms linger or get worse.
Sharp, sudden chest pain that gets worse with deep breathing; fever and chills; headache; weakness; dry cough.	Pleurisy—inflamed lining of lungs.	Call doctor for prompt appointment.
Cough, hoarseness, and lost voice (sometimes); sore throat; fever (sometimes).	Laryngitis—inflamed voice box. May be caused by bacterial or viral infection, or by strained vocal cords.	Call doctor for advice. Avoid talking, drink lots of fluids, and take nonprescription throat lozenges.
Coughing and sneezing, congestion, runny nose, sore throat, headache, aching muscles, fever and fatigue (sometimes).	Flu (see page 95). ■ Cold (see page 93).	Rest, drink lots of fluids, and take over-the-counter painkillers. Don't give aspirin to a child or teenager (see box on Reye's syndrome, page 95).

doctor or pharmacist before using any of these drugs if you are already taking other over-the-counter or prescription medicines.
➤ If you're allergic to insect stings or have severe reactions to some foods, ask your doctor for an emergency kit with an antihistamine and an epinephrine shot. Always carry the kit with you.
➤ If you often have itchy or teary eyes, try over-the-counter eyedrops, or ask your doctor about eyedrops that contain antihistamines or cromolyn sodium.

WHEN TO CALL THE DOCTOR

Call 911 **right away:**
➤ If you get a rapid heartbeat and skin welts along with flushing, itching, dizziness, and trouble breathing. You could be having a potentially fatal reaction called anaphylactic shock (see **shock from allergy,** page 22).

Call 911 or go to an emergency room **right away:**
➤ If it becomes very difficult or painful to breathe. You may be having an attack of **asthma** (see page 88).
➤ If you have severe stomach cramps, vomiting, bloating, or diarrhea. This could signal a reaction to a food.

Call for advice:
➤ If you have recurring allergies. Your doctor may refer you to an allergy specialist, who can test you to find out what causes your attacks. In some cases, allergy shots may tame the body's reaction.

HOW TO PREVENT IT

➤ Try to figure out what you're allergic to so that you can avoid it. (If you're allergic to a common drug such as penicillin, be sure to wear a medical alert tag.)
➤ If you're allergic to cats or dogs, stay away from them—or at least see that your pets are bathed often, and keep them out of your bedroom.
➤ If you're allergic to molds, keep your house clean and dry. Key spots are bathrooms (chiefly shower stalls), refrigerator drip trays, basements, and closets. Use a dehumidifier in muggy weather or if your basement is damp.
➤ If you sneeze and cough year-round, you may be among the millions of people who are allergic to dust mites (tiny bugs that live in house dust). Try to keep your house—your bedroom most of all—free of dust. Encase mattresses in nonallergenic covers. Wash your bedding weekly in hot water (at least 130 degrees); if you keep your water heater set at 120 degrees or lower to protect your children from scalding, try a Laundromat. Leave your floors bare or use washable area rugs instead of

carpets. Avoid upholstered furniture and other dust-catchers. Vacuum often (use a nonporous bag), or better yet, have someone else do it.
➤ If you have a severe food allergy, read package labels. When dining out, ask what's in dishes before you order.
➤ Don't smoke, and avoid smoky places, dust, and insect sprays.

FOR MORE HELP

Key Websites: *www.SavonHealth.com.* For more information on allergies: *www.SavonAllergies.com.*

Organizations: American Academy of Allergy, Asthma and Immunology, 611 E. Wells St., Milwaukee, WI 53202. 800-822-2762, 24-hour recording, or 414-272-6071, M–F 8–5 CST, for questions and information about allergies; *www.aaaai.org.* Staff sends brochures. At Website, click on *Patient/Public Resource Center* and choose any of the topics.

■ American Academy of Otolaryngology–Head and Neck Surgery, 1 Prince St., Alexandria, VA 22314. 703-836-4444, M–F 8:30–5 EST; *www.entnet.org.* Send a business-size self-addressed stamped envelope with a request for a brochure on allergies. At Website, click on *Patient Info,* then *Sinus & Allergy Health Partnership.*

■ Asthma and Allergy Foundation of America, 1233 20th St. NW, Suite 402, Washington, DC 20036. 800-727-8462, M–F 10–3 EST or 202-466-7643m M–F 9-5 EST; *www.aafa.org.* Website lists local support groups, and books, pamphlets, and videos for sale.

■ National Jewish Medical and Research Center, 1400 Jackson St., Denver, CO 80206. 800-222-5864 (Lung Line Information Service), M–F 8–5 MST, or 800-552-5864 (Lung Facts), 24-hour recording that offers information on breathing problems; *www.nationaljewish.org.* Nurses answer questions, make referrals, and send brochures. At Website, click on *Info Center* and do a search for *allergies.*

Websites: The Allergy Learning Lab, *www.allergylearninglab.com.* Set up to be just like a trip to an allergist.

NOSE, THROAT, LUNGS & CHEST

■ National Pollen Network's Allernet, *www.allernet.com*. Provides answers to allergy questions and a directory of allergy specialists.

Books: *Allergies: The Complete Guide to Diagnosis, Treatment, and Daily Management,* by Stuart H. Young, M.D., Bruce S. Dobozin, M.D., and Margaret Miner. Covers the latest advances in allergy treatments. Plume, 1999, $13.95.

■ *Breathe Right Now: A Comprehensive Guide to Understanding and Treating the Most Common Breathing Disorders,* by Laurence A. Smolley, M.D., and Debra Fulghum Bruce. The authors discuss many breathing problems, including allergies. Dell, 1999, $6.50.

■ *The Complete Allergy Book,* by June Engel, Ph.D. Explains causes of allergies and gives tips on avoiding triggers and treating symptoms. Firefly, 1998, $14.95.

Asthma
www.SavonAsthma.com

SIGNS AND SYMPTOMS

Mild or moderate attack:
■ Coughing.
■ Feeling of tightness in the chest.
■ Noisy breathing (wheezing).
■ Trouble catching your breath.

Severe attack:
■ Rapid, shallow breathing.
■ Trouble talking because of rapid breathing.
■ Racing pulse.
■ Panic.

About one person in every 15 has asthma. If you have it, your bronchial tubes—the tiny airways in your lungs—are inflamed and supersensitive. Most of the time you can breathe normally, but not during an asthma attack. During such an episode, the airways swell and fill with mucus, and muscles around them tighten. When that happens, you may cough, wheeze, and feel short of breath (see color illustrations, page 164). Episodes can come on fast and last from a few minutes to a day or longer.

No one knows why some people have asthma and others don't; we do know, though, that most asthma episodes are triggered by things you inhale. Dust, pollen, pet dander (bits of skin), germs, molds, smoke, and chemical fumes can spark an attack. So can exercise, cold air, certain foods—seafood or peanuts, for instance—emotional peaks and dips, a common cold, and pregnancy. About a third of women with asthma find that it gets worse when they're pregnant. For a few people, aspirin and some other painkillers can start an attack.

Asthma is a chronic disease. That means you may have it for the rest of your life, with symptoms that come and go. It often starts during childhood, and it's more common and more serious among African American children than among others. Many youngsters seem to outgrow it, but it can return when they're adults.

Without prompt medical help, severe asthma can be fatal. Once you know how to manage it, though, chances are you can control it by taking medications and by staying away from things that trigger an attack.

WHAT YOU CAN DO NOW

➤ Monitor your breathing regularly with a peak flow meter if your doctor recommends it. A peak flow meter measures how well air moves in and out of your lungs. A dip in your meter's reading may warn you—hours in advance—that an episode is coming. Taking medicine may prevent or ease the attack.

➤ Recognize the signs of an oncoming episode. Many people with asthma learn to detect an episode quickly, so they can take steps to keep it from becoming severe. Typical warning signs include:
■ Tightness in the chest.
■ Scratchy throat and coughing.
■ Feeling very tired.

➤ Keep all your medicines in one place. They may include a bronchodilator—a spray drug to open your airways—in an inhaler that controls the dose. Rinse your mouth with water each time you use it to prevent thrush, a yeast infection (see **fungal infections,** page 153).

During an episode:

➤ Remain calm and quiet. Staying relaxed will help you breathe more easily.

➤ Don't lie down. You can breathe better when you sit upright and lean forward slightly, resting your elbows on a table.

➤ Use your medication exactly as your doctor has told you to. Write down each dose and the time you took it; overdoses can be dangerous.

➤ Ask a friend, coworker, teacher, or family member to stay with you.

WHEN TO CALL THE DOCTOR

Call 911 or go to an emergency room **right away** if you notice any of these signs of troubled breathing:

➤ Difficulty talking because you feel you're suffocating.

➤ Nostrils flaring with the extra effort needed to pull in air.

➤ Skin between the ribs looking sucked-in as you inhale.

➤ Lips and nails tinged blue.

Call for a prompt appointment:

➤ The first time you have long-lasting trouble breathing, with or without coughing and wheezing.

➤ If the medicine your doctor prescribes fails to work as quickly as it's supposed to.

➤ If you cough up green, yellow, or bloody mucus.

➤ If you feel strange new symptoms. These may be side effects of your drugs or may mean your asthma is getting worse.

HOW TO PREVENT IT

Anyone with asthma should be under a doctor's care. New approaches to treatment and a number of new medicines can help prevent or ease episodes, with fewer side effects than before. Also:

➤ Track your attacks by keeping a diary: How frequent? How severe? What happened just before? Notice whether certain foods, drugs, or actions seem to bring on an attack. You can't avoid everything that might bring on an attack. Still, keep an eye on:

■ Pollen and dirty air. When you know that pollution levels are high, keep windows closed and use air conditioning if you have it.

■ Dust. Vacuum often, wearing a dust mask. Or, if you can, ask someone else to do it.

■ Humidity. Dust mites and molds (common allergy triggers) love damp air, so use a dehumidifier to control them. Clean the tank often.

■ Cockroaches. These insects are one of the leading causes of asthma attacks in children. Ward off cockroaches by storing food in airtight containers and wiping up crumbs right away.

■ Dust-catchers in the bedroom, such as large shelves of books. Move them out.

■ Bedding. Use foam-rubber pillows. Avoid wool blankets and down comforters; use washable cotton blankets instead. Wash blankets every week. Wash sheets and pillowcases more often if you can. The wash water should be 130 degrees or hotter to kill mites. (If you keep your water heater set at 120 degrees or lower to protect children from scalding, try a Laundromat.) Use a dryer; pollen sticks to anything that's hung outside.

■ Pets. If being around cats or dogs causes attacks, don't keep pets with hair or fur. If you can't bear to part with Kitty or Fido, try to bathe your pet every week and keep it out of the bedroom.

➤ Don't smoke, and stay out of smoky rooms and away from people who are smoking.

➤ Exercise regularly, but don't overdo it. Swimming is good—unless chlorine in pools bothers you—since the damp air helps ease breathing. If a certain exercise triggers your asthma, try others.

➤ Lower your risk of colds and flu by washing your hands often and getting a flu shot every year.

➤ Learn relaxation methods such as yoga, meditation, or deep breathing; easing stress can reduce the number and strength of attacks (see **relax,** page 303).

FOR MORE HELP

Key Websites: *www.SavonHealth.com.* For more information on asthma: *www.SavonAsthma.com.*

NOSE, THROAT, LUNGS & CHEST

Organizations: Allergy and Asthma Network/Mothers of Asthmatics, 2751 Prosperity Ave., Suite 150, Fairfax, VA 22031. 800-727-8462, M–F 10–3 EST or 202-466-7643 M–F 9-5 EST; *www.aanma. org.* Provides phone information and brochures on asthma.

■ American Lung Association, 1740 Broadway, New York, NY 10019. 800-586- 4872, M–F 9–5 your time; *www.lungusa.org.* Refers you to a local ALA chapter and gives information. At Website, click on *Diseases A to Z,* then *A–Z Listing of Lung Diseases,* then *Asthma.*

■ Asthma and Allergy Foundation of America, 1233 20th St. NW, Suite 402, Washington, DC 20036. 800-727-8462, M–F 10–3 EST; *www.aafa.org.* Website lists local support groups, and books, pamphlets, and videos for sale.

■ National Jewish Medical and Research Center, 1400 Jackson St., Denver, CO 80206. 800-222-5864 (Lung Line Information Service), M–F 8–5 MST; 800-552-5864 (Lung Facts), 24-hour recording that offers information on breathing problems; *www.nationaljewish.org.* Nurses answer questions, make referrals, and send brochures. At Website, click on *Info Center* and do a search for *asthma.*

Websites: Asthma Information Center, *www. mdnet.de/asthma.* A forum for patients and professionals to share the latest information about treatments.

■ Journal of the American Medical Association's Asthma Information Center, *www.ama-assn.org/special/asthma.* Offers in-depth news, medical literature, and clinical guidelines.

■ Yale Pulmonary Medicine Internet Resources, *www.med.yale.edu/library/sir.* Gives a comprehensive list of Internet resources.

Books: *Essential Guide to Asthma,* by the American Medical Association. Pocket Books, 2000, $6.

■ *The American Lung Association Family Guide to Asthma and Allergies: How You and Your Children Can Breathe Easier,* by the American Lung Association Asthma Advisory Group, with Norman H. Edelman, M.D. Gives advice on managing your allergies, including how to allergy-proof your home. Little, Brown, 1998, $13.95.

Bronchitis, Acute
www.SavonBronchitis.com

SIGNS AND SYMPTOMS

■ Hacking dry or wet cough that brings up green, gray, or yellowish mucus.
■ Wheezing and shortness of breath.
■ Pain in the upper chest, made worse by fits of coughing.
■ Fever of 100 degrees or higher.

Acute bronchitis is a swelling in the branches of the windpipe (the bronchial tubes) that carry air to and from the lungs. When these air tubes become irritated and swollen, they produce extra mucus that clogs the airways and causes fits of coughing.

Most people have had an attack of acute bronchitis, which comes on fast and doesn't last long. It often begins when a virus that is causing a cold or throat infection spreads to the airways. The illness can also be brought on by agents such as tobacco smoke, chemical fumes, or dust. If your heart and lungs are healthy, bronchitis most often clears up in a few days and vanishes when the infection that brought it on does.

If bouts of coughing and other signs of bronchitis keep coming back, you may have **chronic bronchitis** (see facing page).

WHAT YOU CAN DO NOW

➤ Take acetaminophen or ibuprofen to fight fever and pain. (Never give aspirin to a child or teenager who has a cold, chicken pox, flu, or any other illness you suspect of being caused by a virus; see box on Reye's syndrome, page 95.)

➤ If you have a lasting dry cough, try an over-the-counter cough medicine. (If you have a cough that is bringing up mucus, don't take medicine labeled as a cough suppressant; doing so could cause mucus to build up in your lungs.)

➤ Stay home in a warm room and rest.

➤ Inhale steam from a vaporizer or a pot of hot water, or take hot showers (see **hints on humidifiers and vaporizers** box, page 92).

This will loosen mucus in your lungs.

➤ Drink a lot of liquids—at least 8 to 10 big glasses a day.

➤ Get a massage for sore back and chest muscles.

WHEN TO CALL THE DOCTOR

➤ If symptoms don't ease in 3 or 4 days, or if your bronchitis keeps coming back.

➤ If the person with bronchitis is an infant or a senior.

➤ If your mucus increases or becomes darker or thicker. You may have a bacterial infection that requires antibiotics.

➤ If you have lung disease or heart disease and you suffer a bronchitis attack.

➤ If you cough up blood or become more short of breath.

➤ If you have a fever of 102 degrees or higher.

HOW TO PREVENT IT

➤ Don't smoke. Avoid smoky places and other places with lots of fumes.

➤ On days with poor air quality, avoid exercise, outdoor work, or long outings.

➤ Keep germs away. Most colds are spread by touch. To help prevent a cold and the bronchitis it can cause:

  ■ Keep your hands away from your face—especially your eyes, nose, and mouth, the main places where cold viruses can get into your body.

  ■ Wash your hands often.

  ■ Clean doorknobs, counters, phones, and hard children's toys with a disinfectant such as Lysol.

  ■ Blow your nose on paper tissues, not cloth handkerchiefs (cold germs can linger on cloth until you wash it).

  ■ Try to stay away from people who are sneezing and coughing.

FOR MORE HELP

Key Websites: *www.SavonHealth.com*. For more information on bronchitis: *www.SavonBronchitis.com*.

Organizations: American Lung Association, 1740 Broadway, New York, NY 10019.

800-586-4872, M–F 9–5 your time; *www. lungusa.org*. Refers you to a local ALA chapter, which provides advice on bronchitis and other lung diseases and referrals to support groups and programs for quitting smoking.

■ National Jewish Medical and Research Center, 1400 Jackson St., Denver, CO 80206. 800-222-5864 (Lung Line Information Service), M–F 8–5 MST, or 800-552-5864 (Lung Facts), 24-hour recording that offers information on breathing problems; *www.nationaljewish.org*. Nurses answer questions, make referrals, and send brochures. At Website, click on *Info Center* and do a search for *acute bronchitis*.

Chronic Bronchitis & Emphysema
www.SavonEmphysema.com

SIGNS AND SYMPTOMS

Chronic bronchitis:

■ Usually begins with a "smoker's cough"—a morning cough that brings up mucus.

■ As the disease goes on, coughing more often and shortness of breath.

■ In the final stages, coughing and wheezing almost nonstop.

Emphysema:

In the early stages, you may have no symptoms. Later symptoms include:

■ A frequent dry cough.

■ Shortness of breath: at first, only with exertion; later, with any activity.

■ In the late stages, chest that is swollen and barrel-shaped from air trapped in lungs.

■ Weight loss.

■ Lung infections that keep coming back.

Chronic bronchitis and emphysema often come on at the same time. ("Chronic" means you may have an ailment the rest of

Hints on Humidifiers & Vaporizers

Humidifiers put cool moisture into the air. Vaporizers make steam. A lot of people with chronic dry noses and throats, sinus problems, or lung ailments use one or the other to boost the moisture in the air so that they can breathe more easily. People who live in dry climates, such as parts of the American Southwest, also find them helpful.

Ask a doctor before using either device, and take extra care when using one in a child's room. Scalding water from a vaporizer can inflict burns, and water and electricity together always pose a danger of shock.

Humid air promotes the growth of both molds and household dust mites, so it can cause problems for people with allergies or asthma. You can also get a problem called "humidifier lung"—an allergic reaction to mold and other organisms that can grow in the device—so clean your humidifier daily using bleach.

For more help: You can order a paper on cleaning humidifiers from the Lung Line Information Service, sponsored by the National Jewish Medical and Research Center, at 800-222-5864, M–F 8–5 MST.

your life, with symptoms that come and go.) Together, they're known as chronic obstructive pulmonary disease, or COPD. They damage the lungs and the bronchial tubes—the branches of the windpipe that carry air to and from the lungs—making it hard to breathe.

Chronic bronchitis: When you cough up mucus for 3 months or more, 2 years in a row, you have chronic bronchitis. It is usually linked to smoking, although dirty air, fumes, dust, and allergies also can play a role. If you don't treat it and you still smoke or breathe fumes, you leave yourself open to other diseases, such as **pneumonia** (see page 97) or emphysema.

Chronic bronchitis affects 14 million Americans. Early treatment—and quitting smoking—can ease symptoms and slow the disease. A small number of cases are fatal.

Emphysema: When the lungs are damaged by tobacco smoke (and often by the coughing of chronic bronchitis), the millions of tiny air sacs inside them can't pass along enough oxygen to the bloodstream. You use more and more energy gasping for breath; you tire quickly and lose weight. Even a short walk may leave you breathless. Because emphysema makes the heart work harder, it can lead to heart disease. It also leaves you open to lung diseases such as pneumonia.

The disease, which can't be cured, most often strikes people over 50, although a small group of those with a defect in their genes may get symptoms in their 20s and 30s. A blood test can tell who has this problem; these people should never smoke.

Emphysema affects nearly 2 million Americans. There are 2 important things to know about it: 1) If you don't smoke, you have very little chance of getting it. 2) If you do smoke, you should quit even if you think you're in good health. Emphysema can sneak up on you because it often has no symptoms in the early stages. By the time most people find out they have it, they have lost 50 to 70 percent of their lung capacity.

A therapist may design a program to help you exercise more. Your doctor may prescribe a bronchodilator—a drug to open your airways—and, in later stages, pure oxygen, which helps some people breathe better.

WHAT YOU CAN DO NOW

➤ Don't smoke, and avoid smoky places. Smoking is the main cause of emphysema and chronic bronchitis. Studies show that giving up tobacco—even after symptoms appear—can slow lung damage.

➤ Get a flu shot every year and a vaccination against pneumonia.

➤ Stay inside if the air is very polluted.

➤ Take good care of yourself to keep up your strength and help your body fight infection.
  ■ Exercise gently but daily in good-quality air.
  ■ Eat right, making sure you get plenty of fruits, grains, and vegetables. They're

loaded with nutrients that may help protect the lungs (see **eat well**, page 296).

(see **eat well**, page 296)

WHEN TO CALL THE DOCTOR

➤ If you have a mild cough that doesn't go away for months.
➤ If you often become breathless after mild exertion, such as climbing a flight of stairs.

HOW TO PREVENT IT

➤ Don't smoke.
➤ Treat bronchitis promptly to guard against emphysema.

FOR MORE HELP

Key Websites: *www.SavonHealth.com*. For more information on emphysema: *www.SavonEmphysema.com*.

Organizations: Agency for Healthcare Research and Quality, 2101 E. Jefferson St., Suite 501, Rockville, MD 20852. 301-594-6380, M–F 9–5 EST; *www.ahcpr.gov.* Call for brochure "You Can Quit Smoking." At Website, click on *Consumer Health,* then *Do You Smoke? Do You Want to Quit?*

■ American Lung Association, 1740 Broadway, New York, NY 10019. 800-586-4872, M–F 9–5 your time; *www.lungusa.org.* Refers you to a local ALA chapter, which provides advice on bronchitis and other lung diseases and referrals to support groups. At Website, click on *Diseases A to Z,* then *Chronic Bronchitis.*

■ National Jewish Medical and Research Center, 1400 Jackson St., Denver, CO 80206. 800-222-5864 (Lung Line Information Service), M–F 8–5 MST, or 800-552-5864 (Lung Facts), 24-hour recording that offers information on breathing problems; *www.nationaljewish.org.* Nurses answer questions, make referrals, and send brochures. At Website, click on *Info Center* and do a search for *chronic bronchitis.*

Book: *Living a Healthy Life With Chronic Conditions: Self-Management of Heart Disease, Arthritis, Diabetes, Asthma, Bronchitis, Emphysema, and Others,* 2nd edition, by Kate Lorig, R.N., Dr.P.H., and Halsted Holman, M.D. Bull Publishing, 2000, $18.95.

Colds
www.SavonColds.com

SIGNS AND SYMPTOMS

■ Runny nose.
■ Sore throat and hoarseness.
■ Watery eyes.
■ Coughing.
■ Low fever, below 100 degrees.

If you have a scratchy throat, runny nose, and cough, you've most likely caught a viral infection of the head and throat known as the common cold. Colds are caused by more than 200 viruses that get into the body chiefly through the nose and tear ducts.

You can't catch a cold from getting your feet wet or sitting in a drafty room—you get it from a virus. But a few simple safety measures can help protect you from this contagious ailment.

WHAT YOU CAN DO NOW

Nobody has found a cure yet for the common cold, but there are things you can do to feel less sick. They start with staying home from work or school for the first 3 or 4 days—not only to rest and recover, but to prevent your cold from spreading to other people as well. Also:

➤ Drink lots of fluids to avoid dehydration.
➤ Take a painkiller for aches and fever. (Never give aspirin to a child or teenager who has a cold, chicken pox, flu, or any other illness you suspect of being caused by a virus; see box on **Reye's syndrome,** page 95.)
➤ If you have a sore throat, try gargling with salt water a few times a day. (Mix 1 teaspoon salt in 8 ounces warm water. Don't swallow.) Sucking on plain hard candy may also help.
➤ To clear up a stuffy nose, try over-the-counter saline drops or sprays. You can also make your own (mix one-half teaspoon salt in 8 ounces lukewarm water). Use a dropper or a bulb syringe to squirt it into your nose 2 to 4 times a day. Or you can put the solution in the palm of your

see box on **Reye's syndrome,** page 95.

NOSE, THROAT, LUNGS & CHEST

hand and sniff it in, a nostril at a time. Wait a few minutes and then blow your nose gently.

➤ Don't smoke, and avoid smoky places.

➤ Try taking a 500-milligram tablet of vitamin C 4 times a day; some researchers say it may shorten your cold and make it milder. But taking too much vitamin C can cause diarrhea.

➤ Use a cool-mist humidifier or a vaporizer or take hot, steamy showers to keep your nasal passages from drying out (see **hints on humidifiers and vaporizers** box, page 92).

WHEN TO CALL THE DOCTOR

Call for a prompt appointment:

➤ If you have a fever of 100 degrees or higher and facial swelling or severe pain in the ears. You may have an **ear infection** (see page 71).

➤ If you have severe throat pain and your throat or tonsils have a white or yellow coating. You may have **tonsillitis** (see page 102) or **strep throat** (see pages 100 and 267).

➤ If you have a severe cough with thick, colored mucus; a cough that lasts more than 10 days; or bluish lips or nails. You may have **pneumonia** (see page 97).

Call for advice:

➤ If you have a headache with pain around the face, a sore upper jaw, or yellow or green mucus coming from your nose or throat; these are signs of a sinus infection (see **sinusitis,** page 98).

➤ If a fever lasts longer than 4 days or goes higher than 102 degrees.

➤ If your cold hasn't improved after 10 days or has gotten worse.

HOW TO PREVENT IT

➤ Most colds are spread by touch. To help prevent a cold:
  ■ Keep your hands away from your eyes, nose, and mouth.
  ■ Wash your hands often.
  ■ Clean doorknobs, counters, phones, and hard children's toys with a disinfectant such as Lysol.

What to Look for in Cold & Cough Medicines

Cold medicines are a $3.1 billion-a-year industry. Many combine far more ingredients than you need, and some may even make you feel worse.

Doctors suggest that you buy generic drugs with only 1 ingredient—such as aspirin, a cough suppressant, or an oral decongestant—rather than brand-name "mega" formulas, which try to tackle many symptoms at once. Here are some drugs that don't really do much to relieve cold symptoms:

➤ **Antihistamines.** Although they help clear up runny noses and sneezing, they can also dry out the nasal passages too much. Also, in older men, they may cause urination problems.

➤ **Expectorants.** There is no proof that these loosen mucus.

➤ **Nasal decongestant sprays.** Although they help shrink swollen nasal passages, they often have a "rebound effect," meaning that the tissues in the nose may swell back up, sometimes even worse than before, after a few days of use.

Cough suppressants (antitussives) also have pros and cons. Some coughs are "productive"—that is, they help bring up mucus from the lungs—so it's better not to suppress them. Dry, hacking coughs, though, are best treated with an antitussive syrup or lozenge. The medicine may make you sleepy, so don't drive if you take it.

Also, don't take decongestants with certain antidepressants (see **drug combinations to avoid,** page 323).

■ Blow your nose on paper tissues, not cloth handkerchiefs (cold germs can linger on cloth until you wash it).

■ Try to stay away from people who are sneezing and coughing.

➤ Since stress, allergies, and menstrual periods may make you more vulnerable to illness, try to get extra sleep—it helps your immune system—and take especially good care of yourself when you're feeling under the weather (see *Staying Healthy*, page 291).

COMPLEMENTARY CHOICES

➤ Echinacea appears to help boost the immune system to fend off colds. Take the herb at the first signs of symptoms. Use echinacea only now and then; its effect on the body seems to fade after about 8 weeks of steady use. It comes as capsules and as a tincture.

➤ Chicken soup really does seem to help. It contains an amino acid that helps clear the lungs. Make your soup as hot, spicy, and garlicky as you can stand.

➤ Try to look on the bright side. Studies show that a positive attitude helps your immune system fight disease.

Reye's Syndrome

This rare disease causes vomiting and sometimes leads to delirium, coma, or even death. Reye's syndrome reached its peak in the late 1970s and early 1980s, with hundreds of cases reported each year, but there are now fewer than 20 cases a year. No age group is immune, although the disease almost always strikes young people, from infants to teens. While its exact causes are unknown, it is connected with aspirin taken during viral infections such as chicken pox and flu.

For this reason, doctors warn that you should never give aspirin to a child or teenager who has chicken pox or any other illness you suspect of being caused by a virus, such as a cold or the flu. Instead, use acetaminophen.

If your child or teenager has a viral infection, begins to vomit, and becomes drowsy, delirious, confused, disoriented, or eager to fight, he or she may have Reye's syndrome. Call your doctor promptly.

FOR MORE HELP

Key Websites: *www.SavonHealth.com*. For more information on colds: *www.SavonColds.com*.

Organization: American Lung Association, 1740 Broadway, New York, NY 10019. 800-586-4872, M–F 9–5 your time; *www.lungusa.org*. Refers you to a local ALA chapter and gives information. At Website, click on *Diseases A to Z*, then *Guidelines for the Prevention and Treatment of Influenza and the Common Cold*.

Books: *Finally . . . The Common Cold Cure*, by Ray Sahelian, M.D., and Victoria Dolby Toews, M.P.H. Gives all-natural remedies for the common cold. Avery, 1999, $9.95.
■ *77 Ways to Beat Colds and Flu: A People's Medical Society Book*, by Charles B. Inlander and Cynthia K. Moran. Bantam, 1996, $4.99.

Flu
www.SavonFlu.com

SIGNS AND SYMPTOMS

■ Fever over 103 degrees.
■ Chills and muscle aches.
■ Fatigue and weakness.
■ Headache and eye pain.
■ Sore throat.
■ Dry cough.

Flu (influenza) is a contagious disease caused by a virus that enters the body through the nose or mouth and often invades the lungs. Flu shows up mainly in winter and early spring, making the rounds of homes, schools, and offices. The virus changes from year to year; some varieties lead to more severe outbreaks than others. Children are more likely than adults to get the flu, but it's most often mild. Older adults and people with lung disease or other chronic illness have a high risk as well; for them the disease is often more severe.

Flus and colds are much alike, but flus are more severe, with higher fevers and aches and pains. A bad case of the flu may send an otherwise healthy person to bed for 3 to 5 days, but he or she will most likely be well within 1 or 2 weeks.

WHAT YOU CAN DO NOW

The more rest you get, the sooner you'll get well. And staying home keeps you from spreading the virus at school or work: Flu is contagious for 3 or 4 days after symptoms appear. To get well quickly:

➤ Drink as many fluids—water, juice, hot tea—as you can. Try some frozen juice bars for variety.

➤ Have chicken soup and bouillon; the heat may relieve the stuffed-up feeling.

➤ Take a painkiller for aches and fever. (Never give aspirin to a child or teenager who has a cold, flu, chicken pox, or any other illness you suspect of being caused by a virus; see box on **Reye's syndrome,** page 95.)

➤ Avoid over-the-counter medicines aimed at treating more than 1 symptom (see box on **cold medicines,** page 94).

➤ Ask your doctor about virus-fighting drugs that can reduce the length and strength of flu. By taking one of them, you may also help family members avoid catching your flu.

WHEN TO CALL THE DOCTOR

Flu is a special danger for people with chronic illness such as respiratory, heart, or kidney disease; cancer; cystic fibrosis; recurring anemia; or diabetes. If you have one of these—or if you are HIV positive—call your doctor at the first sign of flu symptoms.

Call for a prompt appointment:

➤ If you have a fever or chest pain that keeps coming back, or if you cough up mucus that is thick, colored, or bloody; you may have **pneumonia** (see facing page) or **bronchitis** (see page 90).

➤ If you have an earache, facial swelling, drainage from your ear, or severe pain in your face or forehead. These may be symptoms of some other illness, such as **sinusitis** (see page 98) or an **ear infection** (see page 71).

Call for advice:

➤ If you have a fever higher than 102 degrees,

or one higher than 100 degrees for more than 3 to 4 days.

HOW TO PREVENT IT

The flu virus changes every year, so you can't become immune. Also, a flu vaccine might not work if it's designed for a virus different from the one that comes to your area. But if you are over 65 or have a chronic illness, a flu shot every fall is a good idea. Also, consider getting a flu shot if you work in a health care institution, or if you simply can't spare time off to recover from the flu.

➤ If you are pregnant, ask your doctor if you should get a flu shot.

➤ If you are allergic to eggs, or think you are, check with your doctor before getting a flu shot.

➤ Ask your doctor about the new oral vaccines that may help keep you from getting the flu.

The flu virus is spread in the spray from coughs and sneezes, so avoiding people who have the flu may lessen your chances of getting it. Also:

➤ Wash your hands often to reduce your risk of catching a cold or the flu.

➤ Don't smoke, and avoid smoky places.

➤ Keep your immune system healthy by eating well, getting enough sleep, keeping stress levels low, and drinking plenty of water.

FOR MORE HELP

Key Websites: *www.SavonHealth.com.* For more information on flu: *www.SavonFlu.com.*

Organizations: American Lung Association, 1740 Broadway, New York, NY 10019. 800-586-4872, M–F 9–5 your time; *www. lungusa.org.* At Website, click on *Diseases A to Z,* then go to *Guidelines for the Prevention and Treatment of Influenza and the Common Cold.*

■ Centers for Disease Control and Prevention, 1600 Clifton Rd., Atlanta, GA 30333. 888-232-3228 (Voice Information System), 24-hour automated line; *www. cdc.gov.* Choose from several topics about the flu and flu shots. At Website, click on *Health Topics A–Z* and then *Flu.*

Book: *The Natural Way to Beat the Common Cold and Flu: A Holistic Approach for Prevention and Relief,* by Richard Trubo. Berkley Publishing Group, 1998, $6.50.

Pneumonia
www.SavonPneumonia.com

SIGNS AND SYMPTOMS

Common:
- Shaking, chills, and fever as high as 105 degrees.
- Chest pain.
- Mucus that is greenish, greenish-yellow, rust-colored, or streaked with blood.
- Shortness of breath.

Sometimes:
- Sweating, rapid pulse, and rapid breathing.
- Bluish lips and nails.
- Delirium.
- Diarrhea, headache, or pain in the muscles.
- Nausea, vomiting, or pain in the abdomen.

Pneumonia is a severe infection: Parts of the lungs fill with pus or other liquid that clogs air sacs and prevents oxygen from reaching the bloodstream. Symptoms can range from those of "walking pneumonia"—fatigue and congestion that can linger without sending you to bed—to more severe cases that require prompt hospitalization. Call your doctor right away if you think you have any form of the illness.

The most common causes include:
- **Bacteria.** If untreated, bacterial pneumonia can sometimes be fatal, most of all for people with emphysema and other chronic illnesses. It can spread from the lungs to the rest of the body. Bacterial pneumonia is treated with antibiotics.
- **Viruses.** Antibiotics aren't given to anyone who has viral pneumonia, but most people get better with bed rest and care.
- **Fungi.** Certain fungi that cause a mild form of pneumonia in healthy people can cause

severe disease in people with AIDS or other immune system problems. One of the most common causes of pneumonia in people with AIDS is *Pneumocystis carinii*, which is a fungus. It is usually treated with antibiotics, sometimes with steroids such as cortisone.

The people most likely to get severe pneumonia are those under age 2 and over 75, and people with chronic health problems such as heart trouble, cancer, emphysema, HIV, or asthma. The risk is high for people who are bedridden or who have just had surgery, because lying flat on the back makes it harder to cough up mucus.

WHAT YOU CAN DO NOW

- Drink lots of fluids.
- Don't take cough suppressants if you have a wet cough: Coughing up mucus will help you recover.
- Try using a cool-mist humidifier in your bedroom. Clean it daily with bleach, and fill it only with distilled water (see **hints on humidifiers and vaporizers** box, page 92).
- Put hot compresses on your chest. Wet a small towel in hot water, wring it out, and put it in a plastic bag. Wrap it in a cloth before you put it on your skin.
- Don't smoke, and avoid smoky places.
- To prevent a relapse, which can be worse than the first bout, be sure to take all the medicine your doctor prescribes.
- Get plenty of rest and don't rush recovery.

WHEN TO CALL THE DOCTOR

Pneumonia often comes on the heels of some other chest illness, such as a cold or the flu. Call for a prompt appointment if you have been sick and these symptoms appear:
- Change in color of mucus, or mucus streaked with blood.
- Lasting fever higher than 100 degrees, with chills or sweats.
- Shortness of breath, pain when breathing, or both.

If the recently ill person is at high risk (very young, over 65, or someone with a chronic illness), be on guard for the first signs of pneumonia and call a doctor.

NOSE, THROAT, LUNGS & CHEST

HOW TO PREVENT IT

If you are 65 or older you should get the vaccine for bacterial pneumonia as well as a yearly flu shot. If you're younger than 65 and in a high-risk group, talk to your doctor about getting the vaccine. Also:

➤ Don't smoke, and avoid smoke-filled rooms and heavy drinking: These all weaken your ability to fight off disease.

➤ Avoid close contact with people who have a cold, the flu, or any other chest disease.

➤ Eat healthy foods: fruits, vegetables, and grains. Plant-based foods are high in vitamins and fiber (see **eat well,** page 296).

➤ Exercise daily. You'll increase your energy and strength, and build your body's resistance to colds and flu.

➤ If you're bedridden, sit up for 1 or 2 hours after eating so that you don't inhale bits of food; they can lead to pneumonia. If you have just had surgery, ask about breathing exercises to help prevent pneumonia.

FOR MORE HELP

Key Websites: *www.SavonHealth.com*. For more information on pneumonia: *www.SavonPneumonia.com*.

Organizations: American Lung Association, 1740 Broadway, New York, NY 10019. 800-586- 4872, M–F 9–5 your time; *www.lungusa. org*. Refers you to a local ALA chapter. At Website, click on *Diseases A to Z*, then *Pneumonia*.

■ National Jewish Medical and Research Center, 1400 Jackson St., Denver, CO 80206. 800-222-5864 (Lung Line Information Service), M–F 8–5 MST, or 800-552-5864; *www.nationaljewish.org*. Nurses answer questions and send brochures. At Website, click on *Info Center* and do a search for *pneumonia*.

Website: Mayo Clinic Health Oasis; *www. mayohealth.org*. Click on *Search* and type in *pneumonia* for articles and information.

Book: *Pneumonia,* by Simon Godfrey, M.D., Ph.D., and Robert Wilson, M.D. Information about pneumonia and the treatments for it. Blackwell Science, 1996, $14.95.

Sinusitis
www.SavonSinusitis.com

SIGNS AND SYMPTOMS

■ Stuffy nose and trouble breathing, and a cold for longer than a week.

■ Green or yellow nasal discharge, sometimes tinged with blood. It may drip into the back of your throat, making you cough.

■ Pain or pressure in or around the eyes and forehead. The pain may travel to the back of your head and be worse in the morning or when you're leaning forward.

■ Foul smell in your nose, bad breath.

Sometimes:

■ Fever.

■ Pain in the upper jaw or teeth.

Chronic sinusitis:

■ Nasal discharge and sinus congestion that come back or that last for months.

Sinusitis is an inflammation of the sinuses, the air-filled pockets in the bones around the nose and eyes.

When allergies, infections, or smoke, dust, and dirt in the air irritate the inside of your nose, the membranes there swell and clog the tiny openings to your sinuses. Bacteria start to grow in the mucus trapped in the sinuses, causing pressure and pain—sometimes severe—in the forehead and cheeks, or behind and around the eyes.

People who smoke, have allergies, or are often exposed to germs—such as schoolteachers and health care workers—are among the most likely to get sinus infections.

Symptoms of **acute sinusitis** caused by bacteria most often last only a few days if treated with antibiotics. Sinusitis caused by a virus most often goes away by itself. The symptoms of **chronic sinusitis** can be milder than those of the acute form: Chronic sinusitis seldom produces severe headaches. But it can cause congestion and nasal discharge for months or years. Chronic sinusitis occurs when a sinus opening is blocked for a long time, sometimes as a result of small

Your Sinuses

The paranasal sinuses—air spaces in bones around the nose—have 2 main features: They are sound chambers for the voice and they make the skull lighter. Their walls are lined with mucous membranes, which can swell and trap infections.

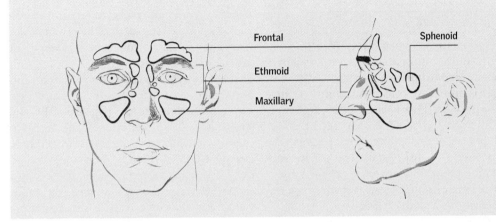

growths in the nose called nasal polyps, or of a deviated septum (in which the wall between the nostrils is crooked, reducing the flow of air).

WHAT YOU CAN DO NOW

➤ Make the air in your home more moist (see **hints on humidifiers and vaporizers** box, page 92).
➤ Inhale steam for relief, take a hot shower, or place a warm, damp cloth over your nose.
➤ Drink plenty of liquids—at least 8 to 10 glasses a day.
➤ Try decongestant pills or nasal sprays. They may help you breathe, but they should not be used for more than 2 days unless a doctor advises you to, because their "rebound effect" can make symptoms worse.
➤ Flush your nose with salt water to wash away mucus and bacteria. You can buy saline solution or make your own: Mix one-half teaspoon salt in 8 ounces lukewarm water. Use a dropper or a bulb syringe to squirt it into your nose 2 to 4 times a day. You can also put the solution in the palm of your hand and sniff it in, a nostril at a time. Wait a moment, then gently blow your nose.

➤ Soothe a throat sore from postnasal drip with a saltwater gargle: Mix 1 teaspoon salt in 8 ounces warm water. Don't swallow.
➤ Take a painkiller to relieve headache. (Never give aspirin to a child or teenager who has a cold, chicken pox, flu, or any other illness you suspect of being caused by a virus; see box on **Reye's syndrome,** page 95.)

WHEN TO CALL THE DOCTOR

Call for a prompt appointment:
➤ If your face swells or your vision blurs; you may have a dangerous infection.
Call for advice:
➤ If symptoms last more than 7 days without getting better. If a bacterial sinus infection goes untreated, it can last for years, causing chronic pain. The postnasal drip of infected mucus can lead to bronchitis, chronic cough, or asthma.

HOW TO PREVENT IT

Since sinus problems often follow ailments such as allergies, colds, or the flu, you should treat those problems to prevent sinusitis.
➤ If you have **allergies** (see page 84), learn their triggers so you can avoid attacks.
➤ Do what you can to prevent **colds** (see page 93) and **flu** (see page 95).

➤ Sleep with your head higher than your body to help your sinuses drain.

➤ Don't smoke, and stay away from smoky places and dirty air, fumes, and dust.

➤ Don't blow your nose hard.

FOR MORE HELP

Key Websites: *www.SavonHealth.com*. For more information on sinusitis: *www.SavonSinusitis.com*.

Organizations: American Academy of Otolaryngology–Head and Neck Surgery, 1 Prince St., Alexandria, VA 22314. 703-836-4444, M–F 8:30–5 EST; *www.entnet.org*. Send a business-size self-addressed stamped envelope with your request for a brochure on sinusitis. At Website, click on *Patient Info* and then *Sinusitis*.

■ National Jewish Medical and Research Center, 1400 Jackson St., Denver, CO 80206. 800-222-5864 (Lung Line Information Service), M–F 8–5 MST, or 800-552-5864 (Lung Facts), 24-hour recording that offers information on breathing problems; *www.nationaljewish.org*. Nurses answer questions, make referrals, and send brochures. At Website, click on *Info Center* and do a search for *sinusitis*.

Sore Throat
www.SavonColds.com

SIGNS AND SYMPTOMS

■ Pain when talking or swallowing.
■ Throat that looks red all over or in streaks when you say "aahhh."
■ Swollen, tender glands in the neck.

Sometimes:
■ Fever.
■ Headache.
■ Earache.
■ Hoarseness or "lost voice."

Strep throat:
■ Sore throat that comes on quickly, with fever, swollen neck glands, headache, or bright red tonsils, sometimes with white pus spots.

Mononucleosis:
■ Same symptoms as strep throat, plus fatigue and loss of appetite.

Most sore throats result from a virus—from flu, a cold, or a sinus infection. Dirty air, allergies, tobacco smoke, and the dry air of winter heating can also bring them on. Even shouting can cause soreness.

A few sore throats come from bacteria—usually streptococcus (strep). **Strep throat** is most common in children (see page 267). Because strep can invade other parts of the body and cause serious trouble such as **rheumatic fever** (see page 265) or a kidney infection—and because it's impossible to find without a test—you should see your doctor promptly if you suspect you have it. A doctor can take a throat culture or give you a rapid strep test. If you have strep, antibiotics should knock it out.

Children often get painful sore throats with **measles** (see page 262) and **chicken pox** (see page 249). A sore throat can also signal problems such as epiglottitis (a serious infection of the larynx) or mononucleosis.

WHAT YOU CAN DO NOW

➤ Drink lots of liquids. Warm ones such as soup or herbal tea are soothing.

➤ Gargle with warm salt water every few hours. (Mix 1 teaspoon salt in 8 ounces warm water. Don't swallow.)

➤ Don't smoke, and avoid smoky places.

➤ Take a nonaspirin painkiller to ease pain and inflammation. (Never give aspirin to a child or teenager who has a cold, chicken pox, flu, or any other illness you suspect of being caused by a virus; see box on **Reye's syndrome,** page 95.)

➤ Suck on throat lozenges or cough drops to keep your throat moist.

➤ Use a vaporizer or humidifier to moisten bedroom air (see **hints on humidifiers and vaporizers** box, page 92).

➤ For laryngitis, rest your voice by not talking or whispering. Don't clear your throat.

WHEN TO CALL THE DOCTOR

Call 911 or go to an emergency room **right**

away:
➤ If you can't swallow liquids or you have trouble breathing.

Call for a prompt appointment:
➤ If you have a fever that's higher than 101 degrees.
➤ If the glands in your neck are swollen.
➤ If your tonsils are bright red or have spots of white pus on them.
➤ If your sore throat lasts longer than the 5-to-7-day span of a cold.

HOW TO PREVENT IT

➤ Don't smoke. Stay away from smoky places and dirty air, fumes, and dust.
➤ Stay away from people who have strep throat or a sore throat.
➤ Do what you can to prevent **colds** (see page 93) and **flu** (see page 95).

FOR MORE HELP

Key Websites: *www.SavonHealth.com*. For more information on sore throats: *www.SavonColds.com*.

Organizations: American Academy of Family Physicians, P.O. Box 11210, Shawnee Mission, KS 66207-1210. 800-274-2237, M–F 8:30–5 CST; *www.aafp.org*. Call for health information. At Website, click on *Patient Information* and then do a search for *sore throat*. ■ American Academy of Otolaryngology–Head and Neck Surgery, 1 Prince St., Alexandria, VA 22314. 703-836-4444, M–F 8:30–5 EST; *www.entnet.org*. Send a business-size self-addressed stamped envelope with your request for a brochure on sore throats. At Website, click on *Patient Info* and then *Sore Throats*.

Swallowing Difficulty
www.SavonOralConditions.com

SIGNS AND SYMPTOMS

■ Pain while swallowing.
■ Trouble getting food to go down.
■ Feeling of a lump in the throat.

Pain and trouble swallowing can signal a disease of the throat or the esophagus, the tube that connects the throat to the stomach (see color illustrations, pages 163 and 174).

Or the problem could be something (such as a fish bone) stuck in the throat. This could become an emergency if it stops a person from breathing (see **choking,** page 18).

If you have problems swallowing, along with a sore throat and maybe a fever and hoarseness, you might have **tonsillitis** (see page 102); an infected larynx, or "voice box" (laryngitis); or an inflamed pharynx, or throat (pharyngitis).

Often, acid pushed up from the stomach can burn the esophagus and produce a feeling like **heartburn** (see page 124). This is called esophagitis; it can also cause chest pain and, rarely, vomiting. Symptoms like these also occur when part of the stomach squeezes up into the chest cavity—a hiatal **hernia** (see page 127)—or when the esophagus is narrowed by a buildup of scar tissue caused by stomach acid.

Other causes of swallowing trouble are cancers of the mouth and esophagus; myasthenia gravis; Lou Gehrig's disease (ALS); **Parkinson's disease** (see page 57); and multiple sclerosis.

WHAT YOU CAN DO NOW

➤ Don't smoke, and avoid smoky places.
➤ For burning pain in the throat that feels like heartburn, take antacids.
➤ For the feeling of a lump in the throat, drink lots of water with meals and practice relaxation techniques to help reduce stress (see **relax,** page 303).

WHEN TO CALL THE DOCTOR

Call 911 or go to an emergency room **right away:**
➤ If something is caught in your throat.

Call for a prompt appointment:
➤ If you have swallowing troubles that last for more than a few days, or if you also are losing weight and vomiting.

Call for advice:
➤ If you suspect you have tonsillitis, laryn-

gitis, or pharyngitis.

➤ If you can swallow food or drink yet still feel as if you have a lump in your throat, even after trying relaxation techniques.

HOW TO PREVENT IT

➤ Don't smoke. Smoking can cause oral cancer and problems of the esophagus.

➤ Take antacids to reduce stomach acid, or acid blockers to cut down on the amount of acid your stomach makes. (See **heartburn,** page 124).

➤ Avoid spicy foods and alcohol, which can worsen heartburn.

➤ If you are overweight, losing weight may help with swallowing and ease heartburn.

FOR MORE HELP

Key Websites: *www.SavonHealth.com*. For more information on swallowing problems: *www.SavonOralConditions.com*.

Organization: National Digestive Diseases Information Clearinghouse, 2 Information Way, Bethesda, MD 20892-3570. 301-654-3810, M–F 8:30–5 EST; *www. niddk.nih.gov/health/digest/nddic.htm*. Ask for the fact sheet on gastroesophageal reflux disease, which includes information about heartburn and hiatal hernias. At Website, click on *Digestive Diseases* and choose from the listed topics.

Book: *Gastrointestinal Health*, by Steven R. Peikin, M.D. A self-help guide for relief from gastrointestinal problems. Harper-Collins, 1999, $15.

Tonsillitis
www.SavonTonsillitis.com

SIGNS AND SYMPTOMS

■ Sore or raw throat.

■ Hoarse or "throaty" voice that gets worse.

More severe cases:

■ Tonsils that are red or have white or yellow spots.

■ Tonsils so swollen that they fill the back of the throat.

■ Tender or swollen lymph glands in the neck.

■ Fever of 100 degrees or higher, headache, or vomiting.

■ Ear or stomach pain.

In children:

■ Not eating because it hurts to swallow.

In adults:

■ Foul-smelling white debris and a burning in the back of the throat.

Thirty years ago, "having your tonsils out" was almost a rite of passage for youngsters. Doctors would remove children's tonsils—pink masses of lymph tissue on both sides of the back of the throat—to prevent tonsillitis, a viral or bacterial infection. Now doctors know that children often outgrow these infections. (Adults can get tonsillitis, too, although it's more common in children.)

Besides, as it turns out, tonsils may actually help the nose and throat fight off infections such as colds, especially in young children. Most doctors now feel that tonsils don't need to be taken out unless they become infected repeatedly and severely enough to make a child miss weeks of school.

WHAT YOU CAN DO NOW

If your child's tonsils are simply red (with no swelling or white or yellow coating) and he or she does not have a fever and doesn't have any trouble swallowing, you can often get good results with home treatment (see **sore throat,** page 100).

➤ Keep your child warm and rested, with a cool-mist humidifier in the bedroom (see **hints on humidifiers and vaporizers** box, page 92).

➤ Give lots of liquids, along with ice cream or frozen yogurt, to soothe the throat.

➤ Use a saltwater gargle to help dull the pain and cleanse the tonsils. (Mix 1 teaspoon salt in 8 ounces warm water. Gargle every few hours. Don't swallow.)

About Adenoids

Tonsillitis should not be confused with enlarged adenoids, which often come along with a tonsil infection. The adenoids are grapelike clusters of tissue in the upper part of the throat where you can't see them, behind the nose. They begin to grow when a child is about 3; when a child is about 5, they begin to shrink, and by the teens they are gone.

A child who snores or breathes through the mouth rather than the nose, and who develops a twangy, nasal voice, may have enlarged adenoids. These can cause sleep apnea, in which the child may stop breathing for several seconds at a time while asleep (see **sleep disorders,** page 286). Call a doctor if any symptoms of enlarged adenoids last for more than a week.

➤ Give acetaminophen for fever and pain. (Never give aspirin to a child or teenager who has a cold, chicken pox, flu, or any other illness you suspect of being caused by a virus; see box on **Reye's syndrome,** page 95.)
➤ Sponge the face with cool water to comfort your child and reduce fever.

WHEN TO CALL THE DOCTOR

In children:
➤ If the tonsils have a white or yellow coating or spots on them. (Use a flashlight to help you look.)
➤ If the tonsils are so swollen that they touch; this may mean a bad infection such as **strep throat** (see page 267).
➤ If a sore throat is severe and lasts more than 2 days.
➤ If your child has a fever above 100 degrees or goes 24 hours without eating.
➤ If your child has greenish, yellowish, or rust-colored mucus or has nausea, skin rashes, chest pain, seizures, inflamed or painful joints, or a fever that returns after being absent for a day or two. These may signal a systemwide staph or other infection.

In adults:
➤ If you have trouble opening your mouth or swallowing, and severe jaw or throat pain.

HOW TO PREVENT IT

Tell children to avoid infections by:
➤ Keeping away from people who are coughing and sneezing.
➤ Not sharing cups or silverware.
➤ Washing their hands often.
➤ Keeping their hands away from their mouths.

FOR MORE HELP

Key Websites: *www.SavonHealth.com.* For more information on tonsillitis: *www.SavonTonsillitis.com.*

Organization: American Academy of Otolaryngology–Head and Neck Surgery, 1 Prince St., Alexandria, VA 22314. 703-836-4444, M–F 8:30–5 EST; *www.entnet. org.* Send a business-size self-addressed stamped envelope with your request for a brochure on tonsillectomy. At Website, click on *Patient Info* and then *Tonsillectomy and Adenoidectomy.*

Website: University of Washington at Seattle Department of Otolaryngology's Tonsillitis and Tonsillectomy page, *www.depts. washington.edu/otoweb/tonsil.html.* Covers tonsillitis and its treatment.

NOSE, THROAT, LUNGS & CHEST

Heart & Circulation

Artery Disease

www.SavonCardiovascular.com

SIGNS AND SYMPTOMS

Artery disease (atherosclerosis) can damage your health before you have any symptoms. That's why it's vital to prevent artery disease, or to find and treat the problem early. Watch for symptoms of the following:

Heart disease:

■ Dull chest pain (angina) or simply a feeling of tightness or heavy pressure. It's most often in the center of the chest but can spread into the arms and jaw. With rest, angina goes away in 30 seconds to 5 minutes.

Heart attack:

Call 911 **right away:**

■ If the pain lasts, gets worse, comes more often, or comes during rest; this could mean you're having a heart attack. Women are less likely than men to have severe chest pain.

Stroke:

Call 911 **right away:**

■ If you lose balance, speech, or vision; or have trouble moving; or have a sudden tingling, numbness, or loss of movement in a limb.

Peripheral vascular disease:

■ Muscle fatigue, weakness, or pain in the buttocks or legs, usually in the calves, when you walk.

■ Cold feet.

■ Discolored skin, sores that won't heal, and sudden sharp pains in the legs or feet when you rest.

The walls of a healthy artery are smooth and elastic, so blood flows freely. But sometimes a substance known as plaque builds up inside an artery; the process is called atherosclerosis. The walls of the vessel thicken and grow rough and stiff, narrowing the artery. (See color illustrations, page 169.)

Plaque deposits build up when a person has high levels of cholesterol in the blood. The problem runs in some families. Lack of exercise, a high-fat diet, smoking, and untreated **high blood pressure** (see page 111) or **diabetes** (see page 277) also increase your chances of having artery disease.

The risk rises with age; heavy people are more at risk than those who are lean; and men are in more danger than women, up to a point: The risk for women goes up sharply once they reach menopause. Women over 35 who smoke and take birth control pills may also face increased risk.

Most of us are likely to have some narrowed arteries by the time we're in our 50s or 60s. But even before symptoms appear, atherosclerosis can make a person feel tired or generally unwell.

When plaque deposits are more advanced, they can cause a number of health problems, including:

Heart disease: This is the leading cause of death in the United States. It occurs when the arteries that supply blood to the heart muscle become narrowed. If these coronary arteries can't supply enough blood to the heart during exertion or strong emotions, your heart complains and you feel chest pain (angina). A heart attack happens when a blood clot forms in a coronary artery and blocks blood flow to a part of the heart. This most often happens

Chest Pain

Never ignore chest pain, especially in an adult. It's hard to tell one kind of chest pain from another, so if it is severe or lasts more than a few minutes, call 911.

SYMPTOMS	WHAT IT MIGHT BE	WHAT YOU CAN DO
Mild to severe pain, pressure, or squeezing in center of chest that may spread to jaw, neck, back, or arms (often left arm); sweating, nausea, or shortness of breath; anxiety.	Heart attack (see page 37).	Call 911 **right away.** If you have aspirin, take a half tablet. (Don't do this if you're already taking a daily aspirin.)
Pain or chest tightness with breathing. In adults: sudden, sharp chest pain with shortness of breath that gets worse. In young people: possibly vague or minor pain that spreads to neck or back with some trouble breathing.	Collapsed lung. Sometimes occurs in young people for no apparent reason, or in adults who have asthma or chronic bronchitis. May follow a recent chest injury.	Call 911 **right away.**
Severe, stubborn, ripping chest pain that may spread to abdomen and upper back; dizziness and fainting.	Aortic aneurysm—weak spot with tear in main artery from heart. Most often caused by artery disease (see facing page) or high blood pressure (see page 111).	Call 911 **right away.** Surgery may be needed to repair aorta.
Sharp chest pain, worse when breathing in; shortness of breath; possibly fever.	Pleurisy—inflamed sac around lungs; often a complication of pneumonia (see page 97) or tuberculosis.	Call 911 or go to emergency room **right away.**
Dull pain, pressure, or squeezing in center of chest that may feel like stomach upset or heartburn; may spread to jaw, neck, back, or arms (usually left arm); brought on or made worse by stress or activity, easing with rest in 30 seconds to 5 minutes.	Angina. ■ Coronary artery disease (see artery disease, facing page, and heart attack, page 37).	Call doctor for prompt appointment, but if symptoms persist 10 minutes or longer, call 911 **right away.**

HEART & CIRCULATION

(continued)

Chest Pain (continued)

SYMPTOMS	WHAT IT MIGHT BE	WHAT YOU CAN DO
Chest pain, trouble breathing, easy fatigue, uneven heartbeat (palpitations), fainting (sometimes).	Problem with heart rhythm. ■ Mitral valve prolapse—heart valve allows blood to leak backward. Affects more women than men; may run in families.	Call doctor for prompt appointment. For mitral valve prolapse, beta-blockers may ease palpitations and chest pain. Antibiotics should be taken before dental work or surgery to prevent infection of heart's lining. **For more help:** American Heart Association, 800-242-8721, hours vary.
Pain or tightening in chest; rapid heartbeat; shortness of breath; numbness or tingling in hands; fear.	Anxiety. ■ Panic attack. ■ Hyperventilation—rapid breathing that lowers level of carbon dioxide in blood (see anxiety and phobias, page 208).	If you can't function as usual, call doctor for advice.
Burning or pressure in chest or upper abdomen, worse on bending over or lying down, especially when stomach is full; belching. Symptoms can resemble those of heart attack.	Heartburn. ■ Esophageal reflux—stomach acid backs up into esophagus when muscle that prevents this becomes weak. ■ Ulcer. ■ Gastritis.	See heartburn, page 124, or ulcers and gastritis, page 134. If you're not sure about the symptoms, call your doctor right away; you may need to be checked for a heart problem.
Severe burning or aching pain on one side of chest that may spread to back, not affected by breathing; followed a few days later by blisters and itchy rash.	Shingles.	See shingles, page 160.
Sharp pain that gets worse with movement or deep breathing, or when area is pressed; may follow severe coughing or sneezing, or chest injury.	Pulled muscle. ■ Inflamed cartilage. ■ Injured rib.	Rest; apply an ice pack (a bag of frozen peas wrapped in a dishcloth works well) several times a day, 10–15 minutes at a time. Take a painkiller—aspirin, ibuprofen, or acetaminophen.

where plaque has built up and damaged the artery's walls.

Stroke: Some types of **strokes** (see page 113) occur when clots form in vessels in the brain or leading to it. As in coronary artery disease, this often happens where the vessel is narrowed by plaque. Another type of stroke happens when a weakened vessel bursts and leaks blood into the brain.

Peripheral vascular disease: This occurs when arteries that go to the arms and legs become narrowed. If untreated it can lead to gangrene and the loss of a limb, most often a leg.

If your doctor suspects you have narrowed arteries, he or she may suggest diet and lifestyle changes, and maybe drugs to reduce high cholesterol or control high blood pressure. A technique called balloon angioplasty can sometimes open blocked arteries, or surgery can bypass them.

WHAT YOU CAN DO NOW

There is no quick fix. But changes in lifestyle can make a big difference. They'll help you prevent artery disease and cut your risk of heart disease, stroke, and other problems. If your arteries have already begun to narrow, these same changes can slow the progress of the disease and even reverse it.

➤ Exercise. Like any muscle, your heart gets stronger with regular work. And a strong heart pumps blood with less effort than a weaker one. Exercise also helps open up clogged arteries, lowers blood pressure, makes clots less likely to form in narrowed arteries, helps keep off extra weight, and reduces stress (see **get some exercise,** page 292).

The idea of exercising may be a little scary if you haven't been active over the years, or if you've been told you have narrowed arteries, but exercise is extra important then. To make it safer and easier:

■ Check with your doctor first if you're at risk for narrowed arteries.

■ Start by being just a bit more active each day. Any exercise is better than none and even brief workouts will lower your blood pressure and cholesterol level. Take the stairs instead of the ele-

vator. Walk your dog for 15 minutes after work. Your dog and your arteries will thank you.

■ When you're used to being more active, add things that make you breathe harder, sweat a bit, and get your heart pumping. Brisk walking, jogging, biking, cross-country skiing, and swimming are all great for your heart. But find something you like—you'll be more likely to stick with it. Take a couple of months to work up to getting exercise 2 or 3 times a week for 20 to 30 minutes at a time.

➤ Eat right. A low-fat, low-cholesterol diet can prevent and even reverse narrowing of arteries (see **eat well,** page 296).

You need some fat and cholesterol to stay healthy. They provide energy and help maintain cell walls. And some vegetable oils, such as canola, safflower, and olive oil, contain substances that help protect the arteries. But when you eat extra fat and cholesterol, you store some of it as body fat, and some of that ends up clogging your arteries.

Build your meals around fruits, vegetables, and grains. They have little fat and no cholesterol and are loaded with vitamins, minerals, and fiber. Fiber is important. It lowers cholesterol and blood pressure and helps keep your arteries open. Foods rich in fiber include apples, oranges, potatoes, squash, peas, carrots, soybeans and other beans, oats, and barley. There are simple things you can do to cut fat and cholesterol:

■ Read food labels to know what you're eating. The important things to look for are calories, calories from fat, total fat, saturated fat, and cholesterol. The American Heart Association says to keep your total fat intake under 30 percent of your daily calories. Of this, only about 8 to 10 percent should come from saturated fat (animal fat). Some experts now think your total fat intake can actually be higher than 30 percent, as long as most of it comes from heart-healthy vegetable oils.

■ If you eat red meat, make it a once-in-a-while treat. Eat no more than 6 ounces of meat, poultry, or fish a day. Keep servings to 3 ounces—a cut of meat about the size of a deck of cards, a skin-less chicken leg or half breast, or three-quarters of a cup of flaked fish.

- Don't fry foods. Bake, broil, steam, or sauté in a nonstick pan.
- If you eat dairy foods, choose the low-fat or nonfat versions.
- Watch out for trans fats, which are found mostly in solid or semisolid (hydrogenated) vegetable oils such as margarine and shortening. These fats, like saturated fats, raise cholesterol levels. If you use margarine, go for soft spreads. When cooking, use liquid vegetable oils instead of shortening. Check package labels and steer clear of foods containing hydrogenated or partially hydrogenated vegetable oil.
- Go easy on eggs—they have lots of cholesterol. Eat no more than 3 or 4 of them in a week.

➤ Don't smoke. With the first puff, your risk for narrowed arteries and heart attack goes way up. A man who smokes a pack a day has twice the risk of a nonsmoker. For a woman, it's even more dangerous—a pack a day increases her risk 5 to 10 times.

The good news: As soon as you stop smoking, your body begins to recover. Within a year, your risk for heart disease drops to half that of a smoker. Fifteen years after stopping, your risk is the same as that of a person who never smoked.

➤ If you have **high blood pressure** (see page 111), do what you can to lower it. Your blood pressure is too high if it's 140/90 or higher. Lose weight if you're overweight, exercise regularly, eat right, and reduce daily stress.

➤ Have your cholesterol level checked. If it's too high, do what you can to bring it down. Best is a total cholesterol reading under 200 milligrams per deciliter of blood. Borderline is 200 to 239. Too high is 240 and over. But total cholesterol tells only part of the story. What's in it also counts. Experts now say it's good to have a high level of high-density lipoprotein (HDL) and a low level of low-density lipoprotein (LDL). Your HDL should make up at least 25 percent of your total cholesterol (at least 40 milligrams per deciliter). Eating right and

exercising will help. If lifestyle changes don't work, your doctor can prescribe medication.

➤ If you're overweight, take steps to lose the extra pounds (see **maintain a healthy weight,** page 295).

➤ Be careful with alcohol. Moderate drinking may help cut the risk of narrowed arteries. But too much can make your heart pump faster and raise blood pressure. It can also damage the heart muscle. What's "moderate"? No more than 2 drinks a day for men, 1 for women. (A drink is a 12-ounce beer, a 5-ounce glass of wine, or a 1.5-ounce shot of hard liquor.)

WHEN TO CALL THE DOCTOR

Call 911 **right away:**

➤ If you feel mild to severe crushing or squeezing pain in your chest, sometimes with nausea, vomiting, sweating, shortness of breath, weakness, or intense feelings of anxiety. You may be having a heart attack.

➤ If you have aspirin, take a half tablet. If the tablet is enteric-coated, crush it first or chew it. Aspirin taken within 24 hours of a heart attack can reduce its severity. **Caution:** Don't do this if you're already taking a daily aspirin.

➤ If you've had chest pain before, but this time it doesn't go away in 5 to 10 minutes.

➤ If you've had chest pain before, but it's getting worse or you have it while resting.

➤ If you have any symptoms of a stroke, such as loss of speech or balance, or numbness.

Call for a prompt appointment:

➤ If you have symptoms of peripheral vascular disease, such as pain in the legs or feet.

HOW TO PREVENT IT

Follow the guidelines in What You Can Do Now, page 107. See **eight ways to feel your best,** page 292, for more details.

➤ Try vitamin E (found in foods such as vegetable oils, wheat germ oil, and almonds), which may help prevent heart attacks (see **the nutrition top ten,** page 298). Experts suggest taking 100 to 400 IU daily. People at high risk of heart problems should aim for 400 to 800 IU.

➤ Consider taking a half or whole aspirin tablet every day if you're a man age 50 or older or a woman past menopause with at least one additional risk factor for heart disease, such as high blood pressure or high cholesterol. This over-the-counter remedy helps prevent heart attacks, as well as strokes caused by blood clots. But aspirin isn't for everyone; check with your doctor before starting this routine.

➤ Enjoy your friends (see **stay involved,** page 303). Friendships can do wonders for your heart. Volunteer, take classes, or join a support group to talk with others who know what you're going through.

COMPLEMENTARY CHOICES

Studies show that several complementary treatments for artery disease may help.

➤ Too much stress is hard on the heart. Do what you can to relax: Try deep breathing, meditation, or simply a "time-out" now and then (see **relax,** page 303).

➤ Rice fermented with red yeast, a spice used in traditional Chinese cooking—it gives Peking duck its unique coloring—contains a natural compound that lowers cholesterol levels. An extract of the substance is sold under the brand name Cholestin.

➤ Garlic—as little as a half a clove per day—and garlic oil capsules may help lower cholesterol.

➤ Ginkgo biloba seems to help improve blood circulation, especially in the brain and lower legs and feet. This herb comes in capsules, tinctures, and extracts.

Don't use any herbal remedy without checking with your doctor, especially if you're already taking medicine for artery disease.

FOR MORE HELP

Key Websites: *www.SavonHealth.com.* For more information on artery disease: *www.SavonCardiovascular.com.*

Organizations: American Heart Association, 800-242-8721, hours vary; *www.americanheart.org.* Staff answers questions and sends out brochures.

■ National Heart, Lung, and Blood Institute Information Center, Box 30105, Bethesda, MD 20824-0105. 800-575-WELL, 24-hour recording, or 301-592-8573, M–F 8:30–5 EST; *www.nhlbi.nih.gov.* Staff answers questions and sends brochures.

Websites: The Franklin Institute Online's The Heart: An Online Exploration, *sln.fi.edu/biosci/heart.html.* This user-friendly tour of the heart and blood system provides links to other heart-related sites.

■ Heart Information Network, *www.heartinfo.org.* A comprehensive online guide to keeping your heart healthy.

Newsletter: *Heart Advisor,* from the Cleveland Clinic Foundation. Call 800-829-2506, M–F 7AM–midnight EST, to subscribe ($32 a year; 12 issues). Information source for heart health and healing.

Books: *Mayo Clinic on High Blood Pressure,* edited by Sheldon G. Sheps, M.D. Kensington, 1999, $14.95.

■ *Her Healthy Heart: A Woman's Guide to Preventing and Reversing Heart Disease Naturally,* by Linda Ojeda, Ph.D. Hunter House, 1998, $14.95.

■ *Dr. Dean Ornish's Program for Reversing Heart Disease,* by Dean Ornish, M.D. A step-by-step guide to reversing heart disease without drugs or surgery. Ivy Books, 1996, $6.99.

Congestive Heart Failure
www.SavonCHF.com

SIGNS AND SYMPTOMS

■ Weakness and fatigue.
■ Shortness of breath, even during light activity or while lying down. This might cause wheezing that is mistaken for asthma.
■ Need to sleep on more pillows than normal or to sleep sitting up.
■ Swelling in the feet, ankles, and legs.
■ Dull ache or pain in the chest.
■ Stubborn cough with foamy, blood-specked mucus.
■ Stomach feels full.
■ Weight gain from fluid buildup.

HEART & CIRCULATION

- Frequent need to urinate, most often at night.
- Swelling of neck veins.
- Nausea, vomiting, loss of appetite.
- Irregular or rapid heartbeat.

Despite its scary name, congestive heart failure is not always a life-threatening disease when the causes are found and treated. It occurs when the heart muscle is damaged, usually by **high blood pressure** (see facing page), a **heart attack** (see page 37), **palpitations** (see page 112), **artery disease** (see page 104), valve problems, or an illness called cardiomyopathy, which may be caused by a virus, alcohol abuse, or inherited heart defects. As a result, the heart can't keep the blood flowing well, causing swelling, most often in the legs and ankles. Sometimes fluid collects in the lungs and makes it hard to breathe. Congestive heart failure also makes it harder for the kidneys to get rid of excess sodium and water, which can make the swelling worse.

Congestive heart failure is the most common reason that people over 65 go to the hospital. With treatment, though, a person who has it can most often go on to lead an active life.

WHAT YOU CAN DO NOW

After diagnosis:
➤ Get plenty of rest at first. Later, as your symptoms ease, staying on the move will help you get better.
➤ To make breathing easier when lying down, raise your head by putting a wedge under your mattress, or use extra pillows.
➤ Put your legs up when sitting.
➤ Eat less salt; it makes you retain fluid and swell. Beware of the hidden salt in fast food and processed food.
➤ Don't eat or drink anything with caffeine; if you're having heart palpitations, caffeine can make them worse.
➤ Use elastic support stockings to control swelling in your legs. Ask your pharmacist about them.

WHEN TO CALL THE DOCTOR

Call 911 **right away:**

➤ If you have severe chest pain or trouble breathing.

Call for a prompt appointment:
➤ If you often become breathless and tired after mild activity.

Call for advice:
➤ If you're being treated for congestive heart failure and your symptoms get worse.
➤ If you gain weight rapidly.
➤ If you notice any unusual swelling in your feet, legs, or neck.

HOW TO PREVENT IT

➤ Eat sensibly and exercise daily to prevent the causes, such as high blood pressure.
➤ If you know you have high blood pressure or heart disease, follow your doctor's advice about treating the problem.
➤ Drink moderately, if at all.

FOR MORE HELP

Key Websites: *www.SavonHealth.com.* For more information on congestive heart failure: *www.SavonCHF.com.*

Organizations: American Heart Association, 800-242-8721, hours vary; *www.american heart.org.* Staff answers questions and sends out literature.

- National Heart, Lung, and Blood Institute Information Center, Box 30105, Bethesda, MD 20824-0105. 800-575-WELL, 24-hour recording, or 301-592-8573, M–F 8:30–5 EST; *www.nhlbi.nih.gov.* Staff answers questions and sends brochures.

Website: Heart Information Network, *www. heartinfo.com.* Scroll to the topic you want. Covers heart news, answers questions about heart disease, and lists resources.

Books: *Living Well, Staying Well,* by the American Cancer Society and the American Heart Association. A guide to heart wellness with practical, step-by-step advice. Times Books, 1999, $14.

- *The Stanford Life Plan for a Healthy Heart,* by Helen Cassidy Page, John Speer Schroeder, M.D., and Tara Coghlin Dickson, M.S., R.D. Covers heart disease and includes more than 200 recipes. Chronicle Books, 1996, $29.95.

High Blood Pressure
www.SavonHBP.com

www.SavonHBP.com

SIGNS AND SYMPTOMS

High blood pressure, or hypertension, is often called the "silent killer." In most cases, there are no clear warning signs, even as the illness harms your health.

Blood pressure refers to the force of blood pushing against artery walls as it courses through the body. It's normal for your blood pressure to rise and fall through the day with changes in your activities and moods. But when it remains high most of the time, it can force your heart to work too hard, which can threaten your health. High blood pressure is the most common of all cardiovascular diseases. It is the leading cause of **heart attack** (see page 37) and **stroke** (see pages 44 and 113).

Blood pressure is measured with a device that records 2 numbers. It's too high if the first number (the peak pressure when your heart beats) is higher than 139 most of the time, or if the second number (the pressure when your heart relaxes between beats) is higher than 89 most of the time. The best is around 110/70.

While the causes of most cases of high blood pressure aren't known, the risk factors are—they include things you can't control and things you can. If high blood pressure runs in your family, your risk is doubled. The risk goes up with age. African Americans have a high risk. If you weigh too much, don't get enough exercise, or are under a lot of stress, you're also at risk. Sometimes high blood pressure can be a sign of other problems, such as **diabetes** (see page 277) or kidney disease.

High blood pressure can be treated with lifestyle changes and, often, with drugs.

WHAT YOU CAN DO NOW

➤ Have your blood pressure checked as often as your doctor advises you to (see **tests,** page 319).

➤ Don't smoke, and avoid smoky places.

➤ Exercise often—try brisk walking, swimming, or biking. If you're not currently active, check with your doctor before start-ing an exercise program (see **get some exercise,** page 292).

➤ Eat no more than 2,000 milligrams of salt a day. (One teaspoon of salt equals about 2,100 mg.) Fresh vegetables and fruits are low in salt; fast food and processed foods contain a lot of it.

➤ Find a healthy outlet for **stress** (see page 218). Try meditation or yoga to **relax** (see page 303).

WHEN TO CALL THE DOCTOR

Call for emergency advice (if you can't get any, call 911 or go to an emergency room):

➤ If you have high blood pressure or suspect you do and you have any of these: recurring headaches, chest pain or tightness, frequent nosebleeds, numbness and tingling, confusion, or blurred vision.

Call for advice:

➤ If you check your blood pressure and it rises and stays high for a number of days.

➤ If you are pregnant and your blood pressure goes up. High blood pressure can harm both you and your unborn child (see **pregnancy,** page 238).

➤ If you have high blood pressure and lifestyle changes don't help.

➤ If you're taking drugs to control your high blood pressure and you start to feel dizzy or sleepy, or you become constipated or impotent. You may need a different drug. But never stop taking your blood pressure medication without telling your doctor; stopping suddenly can cause problems.

HOW TO PREVENT IT

Follow the suggestions in What You Can Do Now. Also:

➤ If you're overweight, try to lose the extra pounds.

➤ If you drink alcohol, drink moderately—no more than 2 drinks a day for men, 1 for women. (A drink is a 12-ounce beer, a 5-ounce glass of wine, or a 1.5-ounce shot of hard liquor.)

➤ If you use birth control pills, give some thought to other methods. The Pill can cause high blood pressure in some women (see **birth control,** page 220).

➤ Make sure you get enough potassium

HEART & CIRCULATION

(orange juice has a lot), magnesium (leafy greens and whole grains), and calcium (leafy greens and dairy products). These minerals help control blood pressure (see **the nutrition top ten,** page 298).

➤ Cut fats in your diet—eat less fatty meat, butter, and whole dairy products, and more vegetables, fruits, and grains (see **eat well,** page 296).

FOR MORE HELP

Key Websites: *www.SavonHealth.com*. For more information on high blood pressure: *www.SavonHBP.com*.

Organizations: American Heart Association, 800-242-8721, hours vary; *www.american heart.org*. Staff answers questions and sends literature, including pamphlets on groups at high risk, such as African Americans and women.

■ Citizens for Public Action on Blood Pressure and Cholesterol, Box 30374, Bethesda, MD 20824. 800-427-6639, M–F 9–4 EST. Call for free educational materials on blood pressure and cholesterol.

■ National Heart, Lung, and Blood Institute Information Center, Box 30105, Bethesda, MD 20824-0105. 800-575-WELL, 24-hour recording, or 301-592-8573, M–F 8:30–5 EST; *www.nhlbi.nih.gov.* Staff answers questions and sends brochures.

Website: Heart Information Network, *www. heartinfo.org*. Click on *Hypertension*. Defines high blood pressure, covers treatment and prevention, and gives links to related articles.

Books: *Alternative Medicine Guide: Heart Disease, Stroke & High Blood Pressure,* by Burton Goldberg. Top physicians explain their safe, nontoxic heart-saving treatments. Future Medicine, 1999, $24.95.

■ *Breathe Well, Be Well: A Program to Relieve Stress, Anxiety, Asthma, Hypertension, Migraine, and Other Disorders for Better Health,* by Robert Fried, Ph.D. John Wiley & Sons, 1999, $14.95.

■ *Good News About High Blood Pressure,* by Thomas Pickering, M.D. New research and treatments. Fireside, 1997, $12.

Palpitations
www.SavonHeart.com

SIGNS AND SYMPTOMS

Rapid heart rate:
■ A nagging awareness of your heartbeat.
■ A fluttering, thumping, pounding, or racing beat.
■ Shortness of breath, chest pain, light-headedness, or fainting.

Slow heart rate:
■ Fatigue, shortness of breath, light-headedness, or fainting.
■ Nausea.

Palpitations are caused by changes in the electrical impulses that control the heart muscle. Nearly everyone has an uneven heartbeat now and then; it's usually harmless. But a frequent or lasting change in the heart's rhythm can cause problems.

The older you are, the greater your chances of having palpitations. Anxiety, stress, thyroid problems, and some drugs, including nicotine, caffeine, and alcohol, can also set them off. But the most important causes are **high blood pressure** (see page 111) and **artery disease** (see page 104). These health problems can damage the heart muscle, causing a "short circuit" in its electrical system.

Mild palpitations can often be controlled with drugs or surgery. Sometimes devices such as pacemakers are put into the chest to control more severe palpitations.

WHAT YOU CAN DO NOW

Call your doctor for a prompt appointment if you have palpitations often—even once a day—if they make you feel dizzy, or if they're bad enough that you become very aware of your heartbeat.

WHAT YOU CAN DO NOW

Call for a prompt appointment:
➤ If you have fainting spells.
➤ If you notice a strange heartbeat and feel light-headed or dizzy.
➤ If you have uneven heartbeats that are intense, painful, or more than fleeting.

➤ If you are taking drugs your doctor has given you for palpitations and you notice a new, uneven heartbeat pattern or you are nauseated, vomit, faint, or have diarrhea or a rash.

HOW TO PREVENT IT

➤ Cut out caffeine (in coffee, tea, chocolate, and caffeinated soft drinks).
➤ Don't smoke, and stay away from alcohol, decongestants, diet pills, and stimulant drugs such as cocaine or amphetamines.

Do what you can to keep your heart in good shape:

➤ Get plenty of exercise, such as brisk walking, jogging, swimming, or bicycling, to help control your resting heart rate (see **get some exercise,** page 292).
➤ Find a healthy outlet for **stress** (see page 218). Try meditation, yoga, or deep breathing (see **relax,** page 303).
➤ Eat balanced, low-fat meals (see **eat well,** page 296). Your doctor may also suggest mineral supplements; calcium, magnesium, and potassium help control the heartbeat (see **the nutrition top ten,** page 298).

FOR MORE HELP

Key Websites: *www.SavonHealth.com*. For more information on heart palpitations *www.SavonHeart.com*.

Organization: American Heart Association, 800-242-8721, hours vary; *www.american heart.org*. Staff answers questions and sends out brochures.

Websites: The Franklin Institute Online's The Heart: An Online Exploration, *sln.fi.edu/biosci/heart.html*. This user-friendly tour of the heart and blood system provides links to other heart-related sites. For more information on palpitations, click on *Search* and type in *arrhythmia*.

■ Heart Information Network, *www.heart info.org*. A comprehensive online guide to keeping your heart healthy.

Stroke
www.SavonStrokes.com

SIGNS AND SYMPTOMS

If you have any of the following symptoms, or if someone with you does, call 911 **right away.**

■ Abrupt weakness or numbness of the face, arm, or leg, often on one side of the body.
■ Sudden trouble seeing or loss of vision—especially in just one eye.
■ Trouble talking or making sense of someone else's speech.
■ Sudden and severe headache.
■ Dizziness or loss of consciousness.

A person has a stroke when blood flow to part of the brain is blocked. A stroke needs treatment right away, since parts of the brain can begin to die within minutes, damaging speech, vision, and movement. Strokes disable more people in the United States than any other cause.

There are three main kinds of strokes:

Cerebral thrombosis, the most common, occurs when a blood clot forms and blocks blood flow in an artery in the brain or leading to it. These clots most often form in arteries narrowed by the fatty substance known as plaque.

Cerebral embolism occurs when a clot forms in some other part of the body, then is carried to the brain.

These 2 types of stroke often occur after a transient ischemic attack (TIA), in which a clot briefly blocks an artery in the brain or leading to it. The symptoms are similar to those of cerebral thrombosis or cerebral embolism, but they usually last only a few minutes. TIAs cause no lasting damage, but they are an important warning sign that you're at risk of a stroke.

Cerebral hemorrhage occurs when a weakened artery in the brain bursts and bleeds into the tissues near it. Sometimes a vessel on the surface of the brain breaks and then bleeds into the space between the brain and the skull. The blood presses on the brain and can cause damage.

The single most important risk factor for stroke is **high blood pressure** (see page 111). Smokers, people over 65, men, African Ameri-

HEART & CIRCULATION

cans, and people with a family history of stroke are all at risk of having a stroke. Women using birth control pills (see **birth control,** page 220) have a greater risk of stroke if they also smoke. They have an even higher risk if they are over 35 or have high blood pressure.

Many people who have had strokes recover fully following physical or occupational therapy combined with other treatments, such as medications to improve circulation and prevent clots, and lifestyle changes to prevent another stroke.

WHAT YOU CAN DO NOW

Get help—call 911 right away—if you are with someone who has symptoms of a stroke. While waiting for help to arrive, follow these steps (for more details, see page 44):

➤ Check the person's **ABCs** (see box on page 12).
➤ Begin **CPR** (see page 14) if the person is not breathing or you can't find a pulse.
➤ If the person is not conscious but is breathing, support the head and roll him or her into the **recovery position** (see box on page 23).
➤ If vomit or fluid is draining from the person's mouth, or he or she is having trouble swallowing, turn the person onto his or her side so the airway isn't blocked. Don't give anything to eat or drink.
➤ If the person is conscious, offer comfort.

WHEN TO CALL THE DOCTOR

Call 911 right away. Don't try to drive the person to an emergency room yourself—wait for help to come, and follow the steps above. The sooner a person gets help, the better his or her chances for recovery. A drug widely used against heart attack—t-PA—can limit the damage from a stroke if it is given within 3 hours.

HOW TO PREVENT IT

➤ If you have high blood pressure (see page 111), do what you can to control it.
➤ Find a healthy outlet for **stress** (see page 218), such as meditation, yoga, or deep breathing (see **relax,** page 303).
➤ Get plenty of **exercise** (see page 292), and

eat plenty of low-fat, high-fiber foods—fresh fruits and vegetables and whole grains (see **eat well,** page 296).
➤ Don't smoke, and avoid smoky places.
➤ If you have **artery disease** (see page 104), your doctor may suggest aspirin or prescription drugs to reduce the chance of clots. Your doctor may also discuss surgery to widen narrowed vessels in your neck.
➤ If you have **diabetes** (see page 277), take steps to control it. This disease can damage blood vessels and increase the risk of stroke.

COMPLEMENTARY CHOICES

See **artery disease,** page 104.

FOR MORE HELP

Key Websites: *www.SavonHealth.com.* For more information on strokes *www.SavonStrokes.com.*

Organizations: American Stroke Association of the American Heart Association, 7272 Greenville Ave., Dallas, TX 75231. 800-553-6321, M–F 7:30–7 CST; *www.strokeassociation.org.* Call for brochures, information, and support groups near you.
■ National Institute of Neurological Disorders and Stroke, Bldg. 31, Room 8A06, 31 Center Dr., MSC 2540, Bethesda, MD 20892-2540. 800-352-9424, M–F 8:30–5 EST; *www.ninds.nih.gov.* Provides free brochures on strokes.
■ National Stroke Association, 800-787-6537, M–Th 8–4:30, F 8–4 MST; *www.stroke.org.* Provides facts about strokes and a list of support groups.

Books: *After Stroke: Enhancing Quality of Life,* by Wallace Sife, Ph.D. Haworth, 1998, $25.
■ *American Heart Association Family Guide to Stroke Treatment, Recovery, and Prevention,* by Louis R. Caplan, M.D., L. Dyken, M.D., and J. Donald Easton, M.D. A source book all about stroke. Times Books, 1996, $15.

Varicose Veins
www.SavonVaricoseVeins.com

SIGNS AND SYMPTOMS

- Swollen, twisted clusters of blue or purple veins.
- Swollen legs.
- Legs ache or feel heavy.
- Itching around affected veins.
- Brown discoloring of skin.
- Sores.

In healthy veins, valves allow blood to flow only one way. Varicose veins form when these valves fail, allowing blood to back up and pool inside the vein, making it swell. These veins can hurt, and they may look bad, but they're rarely harmful.

Varicose veins can occur anywhere on the body, but they show up mostly on the legs, sometimes within patches of thin red capillaries or green veins known as spiders. Hemorrhoids are varicose veins around the anus.

Varicose veins run in families. Women, often those of German or Irish descent, are twice as likely as men to develop them. Anything that puts pressure on the legs, such as standing for a long time, pregnancy, and being overweight, can cause them.

Most varicose veins are near the surface of the skin. Deeper ones can't be seen, but poor circulation can swell, darken, and harden the skin above them. In severe cases, sores may form, often around the ankles. Varicose veins can be removed with surgery or treated with medications.

WHAT YOU CAN DO NOW

- Wear elastic support stockings. They keep blood from pooling in the legs. You can find them at most drugstores.
- If your varicose veins are bothering you, stay off your feet as much as you can. Take breaks often. When you can, sit or lie with your feet above chest level. Sleep with your legs raised to relieve swelling.
- If you have to stand still for a long time, flex your calf muscles and toes. This helps pump blood toward the heart and prevents pooling.

WHEN TO CALL THE DOCTOR

Call for a prompt appointment:
- If you cut a varicose vein—it may bleed heavily. First, lie down, raise the injured leg, and apply gentle, firm pressure with a clean cloth. Get help as soon as you can after the bleeding has slowed.

Call for advice:
- If varicose veins make walking or standing painful.
- If you develop sores.

HOW TO PREVENT IT

The steps in What You Can Do Now will help prevent varicose veins or keep them from getting worse. Also:
- If you are overweight, take steps to lose the extra pounds (see **maintain a healthy weight,** page 295).
- Exercise often. Activities that work the leg muscles, such as walking or jogging, help pump blood toward the heart.
- Don't wear garters, girdles, or other tight clothing.
- Don't cross your legs.
- Avoid long periods of sitting or standing.
- Sit or lie down with your legs at hip level or higher at least twice a day for 30 minutes at a time.

FOR MORE HELP

Key Websites: *www.SavonHealth.com*. For more information on varicose veins: *www.SavonVaricoseVeins.com*.

Organization: National Heart, Lung, and Blood Institute Information Center, Box 30105, Bethesda, MD 20824-0105. 800-575-WELL, 24-hour recording, or 301-592-8573, M–F 8:30–5 EST; *www.nhlbi.nih.gov.* Staff answers questions and sends out brochures.

Book: *Varicose Veins: A Guide to Prevention and Treatment,* reprint edition, by Howard C. Baron, M.D., F.A.C.S., and Barbara Ross. Checkmark, 1997, $14.95.

HEART & CIRCULATION

Stomach, Abdomen & Digestive System

Constipation

www.SavonConstipation.com

SIGNS AND SYMPTOMS

- Dry, overfirm stools that are hard or painful to pass.
- Feeling of fullness after having a bowel movement or of not being able to finish it.
- No bowel movement after 3 days (for adults) or 4 days (for children). How "regular" you are depends on your age, diet, and daily activity. Three bowel movements a week is normal for some, 3 a day for others.
- Swelling, bloating, or pain in the abdomen.

Constipation is a common ailment—and one of the most frustrating. Our modern lifestyle is often at fault: eating fast foods that are low in fiber, drinking too little water, getting too little exercise, and failing to respond right away to the urge to move the bowels. Emotional problems play a role. So do some drugs and food supplements.

Stubborn, chronic constipation may signal a more serious illness, such as **irritable bowel syndrome** (see page 130), **diabetes** (see page 277), or colon cancer.

WHAT YOU CAN DO NOW

Most cases respond to home treatment, such as diet changes and exercise. If constipation isn't caused by disease, simply eating more fiber (found in fruits, vegetables, and whole grains) and drinking lots of water (at least 8 glasses a day) should soften your stools and make you regular once more. Also:

- Don't use over-the-counter laxatives unless your doctor suggests them. You might become hooked. If you must take one, try a bulk-forming psyllium laxative, which is more gentle than other kinds. But don't use a laxative if you have stomach pain, nausea, or vomiting, or if you are pregnant.
- Don't take mineral oil as a laxative unless your doctor advises it.
- If infants under 6 months are mildly constipated, be sure they are getting enough water. Prune juice can help: Start with a half teaspoon. Increase to 4 tablespoons bit by bit. Make sure the infant does not get diarrhea.
- Try strained or whole prunes for adults, older children, and toddlers. (Remove pits for toddlers.)
- Don't use an enema unless your doctor advises you to.

WHEN TO CALL THE DOCTOR

Being constipated every now and then shouldn't send you to the doctor's office, but 2 weeks or more of the problem should. Call for a prompt appointment:

- If you also have fever and lower abdominal pain, and the stools you do have are thin. You may have **diverticulitis** (see page 121).

Call for advice and an appointment:

- If your stools are bloody. This may be from an anal fissure or a **hemorrhoid** (see page 126), but it could also be a sign of colon cancer.
- If you get constipation after taking a new

Abdominal Pain

Abdominal pain is most often a sign of a mild ailment such as indigestion or stomach flu. But severe pain can be an emergency, and long-lasting pain may signal a serious illness.

SYMPTOMS	WHAT IT MIGHT BE	WHAT YOU CAN DO
Sharp, ongoing pain in abdomen that radiates to back and chest; fever; nausea; vomiting; swollen abdomen; sweaty skin.	Pancreatitis—inflamed pancreas. ■ Cholecystitis—inflamed gallbladder.	Call 911 or go to emergency room **right away.** Acute pancreatitis can cause shock, which can be fatal if not treated quickly.
Sharp abdominal pain, perhaps with other acute symptoms.	Intestinal blockage. ■ Appendicitis (see page 24). ■ Pelvic inflammatory disease (see page 236). ■ Heart attack (see page 37). ■ Perforated stomach ulcer (see page 134). ■ Shock from allergy (see page 22). ■ Diabetic emergency (see diabetes, page 277).	■ Poisoning (see page 40). Call 911 or go to emergency room **right away.**
Severe, cramping pain in middle abdomen that radiates to right side or back and often disturbs sleep; nausea; vomiting; gas.	Gallstones (see page 122).	In a first attack, call doctor for emergency advice. If you can't get one, call 911 or go to emergency room. Do not eat or drink anything.
Severe pain in lower side of back that moves toward groin or abdomen; urge to urinate often, or painful or stopped-up urination; murky, smelly, or bloody urine; nausea and vomiting; sweating.	Kidney stones (see page 136). ■ Kidney infection.	Call doctor for prompt appointment. Then drink lots of water to help stone pass, and take a nonaspirin pain reliever if you need to (see pain relief, page 315).
Cramping or pain in abdomen, nausea, diarrhea, vomiting, fever, fatigue, weakness, gas.	Stomach flu (see nausea and vomiting, page 133). ■ Food poisoning (see page 34).	If, with vomiting and pain, you have blurred or double vision, muscle weakness, or trouble speaking or swallowing, call 911 or go to emergency room **right away;** these may be signs of botulism, a sometimes fatal bacterial food poisoning.

STOMACH, ABDOMEN & DIGESTIVE SYSTEM

(continued)

Abdominal Pain (continued)

SYMPTOMS	WHAT IT MIGHT BE	WHAT YOU CAN DO
Pain in upper right abdomen increasing over days, fever, fatigue, nausea and vomiting. Sometimes dark urine, pale stools, yellowed eyes and skin.	Hepatitis (see page 279). ■ Pancreatic cancer.	Call doctor for prompt appointment.
Pain or cramps in abdomen, diarrhea, bloody stool, pus in stool, fever, fatigue, weight loss.	Crohn's disease. ■ Ulcerative colitis. ■ Bacterial dysentery, particularly if you have been overseas.	See inflammatory bowel disease, page 128. If you think you have bacterial dysentery, call doctor for prompt appointment.
Pain that is worse when sore spot on abdomen is touched; severe abdominal cramping, often more painful on the left; nausea; fever; chills; diarrhea, constipation, or thin stools.	Diverticulitis.	See diverticulitis, page 121.
Ache or pain in abdomen or groin when lifting or bending over, swelling or bulge under skin in abdomen or groin.	Hernia.	See hernia, page 127.
Ache or pain in abdomen with diarrhea, constipation, or bouts of both; mucus strands in stool; extreme gas or bloating; nausea, usually after meals; fatigue.	Irritable bowel syndrome.	See irritable bowel syndrome, page 130. (For self-care, also see diarrhea, opposite page, and constipation, page 116.)
Pain in upper abdomen, nausea, vomiting, diarrhea, loss of appetite, burping or gas, heartburn.	Stomach ulcer. ■ Gastritis.	See ulcers and gastritis, page 134.
Pain and cramps after drinking milk or eating other dairy foods, gas and bloating, diarrhea, nausea, rumbling sounds from abdomen.	Lactose intolerance— trouble digesting cow's milk, cheese, butter, ice cream, and other dairy foods.	Eat fewer dairy foods or none. Try soy milk, lactose-free dairy products, and acidophilus yogurt. Lactase enzyme supplements also may help.

A Folk Remedy to Try

An age-old way to get the bowels moving is to mix the juice of a whole lemon into a glass of warm water and drink it in the morning. Or try a glass of water with a teaspoon of apple cider vinegar and a teaspoon of honey mixed in.

prescription drug or food supplements. Changing the dosage may help.

➤ If you are elderly or disabled and haven't had a bowel movement for a week or more. You may have an impacted stool.

➤ If you are losing weight.

➤ If exercise and eating more fiber haven't helped after 2 weeks.

HOW TO PREVENT IT

➤ Exercise. A brisk 30-minute walk every day will help regulate your bowel movements.

➤ Drink plenty of water—at least 8 glasses every day.

➤ Get lots of fiber by eating at least 5 servings a day of fresh fruits, vegetables, and other good sources of fiber, including beans and nuts, bran and other whole-grain cereals, and raw or cooked dried fruits such as raisins and prunes.

➤ Allow enough time for bowel movements. A pattern—the same time every day, after breakfast or dinner—is best. And don't ignore the urge to defecate.

COMPLEMENTARY CHOICES

➤ Try acupressure: Place your fingertips 3 finger widths below the navel and gently press in about an inch. Hold for 3 minutes while taking deep, slow breaths.

FOR MORE HELP

Key Websites: *www.SavonHealth.com*. For more information on constipation: *www.SavonConstipation.com*.

Organizations: American Dietetic Association, 216 W. Jackson Blvd., Chicago, IL 60606-6995. 800-366-1655, M–F 9–4 CST; *www.eatright.org*. Call for a recorded mes-

sage about nutrition or, for a fee, to speak with a registered dietitian who answers questions about constipation and gives names of dietitians near you.

■ International Foundation for Functional Gastrointestinal Disorders, P.O. Box 170864, Milwaukee, WI 53217-8076. 888-964-2001 or 414-964-1799, M–F 8:30–5 CST; *www.iffgd.org*. Offers support and printed advice on bowel disorders.

■ National Digestive Diseases Information Clearinghouse, 2 Information Way, Bethesda, MD 20892-3570. 301-654-3810, M–F 8:30–5 EST; *www.niddk.nih.gov/health/digest/pubs/const/const.htm* for an online brochure on constipation.

Diarrhea
www.SavonDiarrhea.com

SIGNS AND SYMPTOMS

■ Loose, watery stools.
■ Frequent bowel movements.
■ Abdominal pain or cramping.

Diarrhea occurs when stools move faster than usual through the intestines (see color illustration, page 174), before the body can take out the water they contain. Its causes include viruses, a reaction to food, **food poisoning** (see page 34), **stress** (see page 218), too much alcohol, and some drugs, especially antibiotics. Diarrhea can also result from drinking untreated water that contains giardia, a parasite that attacks the intestines, or from other parasites and amoebas.

In some cases, diarrhea may indicate a more serious disease such as **irritable bowel syndrome** (see page 130), **inflammatory bowel disease** (see page 128), **diverticulitis** (see page 121), or colon cancer.

WHAT YOU CAN DO NOW

➤ Don't eat solid food at first. This will let your digestive tract rest.

➤ Don't take over-the-counter antidiarrhea products for the first few hours; let your system get rid of whatever is causing the problem. If you do use such products, don't take

STOMACH, ABDOMEN & DIGESTIVE SYSTEM

Diarrhea in Children

Infants and young children need special care when they have diarrhea. If it's severe, an infant can become very dehydrated in less than a day.

➤ Breast-fed infants should continue regular feedings. If you use formula, ask your doctor about diluting it with water to half strength for 24 to 48 hours. If the diarrhea doesn't improve, try soy-based formula until your child is better.

➤ Don't give soda, fruit juice, or sports drinks to infants or young children. To help prevent dehydration, give child a few sips of a rehydration drink such as Pedialyte or Infalyte every few minutes.

➤ Don't give antidiarrhea medicine to infants or young children.

➤ For older babies, try the BRAT diet—bananas, rice, apple sauce, and toast—to add bulk to the stool; yogurt with active cultures also may help. Don't give babies solid food if they are vomiting.

➤ Call your doctor if you see any signs of dehydration—sticky saliva, lack of tears when crying, weakness, dark yellow urine.

them for more than a day or two without asking your doctor.

➤ Sip clear, warm liquids (water, tea, or broth), sports drinks, or flat sodas (ginger ale, cola, or other sodas that have been left open to lose their fizz). Drink only small amounts for the first few hours, then as much as your stomach can handle.

➤ If your stomach takes the fluids, try eating bland, bulk-adding foods such as bananas, white rice, or toast.

➤ While you are recovering, don't eat dairy foods or fiber-rich foods such as salads and fruit, and don't drink alcohol. Avoid milk for several days: With acute diarrhea, you can temporarily lose the lactase enzymes that help you digest milk, so drinking it will make the problem worse.

➤ If your diarrhea is severe, watch out for dehydration. Signs include dry mouth, sticky saliva, and dark yellow urine in smaller amounts than usual. You can buy rehydration drinks such as sports drinks (or Pedialyte or Infalyte for infants) to help replace lost fluids and minerals—or you can make your own (see box below).

WHEN TO CALL THE DOCTOR

Call for emergency advice (if you can't get any, call 911 or go to an emergency room):

➤ If the diarrhea comes with severe cramping, light-headedness, chills, vomiting, or fever higher than 101 degrees.

➤ If you notice signs of severe dehydration—dry mouth, sticky saliva, dizziness or weakness, and dark yellow urine. Dehydration can be dangerous for older people and for young children.

Call for a prompt appointment:

➤ If stools are bloody or tarry, or contain mucus or worms. (Some medicines and iron may make the stools look black, which isn't anything to worry about.)

Call for advice and an appointment:

➤ If you have diarrhea often, or if you get it while you are taking a medication.

➤ If diarrhea lasts for more than 2 days (1 day for a child under 3, or 8 hours for an infant under 6 months).

➤ If you have been traveling and may have been drinking untreated water.

➤ If diarrhea and constipation come and go in turn for more than a few weeks. You may have **irritable bowel syndrome** (see page 130) or—though less likely—colon cancer.

Rehydration Recipe

To make a rehydration drink at home for anyone older than 12, mix 1 quart water with 1 teaspoon table salt, one-half teaspoon baking soda, 4 teaspoons cream of tartar, and 3 to 4 tablespoons sugar. **Note:** Don't give to children 12 and under. Use only a store-bought drink such as Pedialyte or Infalyte.

STOMACH, ABDOMEN & DIGESTIVE SYSTEM

HOW TO PREVENT IT

➤ Avoid foods you know your body can't handle well.

➤ When traveling in foreign countries, drink only bottled or boiled water or canned drinks. Don't use ice in drinks. Peel fruits and vegetables. Don't eat foods that have been sitting out.

➤ Take *Lactobacillus acidophilus* in liquid or capsules or *Lactobacillus GG* capsules (Culturelle) before meals, especially when you travel to developing countries or have finished a course of antibiotics. These "good" bacteria help fight toxic germs in your gut. Wash capsules down with bottled water; acids in some fruit juices may destroy the beneficial bacteria.

➤ See **nausea and vomiting** (page 133) for tips about food-related diarrhea.

FOR MORE HELP

Key Websites: *www.SavonHealth.com*. For more information on diarrhea: *www.SavonDiarrhea.com*.

Organizations: International Foundation for Functional Gastrointestinal Disorders, P.O. Box 17864, Milwaukee, WI 53217. 888- 964-2001 or 414-964-1799, M–F 8:30–5 CST; *www.iffgd.org*. Provides support and printed advice on bowel problems.

■ National Digestive Diseases Information Clearinghouse, 2 Information Way, Bethesda, MD 20892-3570. 301-654-3810, M–F 8:30–5 EST; *www.niddk.nih.gov/health/ digest/pubs/diarrhea/diarrhea.htm* for facts on diarrhea and how to treat it.

Website: Centers for Disease Control and Prevention's online brochure on chronic diarrhea, *www.cdc.gov/ncidod/dpd/parasites/diarrhea/factsht_chronic_diarrhea.htm*.

Diverticulitis
www.SavonDiverticulitis.com

SIGNS AND SYMPTOMS

■ Abdominal cramping that is most often worse on the lower left side.

■ Nausea.
■ Fever.
■ Diarrhea, constipation, bloody or thin stools, or rectal bleeding.
■ Pain made worse when the sore spot on the abdomen is touched.
■ Gas.

Many people develop small pouches in the colon (the major part of the large intestine)—a fairly harmless condition known as diverticulosis.

But sometimes one or more of the pouches gets inflamed. This is diverticulitis. It can range from mild infection to bowel blockage or breaks in the bowel wall.

People who eat mostly low-fiber foods, are constipated, or use laxatives seem to be at risk of diverticulitis.

Treatment may include bed rest, diet changes, and antibiotics or other drugs. The chances of a full recovery are good if you get prompt medical help. If you don't, diverticulitis can lead to serious problems that need surgery.

WHAT YOU CAN DO NOW

➤ If you have symptoms of diverticulitis, see your doctor.

➤ Never use an enema for this illness.

WHEN TO CALL THE DOCTOR

Call 911 or go to an emergency room **right away:**

➤ If you have sharp abdominal pain and swelling, fever, chills, and nausea or vomiting—even if you think your symptoms are getting better. Peritonitis, a life-threatening infection of the abdominal cavity's lining, could be the problem.

Call for a prompt appointment:

➤ If your stools have blood in them; you may have internal bleeding.

➤ If severe pain lasts despite treatment; you may have another abdominal illness (see **abdominal pain** chart, page 117).

➤ Add whole-grain breads, bran cereals, oatmeal, fresh fruits, and vegetables to your diet. Don't add fiber too fast, though. Too much fiber all at once can create a painful amount of gas.

➤ Be sure you get enough fluids (at least 8 glasses of water a day). If you eat more fiber, be sure to drink at least this much water.

➤ Avoid foods that are hard to digest, such as nuts, seeds, corn, and popcorn.

➤ Heed the urge to have a bowel movement.

➤ Exercise daily to keep the muscles of your abdomen in good shape. This helps you have regular bowel movements.

➤ Don't use laxatives unless your doctor advises them. Eating prunes, drinking prune juice, or taking psyllium (for sale in drugstores as powder or pills) works well.

➤ Don't smoke; smoking can make the problem worse.

➤ Avoid caffeine, and if you drink alcohol, don't drink much.

FOR MORE HELP

Key Websites: *www.SavonHealth.com*. For more information on diverticulitis: *www.SavonDiverticulitis.com*.

Organizations: Intestinal Disease Foundation, 1323 Forbes Ave., Suite 200, Pittsburgh, PA 15219. 412-261-5888, M–F 9:30–5 EST. Offers telephone support, educational programs and brochures, advice on support groups, and names of doctors near you.

■ National Digestive Diseases Information Clearinghouse, 2 Information Way, Bethesda, MD 20892-3570. 301-654-3810, M–F 8:30–5 EST; *www.niddk.nih.gov/health/digest/pubs/divert/divert.htm* for an online brochure about diverticulitis.

Gallstones
www.SavonGallstones.com

SIGNS AND SYMPTOMS

■ Intense pain in the center of the abdomen that radiates to right side or upper right back.
■ Nausea and vomiting.
■ Gas and indigestion.
■ Fever and chills.
■ Yellow-tinged skin and eyes (jaundice).
■ Pale stools or dark urine.

Gallstones are hard lumps of cholesterol or bile salts that collect in the gallbladder. This small pear-shaped organ holds bile, a digestive juice. The stones can be as little as a grain of salt or as large as a lime. Most cause no harm and no symptoms.

A gallstone attack occurs when a stone gets trapped in one of the bile ducts (the tubes that carry bile from the gallbladder to the small intestine). You may have an attack a few hours after a big meal or during the night. Attacks can last several hours. Gallstones may cause jaundice if bile backs up into the liver.

Gallstones may run in families. They are found most often among American Indians and Mexican Americans. You're more likely to have them if you're overweight or obese, eat a lot of fatty foods, or lose a lot of weight quickly. Women are at higher risk than men, especially pregnant women and women who use birth control pills or estrogen replacement therapy. For everyone, risk rises with age.

Treatment for repeated, painful attacks is often surgery to remove the gallbladder. This procedure is simpler for the patient than it used to be, with less pain and a quicker recovery.

WHAT YOU CAN DO NOW

➤ If you have symptoms of a gallstone attack, get medical help right away. In the meantime, do not eat or drink.

WHEN TO CALL THE DOCTOR

Call 911 **right away:**

➤ If you have sudden, squeezing pain in the upper abdomen and are also nauseated, sweating, and short of breath. You may be having a heart attack.

Call for emergency advice (if you can't get any, call 911 or go to an emergency room):

➤ If you think you are having your first gall-stone attack or if you have fever along with the pain.

Call for a prompt appointment:

➤ If you notice a yellow cast to the skin and eyes (jaundice).

➤ If you have been told that you have gall-stones, and you have sharp abdominal pain that lasts more than 2 hours.

HOW TO PREVENT IT

➤ Keep to your ideal body weight (see **maintain a healthy weight,** page 295).

➤ Ask your doctor before trying to lose weight, and diet with common sense.

➤ Some experts say you can cut the risk of gallstones with a diet that is high in fiber and low in fat and cholesterol.

FOR MORE HELP

Key Websites: *www.SavonHealth.com.* For more information on gallstones: *www.SavonGallstones.com.*

Organizations: American Gastroenterological Association, 7910 Woodmont Ave.,

7th Floor, Bethesda, MD 20814. 301-654-2055, M–F 8:30–5 EST; *www.gastro.org/digestinfo.html.* Visit the online Digestive Health Resource Center.

■ National Digestive Diseases Information Clearinghouse, 2 Information Way, Bethesda, MD 20892-3570. 301-654-3810, M–F 8:30–5 EST; *www.niddk.nih.gov/health/digest/pubs/gastn/gallstns.htm* for an online brochure on gallstones.

Book: *Indigestion: Living Better With Upper Intestinal Problems From Heartburn to Ulcers and Gallstones,* by Henry D. Janowitz, M.D. Offers a chapter on the causes of and treatments for gallstones. Oxford University Press, 1994, $11.95.

Gas & Gas Pain
www.SavonGas.com

SIGNS AND SYMPTOMS

■ Burping.
■ Passing gas.
■ Pain or bloating in the abdomen.

Gas and gas pains are normal. They're often caused by air you swallow if you eat and drink too fast. Gas is also made by the food you're digesting. High-fiber foods such as beans, vegetables, fruits, and grains can create a lot of gas. So can dairy foods for some people.

When air goes into your stomach, you may get rid of it by burping, which is natural and healthy—though not always polite. Even less polite is passing gas through the anus (flatulence). But what many people think of as lots of gas may be normal. In fact, most adults pass gas from 8 to 20 times a day.

WHAT YOU CAN DO NOW

➤ Try teas made with anise, peppermint, chamomile, or fennel to relieve gas pains.

➤ Take simethicone to help reduce gas.

➤ If you need to release gas, do it—even if you have to leave the room.

Gallstones

Stones may cause no symptoms if they stay in the gallbladder or travel freely through the bile duct. Trouble occurs when they get stuck in the duct.

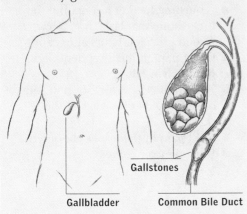

Gallstones

Gallbladder   Common Bile Duct

STOMACH, ABDOMEN & DIGESTIVE SYSTEM

➤ If you have severe gas pains, try lying on your back and pulling your legs up to your chest. It's easier to expel the gas this way.

WHEN TO CALL THE DOCTOR

Call for emergency advice. If you can't get any, call 911 or go to an emergency room:

➤ If you have severe pain that starts close to the navel and moves to the lower right area of the abdomen; this could be a sign of **appendicitis** (see page 24).

Call for a prompt appointment:

➤ If you notice pain in the upper right part of the abdomen; this may be a sign of a gallbladder problem (see **gallstones,** page 122) or an **ulcer** (see page 134).

Call for advice:

➤ If you have long-lasting bloating for more than 3 days for no known reason.

➤ If you have less pain in the lower abdomen after passing gas or having a bowel movement; you may have **irritable bowel syndrome** (see page 130).

➤ If you have gas often, have lost weight, and have oily, light-colored, bad-smelling bowel movements; you could be unable to digest fat.

HOW TO PREVENT IT

You can most likely avoid too much gas and gas pains simply by changing your diet. Keep in mind, though, that the high-fiber foods that often cause gas are also those most vital to a healthy diet. Rather than cutting down on fruits, vegetables, beans, and whole grains, try these changes:

➤ Buy dry beans rather than canned. Soak them overnight in water, then pour out the water and replace it with fresh water for cooking. Make sure to cook the beans until they're soft.

➤ If you do use canned beans, rinse them first. Adding Beano, an over-the-counter digestive aid, also helps.

➤ For a good source of protein, try tofu, a soy food; it's easier to digest than many beans are.

➤ Drink plenty of fluids.

➤ Avoid foods and snacks sweetened with fructose (fruit sugar) or sorbitol (an artifi-

cial sweetener). Both can increase gas.

➤ Eat slowly, chew your food well, and don't overeat. (It may take 20 to 30 minutes to feel full.)

➤ Take a walk after meals. Mild exercise improves digestion and helps move gas through your system more quickly.

➤ Avoid carbonated drinks and don't chew gum or drink through a straw; these may put extra air into your stomach.

FOR MORE HELP

Key Websites: *www.SavonHealth.com.* For more information on gas pain: *www.SavonGas.com.*

Organizations: American Dietetic Association, 216 W. Jackson Blvd., Chicago, IL 60606-6995. 800-366-1655, M–F 9–4 CST; *www.eatright.org.* Call for a recorded message about nutrition or, for a fee, to speak with a registered dietitian who answers questions about gas and gives you names of dietitians near you.

■ National Digestive Diseases Information Clearinghouse, 2 Information Way, Bethesda, MD 20892-3570. 301-654-3810, M–F 8:30–5 EST; *www.niddk.nih.gov/health/digest/pubs/gas/gas.htm* for an online bro- chure on gas and dietary advice.

Heartburn
www.SavonHeartburn.com

SIGNS AND SYMPTOMS

■ A burning feeling just behind the breastbone that lasts from a few minutes to a few hours after eating.

■ Chest pain, often after bending over or lying down.

■ Burning in the throat; or hot, sour, or salty fluid at the back of the throat.

■ Mild pain in the upper abdomen.

■ Burping (sometimes).

Heartburn has nothing to do with the heart. Also known as acid indigestion and sometimes gastroesophageal reflux disease, heartburn is caused by stomach acid backing up into the lower esophagus (the muscular tube that leads from the throat to the stomach).

It can be triggered by overeating or by too much pressure on the abdomen, often from being overweight or pregnant. A hiatal **hernia** (see page 127) that squeezes part of the stomach up through the diaphragm can also cause it. Eating spicy, acidic, or fatty foods can lead to heartburn, as can drinking alcohol. So can certain medicines such as aspirin, ibuprofen, and some antibiotics and other prescription drugs. Smoking also prompts the release of stomach acid.

Heartburn is common. If you have it often, it may cause serious problems, such as bleeding or scarring in the esophagus. It isn't dangerous, though, if it happens only once in a while. Medication or changes in your lifestyle will most likely take care of it.

WHAT YOU CAN DO NOW

Many doctors advise taking over-the-counter aids such as antacids or acid blockers for heartburn that happens now and then. Take them before eating if you get it often. But check with your doctor before taking antacids if you have **high blood pressure** (see page 111), an irregular heartbeat, kidney disease, intestinal problems, chronic heartburn, or any symptoms of **appendicitis** (see page 24). Pregnant women and nursing mothers should ask their doctors before taking any medicine, including antacids.
Try these treatments instead of medications:
➤ Drink 1 teaspoon baking soda mixed into 1 cup water.
➤ Avoid lying down for 2 to 3 hours after eating. If you must recline, lie on your left side; in this position, your stomach is lower than your esophagus, so the acids are less likely to back up.
➤ Don't exercise for an hour after eating.
➤ Don't smoke. Avoid smoky places.
➤ Cut down on coffee and alcohol.
➤ Raise the head of your bed 4 to 6 inches by putting something such as bricks or

phone books under the legs, or by placing a foam-rubber wedge under your pillows.
➤ Don't wear tight clothes such as girdles, snug jeans, or belts.

WHEN TO CALL THE DOCTOR

Call 911 **right away:**
➤ If you have sharp chest pain or pain that goes into your arms and shoulders. This could signal a heart attack.
Call for advice:
➤ If you've tried the tips above, but your symptoms persist.

HOW TO PREVENT IT

Many of the treatments for heartburn will also help prevent it. In addition:
➤ Keep to your ideal body weight (see **maintain a healthy weight,** page 295).
➤ Avoid foods and drinks that can set off the problem. These may include tomatoes, citrus fruits, garlic, onions, chocolate, coffee and tea, alcohol, peppermint-flavored food, and carbonated drinks.
➤ Cut down on dishes that are high in fats and oils.
➤ Eat small meals often (4 or 5 a day) instead of 3 large ones.
➤ Avoid eating just before bedtime or before you exercise.
➤ Get plenty of rest and exercise.
➤ Don't smoke. Nicotine prompts the release of stomach acid, and relaxes a muscle that allows gastric juice to back up from the stomach into the esophagus.
➤ Avoid aspirin, ibuprofen, and other non-steroidal anti-inflammatory drugs. Try acetaminophen (see **pain relief,** page 315).

COMPLEMENTARY CHOICES

➤ For quick relief, drink ginger tea or take capsules of gingerroot.
➤ Drink teas of aromatic herbs such as catnip and fennel.
➤ Try stress-reduction techniques such as yoga and meditation. Acupuncture may also be helpful. (See **how to choose a natural healer,** page 310.)

STOMACH, ABDOMEN & DIGESTIVE SYSTEM

FOR MORE HELP

Key Websites: *www.SavonHealth.com.* For more information on heartburn: *www.SavonHeartburn.com.*

Organizations: American Dietetic Association, 216 W. Jackson Blvd., Chicago, IL 60606-6995. 800-366-1655, M–F 9–4 CST; *www.eatright.org.* Call for a recorded message about nutrition or, for a fee, to speak with a registered dietitian who answers questions about heartburn and gives you names of dietitians near you.

■ National Digestive Diseases Information Clearinghouse, 2 Information Way, Bethesda, MD 20892-3570. 301-654-3810, M–F 8:30–5 EST; *www.niddk.nih.gov/health/digest/pubs/hearbrn/heartbrn.htm* for an online brochure about heartburn (gastroesophageal reflux disease). Call or write for a free fact sheet.

Book: *The Fire Inside,* by M. Michael Wolfe, M.D., and Thomas Nesi. Provides facts and advice on heartburn. W. W. Norton, 1996, $23.

Hemorrhoids
www.SavonHemorrhoids.com

SIGNS AND SYMPTOMS

■ Stools with red blood, or blood on toilet paper or in toilet bowl.
■ Painful bowel movements.
■ Lump near the anus, or a swelling that hurts.
■ Itching in or near the anus.
■ Mucus coming from the anus.

Hemorrhoids are inflamed or swollen veins either inside or outside the anus. Also known as piles, they may result from straining to pass hard stools during bouts of **constipation** (see page 116). Other causes may include your genes, aging, pregnancy, chronic diarrhea, and the overuse of laxatives. The pain often lingers for many days and recurs. Still, home treatment can help.

WHAT YOU CAN DO NOW

➤ Try a sitz bath: Sit in warm water for 10 to 15 minutes every few hours. After a bowel movement is a good time.
➤ Bathe often so your anus stays clean, but be careful when washing the area. Don't scrub the skin. Pat dry.
➤ Wipe gently. Try cotton balls, alcohol-free baby wipes, or damp toilet paper. Avoid scented or colored toilet paper.
➤ Many times a day, dab hemorrhoids on the outside of the anus with witch hazel or soothe them with a cold compress.
➤ To ease painful bowel movements, place a bit of petroleum jelly inside and around the edge of the anus.
➤ Try an over-the-counter stool softener.
➤ Use suppositories for pain, but avoid ointments with a local numbing agent (you'll see "caine" in the name or on the label). These can cause more soreness.
➤ Don't scratch hemorrhoids. You'll make them worse. Try 0.5 percent hydrocortisone cream, sold in drugstores, to relieve itching.

WHEN TO CALL THE DOCTOR

➤ If bleeding persists for more than a few days. You could have a more serious problem, such as colon cancer.
➤ If you have lasting or severe pain. You may need outpatient surgery to remove or shrink the hemorrhoids.

HOW TO PREVENT IT

➤ For softer, more easily passed stools, eat plenty of fruits, vegetables, bran cereals, and whole grain bread. (If you are pregnant, ask your doctor before making any changes in your diet.) Drink lots of liquids (at least 8 big glasses a day) such as water or fruit and vegetable juices.
➤ Cut back on meat, animal fat, and alcohol.
➤ Set a regular time for your bowel movements. Also, don't sit on the toilet for more than 5 or 10 minutes.
➤ If you sit all day at work, take breaks to walk around. Long periods of sitting reduce blood flow around the anus.
➤ Don't sit on a "doughnut" cushion; these can trap blood in the swollen veins.

FOR MORE HELP

Key Websites: *www.SavonHealth.com*. For more information on hemorrhoids: *www.SavonHemorrhoids.com*.

Organizations: American Dietetic Association, 216 W. Jackson Blvd., Chicago, IL 60606-6995. 800-366-1655, M–F 9–4 CST; *www.eatright.org*. Call for a recorded message about nutrition or, for a fee, to speak with a registered dietitian who answers questions about hemorrhoids and gives you names of dietitians near you.

■ American Gastroenterological Association, 7910 Woodmont Ave., 7th Floor, Bethesda, MD 20814. 301-654-2055, M–F 8:30–5 EST; *www.gastro.org/digestinfo.html*. At Website, click on *Hemorrhoids.*

■ National Digestive Diseases Information Clearinghouse, 2 Information Way, Bethesda, MD 20892-3570. 301-654-3810, M–F 8:30–5 EST; *www.niddk.nih.gov/health/digest/pubs/hems/hemords.htm* for an online brochure on hemorrhoids.

Hernia
www.SavonHernia.com

SIGNS AND SYMPTOMS

■ Swelling under the skin in the abdomen or groin. May be tender. May not show when you lie down.

■ Fullness or heaviness in the abdomen, sometimes with constipation.

■ While lifting or bending, pain or ache in groin or abdomen.

■ In severe cases, pain in the abdomen, nausea, and vomiting.

■ Chronic heartburn, belching, or stomach fluids backing up into the throat. These could signal a hiatal hernia, which occurs when part of the stomach or lower esophagus squeezes into the chest cavity.

A hernia is a bulge, often visible, that is caused by a lump of tissue poking through a hole or weak area in a nearby muscle. Although hernias can occur in many

An Abdominal Exercise

Here's a quick and easy exercise you can do every day to strengthen your stomach muscles and help prevent abdominal hernias: Lie down with knees bent and feet flat on the floor. Cross your arms over your chest. Raise your shoulders a couple of inches off the floor; hold for a count of 5; lie back down. Repeat 5 times at first, more after a few weeks when you're stronger.

places in the body, they are most common in the abdominal wall. Pressure on a weak point—from extra body weight, from lifting a heavy object, or from straining during bowel movements—can force a split in an abdominal muscle, or between muscles. This allows part of an internal organ to push its way through.

Ninety percent of all abdominal hernias occur in men. Some people are born with a weakness in the muscle, which allows a hernia to form. More often, it occurs later in life. Poor diet, excess pounds, smoking, and muscle strain or overexertion can all make hernias more likely.

Most hernias can simply be pushed back into place, by you or by a doctor. But they will protrude again. If the hernia is part of an intestine poking through the abdominal wall, the intestine could become blocked; the result will be pain, nausea, and vomiting. Another danger is a strangulated hernia, when tissue around the bulging organ squeezes it and cuts off its blood supply. If the hernia isn't treated, a serious infection can destroy tissue in the bowel.

The 4 types of abdominal hernia that occur most often are: *Inguinal,* in the groin. Pain is rarely the main symptom, though you may have a heavy feeling in the groin after standing up for a while. *Femoral,* also in the groin but slightly lower than the inguinal; it may cause no symptoms and give no trouble unless it becomes blocked or strangulated. *Paraumbilical,* near the navel. It may or may not be painful. *Epigastric,* between the breastbone and the navel; part of the sheet of fat that covers the intestines pushes through a weak point between muscles. The lump is most often small, but it may be sore.

In many cases, even hernias that aren't serious slowly get worse and may require surgery.

WHAT YOU CAN DO NOW

➤ Call your doctor if you think you may have a hernia. Some hernias need care right away.

➤ Don't strain or lift anything heavy.

WHEN TO CALL THE DOCTOR

Call 911 or go to an emergency room **right away:**

➤ If you have a hernia, and you are nauseated and vomiting or can't have a bowel movement or pass gas. You may have a blocked or strangulated hernia.

Call for advice:

➤ If you suspect you have a hernia.

HOW TO PREVENT IT

➤ If you are overweight, lose some weight to ease the pressure on your abdominal muscles.

➤ Avoid lifting heavy objects.

➤ Don't strain when having a bowel movement (see **constipation,** page 116).

➤ Eat well to avoid constipation.

➤ Don't smoke, and avoid smoky places. Chronic coughing from smoke or other agents makes a hernia more likely and also can make one recur.

➤ Do gentle exercises daily to tone and strengthen your abdominal muscles.

FOR MORE HELP

Key Websites: *www.SavonHealth.com.* For more information on hernia: *www.SavonHernia.com.*

Organizations: The Hernia Hotline, 800-437-6427, M–F 8:30–4:30 EST. Sends a brochure on hernias and lists doctors.

■ National Digestive Diseases Information Clearinghouse, 2 Information Way,

Bethesda, MD 20892-3570. 301-654-3810, M–F 8:30–5 EST; *www.niddk.nih.gov/health/digest/summary/-inhernia/inhernia.htm* for an online brochure on inguinal hernias.

Website: Hernia Resource Center, *www.herniainfo.com.* Answers common questions about hernias, talks about surgery options, and lists doctors near you.

Book: *Indigestion: Living Better With Upper Intestinal Problems,* by Henry D. Janowitz, M.D. Covers hernias. Oxford University Press, 1994, $11.95.

Inflammatory Bowel Disease
www.SavonIBD.com

SIGNS AND SYMPTOMS

Most common:
■ Abdominal pain (in Crohn's disease, often in the lower right side of the abdomen; in ulcerative colitis, in the left side).
■ Stubborn, severe diarrhea.
■ Awakening during the night for bowel movements.
■ Bloody stools or rectal bleeding.

Less common:
■ Pus or mucus in stools.
■ Fever.
■ Fatigue and weakness.
■ Skin rashes.
■ Arthritis-like pains in the joints.
■ Weight loss.

Inflammatory bowel disease (IBD) is the name given to a group of chronic intestinal ailments. They share a number of symptoms and complications. The most common are Crohn's disease and ulcerative colitis.

In Crohn's disease, parts of the digestive tract (see color illustration, page 174) become inflamed, making digestion hard and weakening the body. In ulcerative colitis, tiny sores in the colon flare up and sometimes cause bloody stools or painful attacks

Do You Have a Parasite?

Parasitic illnesses such as giardiasis or amebiasis can cause symptoms much like those of IBD. So can certain bacterial illnesses. Parasites and bacteria often enter the body through bad food or water. If you have been traveling, camping, or drinking untreated water, or have any other reason to suspect an intestinal parasite, ask your doctor about a stool test.

of diarrhea. Both can be serious, but only in rare cases are they fatal.

The cause of IBD is unknown. Anyone can get it, including young children, but most cases occur in people ages 15 to 40. Although there is no known cure, new treatments are being tested. Minor changes in diet and the right medication can often control the symptoms. Some severe cases of IBD call for surgery to remove the diseased part of the bowel.

Both the symptoms and the severity of IBD are hard to predict. See your doctor if you suspect you have IBD; proper treatment can keep it under control.

WHAT YOU CAN DO NOW

➤ If you have many bouts of diarrhea, be careful not to let yourself get dehydrated (see **diarrhea,** page 119).
➤ Maintain a balanced diet. Diarrhea and poor digestion rob the body of vital fluids and nutrients.
➤ Avoid foods that irritate the colon. If you suspect a food, don't eat it for 10 to 30 days. Then try it. If your symptoms flare up, stay away from that food. (Common irritants are spicy or high-fiber foods, dairy products, eggs, and wheat.)
➤ Avoid alcohol.
➤ Avoid aspirin, ibuprofen, and other anti-inflammatory drugs.
➤ Because you may be at greater risk of colon cancer, talk about routine screening with your doctor (see **tests,** page 319).
➤ Reduce **stress** (see page 218).

WHEN TO CALL THE DOCTOR

Call for a prompt appointment:
➤ If you have a sudden attack of abdominal pain, fever, and the urge to pass gas or to have a bowel movement. You may be in the first stages of **appendicitis** (see page 24).
➤ If you have rectal bleeding with clots of blood in your stool; this could be a severe stage of colitis.
Call for advice:
➤ If diarrhea lasts more than 48 hours. You may be at risk of dehydration.
➤ If you have the most common signs of IBD. These could point to other ailments as well, such as the less serious **irritable bowel syndrome** (see page 130).

HOW TO PREVENT IT

There is no known way to prevent Crohn's disease or ulcerative colitis. But it may help to stay away from foods that have given you trouble (see What You Can Do Now, left).

FOR MORE HELP

Key Websites: *www.SavonHealth.com*. For more information on inflammatory bowel disease: *www.SavonIBD.com*.

Organizations: Crohn's and Colitis Foundation of America, 386 Park Ave. S., New York, NY 10016. 800-932-2423, M–F 9–5 EST; *www.ccfa.org*. Offers referrals to specialists and support groups. Ask for a free fact packet.

■ Intestinal Disease Foundation, 1323 Forbes Ave., Suite 200, Pittsburgh, PA 15219. 412-261-5888, M–F 9–5 EST. Provides telephone support, educational programs and readings, advice on support groups, and lists of doctors.

Books: *Inflammatory Bowel Disease: A Guide for Patients & Their Families*, 2nd edition, by Stanley H. Stein, M.D., and Stephen B. Hanauer, M.D., F.A.C.P. The official patient guide of the Crohn's and Colitis Foundation of America. Lippincott, Williams & Wilkin, 1998, $22.

■ *Your Gut Feelings*, by Henry D. Janowitz, M.D. Covers intestinal problems, including inflammatory bowel disease. Oxford University Press, 1994, $13.95.

STOMACH, ABDOMEN & DIGESTIVE SYSTEM

Irritable Bowel Syndrome

www.SavonIrritableBowelSyndrome.com

SIGNS AND SYMPTOMS

Symptoms of irritable bowel syndrome (IBS) can differ greatly from one person to another but may include:

- Diarrhea or constipation, or both back and forth over a few months.
- Mucus strands in stools.
- Abdominal cramps or pain.
- Lots of gas or bloating.
- Nausea, most often after eating.
- Headaches, fatigue, feeling anxious or depressed.
- A feeling that bowel movements aren't complete.

As you digest your food, your intestinal tract moves it along with waves of muscle contractions. Irritable bowel syndrome occurs when these movements lose their rhythm and upset the process. IBS, also called spastic colon, is the most common digestive ailment, affecting at least 10 to 15 percent of adults at some time. It does not lead to any fatal bowel diseases. It can be hard to treat, though, because no one is sure what causes it. Some experts think it is brought on—or made worse—by **stress** (see page 218) or by a poor diet. There also appears to be a link between IBS and **panic disorder** (see page 208).

WHAT YOU CAN DO NOW

If you have symptoms of IBS, see your doctor. He or she may want you to have some tests, such as a barium enema and X-ray, to rule out more serious ailments (see **abdominal pain** chart, page 117). In the meantime, self-care can help:

- If you have **constipation** or **diarrhea,** see page 116 or 119.
- Keep a record of what you eat and note which foods seem to cause problems. Avoid those foods if you can.
- Change your diet. Cut down on fatty foods. See if it helps to avoid items that can cause

problems, such as eggs, dairy foods, spicy foods, cabbage and broccoli, caffeine, and diet foods with sorbitol (an artificial sweetener).

- Try slowly adding more high-fiber foods to your diet (raw fruits and vegetables, bran, whole wheat, and beans). Some people find this helps, but others find it can make the problem worse.
- Eat smaller meals 4 or 5 times a day to make digestion easier.
- Don't smoke. Avoid smoky places.
- Include exercise and relaxation in your daily life.
- Seek therapy or try a stress-reduction program if you suspect that stress is a cause of the problem (see **is stress putting your health at risk?** page 302).

WHEN TO CALL THE DOCTOR

Call for a prompt appointment:

- If you notice pain in your lower left abdomen, with fever and maybe a change in your bowel movement pattern; **diverticulitis** may be the problem (see page 121).
- If you get a fever with diarrhea, or you wake up during the night with diarrhea and you have been losing weight. These may be signs of **inflammatory bowel disease** (see page 128).

Call for advice and an appointment:

- If your stools have blood or mucus, if your stools look different, or if you notice a change in how often you have bowel movements. You may have colon polyps or colon cancer.
- If any bowel problems get in the way of your normal daily life.

HOW TO PREVENT IT

- The causes of irritable bowel syndrome are unknown, so the best approach is to take care of yourself by eating well and easing stress.

COMPLEMENTARY CHOICES

- Take 1 or 2 coated peppermint-oil capsules between meals, 3 times a day, or drink peppermint tea.
- Take gingerroot capsules or drink ginger

Rectal Bleeding & Itching

Itching and bleeding in and around the anus often signal an ailment you can cure fairly easily with home care or some help from your doctor. Even blood on the stools doesn't always mean a bad illness. Some bleeding and itching, however, does require prompt medical help.

SYMPTOMS	WHAT IT MIGHT BE	WHAT YOU CAN DO
Bloody stools, painful abdominal cramping and swelling, nausea and vomiting, constipation, weakness or dizziness.	Intestinal obstruction—blockage of small or large intestine. ■ Scarring from abdominal surgery. ■ Strangulated hernia (see page 127). ■ Colon cancer. ■ Diverticulitis (see page 121). ■ Object in digestive tract.	Call 911 or go to emergency room **right away.**
Bright red bleeding from the rectum after injury, anal intercourse, or putting an object into rectum.	Tear in sphincter muscle or skin around anus.	Call doctor for emergency advice. If you can't get one, call 911 or go to emergency room **right away.**
Watery diarrhea with blood, mucus, or pus; abdominal cramps or pain; nausea and vomiting; fever; muscle aches or pain; rapid dehydration and weight loss.	Dysentery—bacterial infection of intestinal tract. You can catch it from others and pass it on to someone else.	Call doctor for prompt appointment. Drink lots of fluids, and don't take over-the-counter stomach medications.
Painful anal itching at night, often in children; restless sleep and bad temper.	Pinworms—common intestinal parasites.	Call doctor for advice and appointment. If you're given antiworm medication, follow directions carefully.
Painful or hard bowel movements, soreness in rectal area, blood or mucus from rectum, abdominal cramps, constipation.	Proctitis—swelling of rectum and anal tissues. ■ Bacterial or viral infection. ■ Inflammatory bowel disease (see page 128). ■ Sexually transmitted disease (see chart, page 221). ■ Colon cancer. ■ Injury from anal intercourse.	Call doctor for advice and appointment. Take warm baths often to ease pain. Eat high-fiber foods and drink at least 8 glasses of water a day to soften stools.

(continued)

STOMACH, ABDOMEN & DIGESTIVE SYSTEM

Rectal Bleeding & Itching (continued)

SYMPTOMS	WHAT IT MIGHT BE	WHAT YOU CAN DO
Bloody stools, diarrhea that won't go away, nausea, cramps or pain in lower right side of abdomen.	Crohn's disease.	See inflammatory bowel disease, page 128.
Repeated bouts of diarrhea with mucus and blood, pain in left side of abdomen that lessens after bowel movements.	Ulcerative colitis.	See inflammatory bowel disease, page 128.
Itching in anal area or bright red blood in stool, pain during or after bowel movements.	Inflamed blood vessels in anus (see hemorrhoids, page 126). ■ Split or tear in skin around anus (anal fissure). ■ Psoriasis (see page 159).	Take warm baths, especially after painful bowel movements. Include lots of fiber and plenty of fluids in diet (see constipation, page 116). See doctor if it persists.
Itching around anus.	Often no clear cause. In older people, may be dry skin that comes with aging.	After bowel movements, gently clean anal area with moist, undyed tissue or baby wipes. Avoid soap, which can make itching worse.

tea to soothe the intestinal tract. Chamomile, valerian, and rosemary teas also help reduce spasms.

➤ Practice relaxation techniques such as yoga and meditation. Acupressure and acupuncture may also reduce symptoms. (See page 310 for tips on finding a reliable acupuncturist.)

FOR MORE HELP

Key Websites: *www.SavonHealth.com*. For more information on irritable bowel syndrome: *www.SavonIrritableBowelSyndrome.com*.

Organizations: American Gastroenterological Association, 7910 Woodmont Ave., 7th Floor, Bethesda, MD 20814. 301-654-2055, M–F 8:30–5 EST; *www.gastro.org/digestinfo.html*. At Website, click on *Gas in the Digestive Tract*.

■ International Foundation for Functional Gastrointestinal Disorders, P.O. Box 170864, Milwaukee, WI 53217-8076. 888-964-2001, M–F 8:30–5 CST; *www.iffgd.org*. Provides support and brochures on bowel problems.

■ Intestinal Disease Foundation, 1323 Forbes Ave., Suite 200, Pittsburgh, PA 15219. 412-261-5888, M–F 9–5 EST. Offers telephone support, educational programs and fact packets, advice on support groups, and names of doctors near you.

■ National Digestive Diseases Information Clearinghouse, 2 Information Way, Bethesda, MD 20892-3570. 301-654-3810, M–F 8:30–5 EST; *www.niddk.nih.gov/health/digest/pubs/irrbowel/irrbowel.htm* for an online brochure on irritable bowel syndrome.

Newsletter: *Nutrition Action*, from the Center for Science in the Public Interest, 1875 Connecticut Ave. NW, Suite 300, Washington, DC 20009-5728. 202-332-9110,

M–F 9–5 EST; *www.cspinet.org*. $24 per year (10 issues). Offers clear, useful advice on good nutrition and diet.

Books: *Good Food for Bad Stomachs,* by Henry D. Janowitz, M.D. Provides sample dietary programs to help avoid irritable bowel syndrome and other intestinal problems. Oxford University Press, 1998, $13.95.

■ *Your Gut Feelings,* by Henry D. Janowitz, M.D. Facts about intestinal problems, including irritable bowel syndrome. Oxford University Press, 1994, $13.95.

Nausea & Vomiting
www.SavonNauseaandVomiting.com

SIGNS AND SYMPTOMS

Nausea and vomiting sometimes happen with:
■ Diarrhea.
■ Abdominal cramps or pain.
■ Fever, weakness, and fatigue.
■ Headache.
■ Loss of appetite.

Although nausea and vomiting are common and usually aren't serious, they can worry you. In children and young adults, they most often result from the viral infection commonly called stomach flu. In these cases, vomiting and diarrhea often go away within 2 or 3 days, but weakness and fatigue may last about a week.

In older people, medicines and ulcers are more often the culprits (see **ulcers and gastritis,** page 134). Less common causes are bacterial and parasitic infections (see **do you have a parasite?** box, page 129), food **allergies** (see page 84), and drinking too much alcohol.

Another cause is **food poisoning** (see page 34), which you can get from eating food tainted with viruses, bacteria, or chemicals. In this case, you could also have abdominal cramps and diarrhea, headache, dizziness, or fever and chills. The vomiting may leave you dehydrated.

Mild food poisoning lasts only a few hours or at worst a day or two, but some types—such as botulism and certain forms of chemical poisoning—are severe and may be fatal unless you get prompt treatment.

WHAT YOU CAN DO NOW

If you think you might have severe food poisoning or chemical poisoning:
➤ Call the local poison control center listed in the front of your phone book. Trained staff members can help you decide whether you need medical help. (If you can't find the local center in your phone book, call information, a local hospital, or 911.)
➤ For food poisoning, ask others who ate the same food whether they got sick. Try to get a sample of the food, which can be tested if your symptoms get worse or don't go away.

If you have mild vomiting and diarrhea:
➤ It's best not to take over-the-counter antinausea or antidiarrhea medication for 24 hours, unless a doctor advises it. Vomiting and diarrhea are the body's way of getting rid of whatever is causing the problem. But if you do need relief after a few hours, it's safe to take Pepto-Bismol (it will turn your stools black). Also, children may need medication because they become dehydrated more quickly.
➤ Sip clear fluids. Suck on ice chips or Popsicles if nothing will stay down.
➤ Once you can keep fluid in your stomach, drink clear liquids for the next 12 hours or so. Then, for a full day, eat bland foods—such as rice, cooked cereals, baked potatoes, and clear soups—if your stomach will take them.
➤ Watch for signs of dehydration, especially in infants, children, and older adults. You can lose lots of fluid from repeated vomiting. Symptoms include dry mouth, sticky saliva, dizziness or weakness, dark yellow urine, and sometimes extreme thirst. For advice about replacing lost fluids, see **diarrhea,** page 119. If you can't keep liquids down and are becoming badly dehydrated, you will need to go to a hospital to get enough fluids into your body.
➤ Get plenty of rest until symptoms are completely gone.

STOMACH, ABDOMEN & DIGESTIVE SYSTEM

WHEN TO CALL THE DOCTOR

Call 911 or go to an emergency room **right away:**

➤ If, along with vomiting and abdominal pain, you have blurred vision; muscle weakness; a hard time breathing, speaking, or swallowing; or trouble moving or feeling your muscles. These may be signs of botulism, a rare but sometimes fatal type of bacterial food poisoning.

➤ If you have symptoms of chemical food poisoning—vomiting, diarrhea, sweating, dizziness, very teary eyes, great amounts of saliva, mental confusion, and stomach pain—about 30 minutes after eating. Pesticides or tainted food may be to blame. This type of poisoning can be deadly.

➤ If you vomit blood or anything that looks like coffee grounds. These are signs of bleeding in the esophagus or stomach.

Call for a prompt appointment:

➤ If you have bloody or black, tarry stools. This can signal internal bleeding.

➤ If you develop signs of dehydration—dry mouth, sticky saliva, dizziness or weakness, dark yellow urine, and, sometimes, extreme thirst. Dehydration is very serious in infants.

➤ If you have intense pain or swelling in the abdomen, rectum, or anus. You may have an abdominal disorder (see **abdominal pain** chart, page 117).

Call for advice:

➤ If your symptoms come back after treatment; you may have another problem such as an intestinal parasite (see **do you have a parasite?** box on page 129).

➤ If your vomiting and diarrhea are severe and last longer than 2 or 3 days.

➤ If you have a fever of 101.5 or higher.

➤ If you think a prescribed drug might be the cause.

HOW TO PREVENT IT

To avoid catching viral stomach flu:

➤ Keep your immune system strong with plenty of rest, exercise, and a healthy diet.

➤ Wash your hands often.

To prevent food poisoning:

➤ Don't thaw frozen meat on the kitchen counter. Let meat thaw in the refrigerator, or thaw it quickly in a microwave oven and cook it right away. Be sure that frozen food (especially poultry) is fully thawed or defrosted before cooking. This will help it cook all the way through so that the heat can kill any bacteria.

➤ Quickly refrigerate food that can spoil. Set your refrigerator at 37 degrees, and never eat cooked meat or dairy foods that have been out of a refrigerator longer than 2 hours.

➤ Avoid raw meat, fish, or eggs. Cook all these foods well.

➤ At picnics (or anywhere else), don't eat moist foods that have been out 2 hours or more, or long enough to become warm.

➤ Using soap and hot water, wash your hands and any utensils, cutting boards, or countertops that are touched by uncooked meat, fish, or poultry.

➤ Be sure that all members of your household wash their hands with soap and water after using the toilet and before fixing food or eating.

➤ Don't eat any food that looks or smells spoiled, or any food in bulging cans or cracked jars—a sign that the contents have gone bad.

➤ Don't eat any wild berries, mushrooms, or other plants unless you know for sure what they are.

Ulcers & Gastritis
www.SavonGastritis.com

SIGNS AND SYMPTOMS

- Pain in the upper abdomen.
- Nausea.
- Vomiting.
- Loss of appetite.
- Belching or gas.
- Heartburn.
- Dark or bloody stools.

Stomach ulcers are sometimes called peptic ulcers. They are holes or breaks in the lining of the stomach, in the esophagus (the tube between the throat and the stomach), or in the duodenum (the upper part of the small intestine). Experts used to blame most ulcers on stress, but now the prime suspect is a germ—a common bacterium called *Helicobacter pylori*. Overuse of painkillers such as aspirin and ibuprofen can also cause ulcers. Other factors may include:

➤ **Stress** (see page 218).
➤ Smoking and heavy drinking.
➤ Too much stomach acid.
➤ Too little mucus to protect the stomach lining.

Stomach ulcers are fairly easy to treat. If bacteria are the problem, antibiotics (sometimes with another drug) will take care of them.

The bacteria that cause ulcers can also cause gastritis—inflammation of the stomach lining. In some people, but not all, gastritis may cause symptoms that are like those of indigestion, such as upper abdominal pain, nausea, and vomiting.

Although the symptoms are like those that some people get from overeating or from eating fatty or spicy foods, gastritis is not caused by any of these things.

Your doctor may advise over-the-counter antacids or acid blockers for gastritis that isn't too serious. If he or she suspects bacteria, you will most likely need antibiotics. Untreated gastritis can cause severe damage.

WHAT YOU CAN DO NOW

➤ Don't take aspirin, ibuprofen, or other non-steroidal anti-inflammatory drugs. Try acetaminophen instead (see **pain relief** box, page 315).
➤ Drink lots of water and other liquids to prevent dehydration, but avoid milk, which can increase acid.
➤ Take antacids or acid blockers.
➤ Eat smaller meals and eat more often. Stay away from any foods that cause symptoms.
➤ Don't drink alcohol, or don't drink much.
➤ Don't smoke. Avoid smoky places.
➤ Do relaxation or stress-reduction exercises (see **relax,** page 303).

WHEN TO CALL THE DOCTOR

Call 911 or go to an emergency room **right away:**

➤ If you throw up blood or anything that looks like coffee grounds. This is a sign of bleeding in the esophagus or stomach.
➤ If you faint or feel faint, chilly, or sweaty. These may signal blood loss, one cause of shock (see **shock,** page 22).

Call for a prompt appointment:

➤ If you have sharp pain with ulcer symptoms. The ulcer may be perforated—making holes or rips in your stomach or upper intestine.
➤ If you have an ulcer and are weak and pale. You could have anemia from a bleeding ulcer.
➤ If your stools are deep red or black, or have blood on them. These can be signs of internal bleeding.

Call for advice and an appointment:

➤ If you have sharp stomach pain.
➤ If you have symptoms of a stomach ulcer or gastritis that last more than 2 weeks.

HOW TO PREVENT IT

➤ Cut down use of aspirin and ibuprofen.
➤ Avoid foods that upset your stomach.
➤ Do what you can to reduce stress.
➤ To prevent an ulcer from coming back, follow your doctor's advice about any ulcer drugs you are taking.

FOR MORE HELP

Key Websites: *www.SavonHealth.com*. For more information on ulcers and gastritis: *www.SavonGastritis.com*.

Organization: National Digestive Diseases Information Clearinghouse, 2 Information Way, Bethesda, MD 20892-3570. 301-654-3810, M–F 8:30–5 EST; *www.niddk.nih.gov/health/digest/pubs/ulcers/ulcers.htm* for an online brochure on ulcers. Call or write for a free fact sheet and packet on gastritis and the helicobacter bacterium.

Website: Centers for Disease Control and Prevention's fact sheet on peptic ulcers, *www.cdc.gov/ncidod/dbmd/hpylori.htm*.

Book: *Indigestion: Living Better With Upper Intestinal Problems,* by Henry D. Janowitz, M.D. Covers signs and treatment of ulcers. Oxford University Press, 1994, $11.95.

STOMACH, ABDOMEN & DIGESTIVE SYSTEM

Urinary System

Kidney Stones
www.SavonKidneyDiseases.com

SIGNS AND SYMPTOMS

- Sharp pains that come in waves—often on one side of the body—and start in the back below the ribs, then move toward the groin.
- In men, pain in testicles and penis.
- Trouble urinating.
- Urge to urinate often, but trouble passing more than small amounts of urine at a time.
- Dark urine or blood in the urine.
- Nausea and vomiting.

You may have a kidney infection if you also have:

- Fever.
- Pain when you urinate.
- Cloudy urine.

Kidney stones are hard lumps in the kidneys, most often made of excess calcium. The two kidneys filter waste products out of the blood and mix them with water to make urine. Stones that form in a kidney must pass through one of the tubes (ureters) that connect the kidneys to the bladder (see illustration, page 138). From there, the stones can pass out of the body with the urine.

Some stones aren't a problem. But most cause intense pain as they move from a kidney to the bladder—a journey that can take hours, days, or weeks. The pain and other symptoms go away once you pass the stone.

Sometimes a stone gets trapped in a tube leading to the bladder, blocking the flow of urine. Doctors can often destroy such stones with bursts of shock waves that turn the stones into powder, which is then washed out with the urine.

Kidney stones tend to run in families. They're also more common in men than in women. People with **irritable bowel syndrome** (see page 130), Crohn's disease (see **inflammatory bowel disease,** page 128), gout (see **arthritis,** page 182), and chronic urinary tract infections (see **painful urination,** page 138) are among the most likely to get them. Kidney stones are also more common in hot climates than in cool ones: When people sweat a lot and don't drink enough liquid, their urine builds up more of the waste products that turn into stones.

Some researchers think that a bacterium in some people's kidneys may start the stone formation. Further studies could lead to new approaches in preventing kidney stones.

WHAT YOU CAN DO NOW

- ➤ If you're having a kidney stone attack, drink lots of water—at least 8 to 10 large glasses a day. This will help flush the stone out of your system and help keep new ones from forming.
- ➤ Take an over-the-counter painkiller or one prescribed by your doctor (see **pain relief,** page 315).

WHEN TO CALL THE DOCTOR

- ➤ If you feel waves of sharp pain in your back, abdomen, or side.
- ➤ If you have trouble urinating.
- ➤ If you see blood in your urine.
- ➤ If you have fever with your symptoms.

Urinary Problems

Don't ignore these problems. Most can be treated and, with the right care, prevented.

SYMPTOMS	WHAT IT MIGHT BE	WHAT YOU CAN DO
Passing no urine or very little; weight gain and swelling of ankles and face.	Advanced kidney disease. ■ Kidney failure—when both kidneys stop working. ■ Blockage of the tubes that carry urine to the bladder.	Call 911 **right away** if you also have chest pains or trouble breathing. Otherwise, call doctor for prompt appointment.
Urge to urinate often, with extreme thirst.	Diabetes (see page 277). ■ Disorder of pituitary gland, which regulates body's fluid balance.	Call doctor for prompt appointment if you also have fever, chills, nausea, vomiting, low back pain, or extreme thirst. You may also have a kidney infection.
Urge to urinate often, but with only small amounts passed each time.	Infection of bladder or tube that carries urine out of body. ■ Prostate problem (see page 228). ■ Kidney stone (see facing page). ■ Sexually transmitted disease (see chart on page 221). ■ Interstitial cystitis— inflamed bladder wall.	Call doctor for prompt appointment if you also have fever, chills, nausea, vomiting, low back pain, or extreme thirst. You may also have a kidney infection. See painful urination, page 138.
Pain when you urinate.	Infection of bladder or tube that carries urine out of body (see page 175). ■ Kidney stone (see facing page) or other kidney disease. ■ Sexually transmitted disease (see chart on page 221). ■ Pelvic inflammatory disease (see page 236). ■ Prostate problem (see page 228). ■ Vaginal problem (see page 244).	Call doctor for prompt appointment when acute pain starts or when it hurts to urinate. See also painful urination, page 138.
Blood in urine.	Kidney stone (see facing page) or other kidney disease. ■ Prostate problem (see page 228). ■ Bladder infection. ■ Bladder or kidney cancer. ■ Injury to kidneys or bladder.	Call doctor for prompt appointment. See also painful urination, page 138.

URINARY SYSTEM

HOW TO PREVENT IT

Kidney stones can come back. To help prevent them:

➤ Drink at least 3 quarts of water a day—12 8-ounce glasses—and more in hot weather. Drink enough so that your urine has no color.

➤ Ask your doctor about drugs or diet changes that might help.

FOR MORE HELP

Key Websites: *www.SavonHealth.com.* For more information on kidney stones: *www.SavonKidneyStones.com.*

Organizations: National Kidney Foundation, 30 E. 33rd St., New York, NY 10016. 800-622-9010, M–F 8:30–5:30 EST; *www.kidney.org.* Call or write for a brochure on kidney stones.

■ National Kidney and Urologic Diseases Information Clearinghouse, 3 Information Way, Bethesda, MD 20892-3580. 301-654-4415, M–F 8:30–5 EST; *www.niddk.nih.gov.health/kidney/nkudic.htm.*

Kidney Stones

A stone can hurt when it passes through a ureter, the tube that leads from each kidney to the bladder.

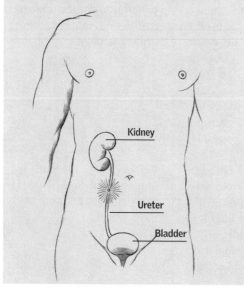

Kidney

Ureter

Bladder

Offers facts about kidney ailments.

Book: *The Kidney Stones Handbook: A Patient's Guide to Hope, Cure, and Prevention,* revised, by Gail Savitz and Stephen W. Leslie, M.D. Four Geez Press, 1999, $17.95.

Painful Urination
www.SavonPainfulUrination.com

SIGNS AND SYMPTOMS

■ Burning or stinging when urinating.

■ Urge to urinate often, but with only small amounts passed each time.

■ Cloudy, strong-smelling, or bloody urine.

■ Yellow discharge from the urinary tube (urethra).

■ Pain in the lower abdomen or lower back.

■ In women, pain during intercourse.

Many problems can make urination painful, but urinary tract infections are the most common.

Although normal urine contains no bacteria, bacteria always live on your skin and in the anal area. These germs can get into the urinary tract and travel up the tube (urethra) between the bladder and the outside of the body. They can then grow in the bladder and cause pain, swelling, and redness. This infection is called cystitis. It's the most common urinary tract infection.

The urethra itself can get infected; so can the kidneys if bacteria reach them.

Adult women are more likely than others to get urinary tract infections. Sexually active women are most at risk. That's because the urethra is near the vagina; during intercourse, germs can move into the urethra, and then to the bladder. Women who use a diaphragm may be more likely than others to get these infections because the device can irritate the urethra.

People with diabetes and weakened immune systems also have a higher risk of infection. So do those with kidney stones or other urinary problems (see **diabetes,** page 277, and

kidney stones, page 136), and people who must use catheters. Risk of a urinary tract infection goes up as you grow older.

Though these infections can be painful, they are easy to cure with antibiotics.

WHAT YOU CAN DO NOW

➤ Drink lots of water in the first 24 hours—at least 8 to 10 glasses, more if you can. Doing so will dilute your urine and help wash out the germs. (But don't drink lots of water if you're going to see the doctor. This can dilute any urine samples you may be asked to give, making it harder to find the cause of your problem.)
➤ When you have symptoms, avoid juices high in acid, such as cranberry juice.
➤ Stay away from drinks with caffeine or alcohol in them, and foods with a lot of spices such as black pepper.
➤ Take a hot bath or use a heating pad to help relieve pain or itching.
➤ Don't have intercourse until all of your symptoms are gone.

WHEN TO CALL THE DOCTOR

Call for a prompt appointment:
➤ If you have a sharp pain that comes in waves, starting in the back below the ribs and moving toward the groin. You may have a kidney stone.
➤ If you have a fever that gets worse quickly, with sudden, intense pain in your back near or above your waistline. You may have a kidney infection.
➤ If your urine looks bloody or very cloudy.
➤ If you have painful urination and any discharge from the penis or vagina that seems strange. You may have a **sexually transmitted disease** (see chart, page 221).
➤ If you are a woman and it hurts to urinate, and you have tenderness and a dull ache or pain in your lower back and abdomen, have pain during intercourse, or sometimes miss menstrual periods or have very heavy ones. You may have endometriosis (see **menstrual irregularities chart,** page 233) or **pelvic inflammatory disease** (see page 236).
Call for advice and an appointment:

If You're Pregnant

Urinary tract infections in pregnant women sometimes move up to the kidneys, where they can become dangerous. For this reason, many doctors agree that it is wise to have regular urine tests during pregnancy. If you are pregnant and you're finding it painful to urinate or you have any of the other symptoms listed on page 138, call your doctor for a prompt appointment.

➤ If you are a man and painful urination is accompanied by a frequent need to urinate, an interrupted urinary stream, painful ejaculation, or pain in the pelvis or lower back. You may have a **prostate problem** (see page 228).
➤ If it is painful to urinate or you have other symptoms of a urinary tract infection.
➤ If your symptoms don't go away or if they come back despite treatment.

HOW TO PREVENT IT

➤ Drink 8 glasses of fluids—mostly water— each day. Cranberry juice can help keep an infection from starting, but only if you drink at least a *quart* every day.
➤ Try supplements of vitamin C (ascorbic acid); they may slow bacterial growth.
➤ Urinate when you have the urge to go. Empty your bladder every time.
➤ Wash before and after sex. Ask your partner to do the same.
➤ Urinate right after sex; this helps flush out bacteria that may have entered the urinary tract.
➤ Take showers instead of baths.
➤ Don't use bubble bath or scented soaps. Use a mild, scent-free detergent to wash underwear; scented or harsh products can irritate the skin around the urethra.
➤ Wear cotton-crotch underwear and loose-fitting clothes.
➤ Wash genitals with plain water once a day.
For women:
➤ If you use a diaphragm, wash it after each use with warm, soapy water, then rinse and dry it. If you continue to have infec-

URINARY SYSTEM

tions, ask your doctor to help you make sure the diaphragm fits well. If a different size doesn't help, try using another type of birth control.

➤ To keep the urinary tract free of bacteria, always wipe yourself from front to back after using the toilet.

COMPLEMENTARY CHOICES

➤ Nettle, an herb, may help relieve inflammation. To make an infusion, mix 1 teaspoon dried, crushed nettle leaves or root in 1 cup boiling water; let cool. The usual dose is 1 tablespoon every 1 to 2 hours.

➤ Washing the genitals with a solution of the herb goldenseal before and after sexual activity may help ease symptoms and fight the infection. Mix 2 teaspoons of the herb per cup of water, bring to a boil, and simmer for 15 minutes. Cool to room temperature before using.

FOR MORE HELP

Key Websites: *www.SavonHealth.com*. For more information on painful urination: *www.SavonPainfulUrination.com*.

Organizations: The American Foundation for Urologic Disease, 1128 N. Charles St., Baltimore, MD 21201. 800-242-2383 or 410-468-1800, M–F 8:30–5 EST; *www.afud. org.* Write or call for brochures.

■ Interstitial Cystitis Association of America, 51 Monroe St., Suite 1402, Rockville, MD 20850. 800-435-7422, M–F 9–5 EST; *www.ichelp.org.* Call or send a business-size self-addressed stamped envelope for information on cystitis.

■ National Institute of Diabetes and Digestive and Kidney Diseases, 301-496-3583, M–F 8:30–5 EST; *www.niddk.nih. gov.* Sends information on kidney and urinary tract problems. At Website, click on *Health Information,* then on *Urologic Diseases,* and choose from list of topics.

Books: *You Don't Have to Live With Cystitis,* by Larrian Gillespie, M.D. Offers approaches that can put a stop to urinary tract infections. Avon Books, 1996, $12.

■ *Overcoming Bladder Disorders,* by Rebecca

Chalker and Kristene E. Whitmore, M.D. A practical guide for people who have chronic urological disorders. HarperCollins, 1991, $14.

Urinary Incontinence
www.SavonIncontinence.com

SIGNS AND SYMPTOMS

■ Leaking a small amount of urine when coughing, exercising, laughing, or in any other way putting pressure on the bladder.

■ Urge to urinate that you can't control.

■ Urinating without knowing it.

More than 10 million people in the United States, mostly older men and women, have trouble holding the flow of urine. This problem is called urinary incontinence. Most of the several types can be helped or cured.

In *stress incontinence,* the muscles that close the tube (urethra) that carries urine outside the body sometimes get weak. When you sneeze, cough, or in any other way put pressure on the bladder, a little urine escapes. Childbirth or being overweight can weaken these muscles and cause this problem.

In *urge incontinence,* also called irritable bladder, you may not be able to control the need to urinate. This problem is sometimes caused by a urinary tract infection, or by **stroke** (see pages 44 and 113), **Alzheimer's disease** (see page 48), or **Parkinson's disease** (see page 57).

With *overflow incontinence,* you no longer feel when it's time to urinate. Rather than being wholly emptied several times a day, your bladder is always a little full. Then urine leaks out in dribbles. This problem may be linked to **diabetes** (see page 277), nerve problems, or an enlarged prostate gland that blocks the flow of urine (see **prostate problems,** page 228). In women, it may result from a large fibroid or ovarian tumor.

Sometimes the cause of incontinence is a short-term problem and easy to cure. It may be the first and only symptom of a urinary tract infection (see **painful urination,** page 138), so clearing up the infection will often cure the incontinence. Some drugs, such as sleeping pills, diuretics, and tranquilizers, can make it hard to control your bladder. The problem may go away if your doctor prescribes a different drug.

Incontinence seldom poses a health risk, but you do need to take steps to treat it. Even if it can't be cured, it can almost always be controlled so that it stops being a problem in your daily life.

WHAT YOU CAN DO NOW

➤ Stay engaged with life and keep on doing the things you like. Don't withdraw from others.
➤ When you go out, wear underwear that absorbs moisture. But don't wear it for too long; these garments can cause rashes.
➤ Cross your legs when you feel a sneeze coming on. It's a safe, simple way to prevent stress incontinence.
➤ Avoid drinks with caffeine. They can irritate the bladder.
➤ Don't drink a lot of liquid when you're away from home.
➤ Wear clothing that's easy to take off.
➤ Keep a diary—note when you lose control, how much urine is lost, and what you were doing at the time. It will help you and your doctor devise the best treatment plan.
➤ Try bladder training:
  ■ Go to the bathroom every hour, even if you don't feel the need. Stretch the time between visits by 15 to 30 minutes every 2 days. Slowly work up to 3 or 4 hours between visits.
  ■ If you need to urinate between visits, relax where you are until the urge is gone, then find a bathroom.
  ■ Practice "double voiding." Empty bladder, then relax a moment and try again.

WHEN TO CALL THE DOCTOR

➤ If you have any bladder control problems.
➤ If you have signs of an infection, such as fever, or pain when you urinate.
➤ If you think a drug may be causing your incontinence.

HOW TO PREVENT IT

➤ Practice Kegel exercises, which tone the muscles that control the flow of urine: As you start and stop the flow, try to sense which muscles you're working. Later, contract and release them—at least 15 to 20 squeezes, 3 times a day. After some practice, tighten the muscles for at least 10 seconds each time. Kegels are private: You're the only one who will know you're doing them.
➤ Exercise often, and try to lose any extra pounds. Excess body weight puts pressure on the bladder muscles.
➤ Eat a lot of fresh fruits, vegetables, and whole grains to avoid constipation. Straining can weaken bladder muscles.
➤ Ask your doctor about biofeedback.

FOR MORE HELP

Key Websites: *www.SavonHealth.com*. For more information on urinary incontinence: *www.SavonIncontinence.com*.

Organizations: The American Foundation for Urologic Disease, 1128 N. Charles St., Baltimore, MD 21201. 800-242-2383 to order brochures, or 410-468-1800 to speak with someone, M–F 8:30–5 EST; *www.afud.org*. Call or write for a copy of "Answers to Your Questions About Urinary Incontinence" or "Freedom From Overactive Bladder."

■ National Association for Continence, P.O. Box 8310, Spartanburg, SC 29305. 800-252-3337 or 864-579-7900, M–F 8–5 EST; *www.nafc.org*. An educational material and advocacy information clearinghouse for urinary incontinence.

■ Simon Foundation for Continence, P.O. Box 835, Wilmette, IL 60091. 800-237-4666, or 847-864-3913, M–F 8:30–5 CST; *www.simonfoundation.org*. Staff members answer questions and send brochures on incontinence.

Books: *The Urinary Incontinence Sourcebook*, by Diane Kaschak Newman, R.N.C., M.S.N., and Mary Dzurinko. Gives information about the physiology, prevention, and treatment of urinary incontinence problems. Lowell House, 1999, $19.95.

■ *7 Steps to Normal Bladder Control*, by Elizabeth Vierck. Provides step-by-step instructions on how to reclaim bladder control. Harbor, 1998, $16.95.

Skin, Scalp & Nails

Acne

www.SavonAcne.com

SIGNS AND SYMPTOMS

- Ongoing outbreaks of reddish blemishes on the face and sometimes on the chest, shoulders, neck, upper back, or buttocks.
- Spots that have a dark, open center (blackheads).
- Bumps under the skin (whiteheads).
- Whiteheads that rupture (pimples).
- Boil-like lumps (nodules).

Acne is an outbreak of pimples, blackheads, whiteheads, or boils. It seems to be linked to too much sebum, the oil that keeps your skin moist. Sebum can plug a hair follicle, forming a whitehead or blackhead. Bacteria that grow behind the plug can cause a pimple or, rarely, a boil or cyst.

Acne is most common among teenagers, but anyone at any age can get it. You may develop acne:

- If you have a family history of acne.
- If your male hormones (both men and women have them) increase, chiefly during puberty.
- If you take certain drugs, such as lithium or corticosteroids (anti-inflammatories).
- If you use creams, oils, makeup, or other products that block the skin's pores.
- If you're a woman, when you undergo hormonal changes from menstrual periods, pregnancy, or the Pill.

No matter what people say, stress, poor cleaning habits, and a poor diet don't seem to cause acne, although they can make it worse. You can also get acne-like outbreaks if you have **allergies** to some foods (see page 84).

WHAT YOU CAN DO NOW

- Wash the affected area twice a day with mild, oil- and scent-free soap. Don't wash too often—your acne may get worse. Try astringents such as witch hazel if you have very oily skin or an oily "T zone" (forehead, nose, and chin).
- Shampoo your hair often. Oily hair may make the acne worse. Keep long hair off your face and shoulders.
- Shave as seldom as possible. Men with acne should take care to avoid nicking pimples. If you have severe acne, always use a fresh blade to avoid infection.
- Use only hypoallergenic, scent-free makeup made for acne-prone skin. Remove all makeup before going to bed.
- Try an over-the-counter treatment with benzoyl peroxide (a germ-killing agent) or salicylic acid (a mild peeling agent that helps unblock pores).
- After exercising, wipe off your sweat with a moist towel, or take a shower or bath. Do the same if you sweat a lot during the day.
- Wear a sunscreen, but choose one with care. If you have oily skin or sweat a lot, heavy sunscreens with coconut oil and cocoa butter may make your acne worse. Use sunscreen that's "non-comedogenic" (won't clog pores).
- Don't rest your face in your hands while reading, working, or watching TV.
- Avoid propping the phone against your

Rashes

The causes of rashes range from minor to serious. This chart includes some of the most common, as well as some that could be fatal. If your child has a rash, or if you and your child have the same rash, see the **children's rashes** chart (page 247).

SYMPTOMS	WHAT IT MIGHT BE	WHAT YOU CAN DO
Itchy red bumps anywhere on body; swelling of eyes, lips, and tongue; weakness; shortness of breath; sweating; rapid heartbeat.	Shock from allergy—severe, sudden reaction (that may be fatal) to foods, drugs, or insect bites (see pages 22 and 25).	Call 911 **right away.**
Bumpy, deep red or purplish rash; fever; stiff neck; headache; sensitivity to light.	Meningitis (see page 55).	Call 911 or go to emergency room **right away.**
Rash that looks like sunburn, often on palms of hands or soles of feet; sudden high fever (above 102); vomiting and diarrhea; headache; weakness; fainting; dizziness; confusion.	Toxic shock syndrome (see page 243).	Call 911 or go to emergency room **right away.** If you are using a tampon, menstrual sponge, diaphragm, or cervical cap, remove immediately after calling.
Itchy, raised red or pink patches (sometimes with white centers) that may come and go, anywhere on body.	Hives (see page 155).	Call 911 or go to emergency room if you also have wheezing, dizziness, and trouble breathing. This may be shock from allergy (see page 22).
First, rash that often begins at ankles or wrists, then moves to torso, face, and elsewhere. Often with headache, chills, and fever. Next, rash turns deep red, then looks like red pinpricks.	Rocky Mountain spotted fever. Caused by microorganism that enters body through tick bite. Illness gets its name from place where first reported. Now widespread (see tick bites, page 45).	Call doctor for prompt appointment. Can be fatal if untreated. Ask for test for Rocky Mountain spotted fever and also for Lyme disease (see next page of chart).
Butterfly-shaped red rash on cheeks and nose, fever, fatigue, joint pain, swelling.	Lupus (see page 284).	Call doctor for prompt appointment.

(continued)

SKIN, SCALP & NAILS

Rashes (continued)

SYMPTOMS	WHAT IT MIGHT BE	WHAT YOU CAN DO
Red rash, often with bull's-eye shape, spreading several inches from tick bite. Followed within a month by fever, headache, lethargy, and joint pain.	Lyme disease (see page 285). Caused by micro-organism that enters body through tick bite (see tick bites, page 45).	Call doctor for prompt appointment. Get tested for Lyme disease and also for Rocky Mountain spotted fever. If you can find tick, remove with tweezers; don't squeeze or twist it.
Burning or tingling skin followed by painful, blistery red rash; most often on only one side of torso, buttocks, or face.	Shingles (see page 160).	Call doctor for prompt appointment.
Thick patches of itchy red skin anywhere on body, or blisters with severe itching.	Eczema (see page 152). ■ Dermatitis (see page 149). ■ Poison oak or ivy (see page 151).	Call doctor for advice and appointment.
Raised patches of itchy pink skin with white scales, often on knees, elbows, and scalp.	Psoriasis (see page 159).	Call doctor for advice and appointment.
Small, pus-filled, pimple-like bumps anywhere on body, but most often on the thighs, buttocks, groin, scalp, armpits, and face.	Folliculitis—bacterial infection of hair follicles (see boils, page 146). May be caused by shaving or by clothing that rubs against skin.	Use over-the-counter anti-bacterial soap or cream. If infection gets worse or lasts after 2 weeks of home care, call doctor for advice and appointment.
Itchy, red, flaky, or scaly patches that appear on just one part of body; can affect feet, genitals, skin, and nails.	Fungal infection (see page 153). Could be ringworm—infection that can be caught from another person or even from dog or cat; common in children.	Use over-the-counter anti-fungal powders and creams. If rash gets worse or lasts after 2 weeks of home care, call doctor for advice and appointment.
Extreme itching (most often at night); rough, red rash in folds of body—between fingers, on wrists, elbows, breasts, buttocks, or waist.	Scabies (see page 157).	Call doctor for advice and appointment.

What Is Rosacea?

Rosacea (rose-AY-sha) is a rash caused by the swelling of the tiny blood vessels under the skin of the cheeks, nose, and forehead. It can cause an enlarged red nose, puffy cheeks, and a lasting blush on other parts of the face. Because red, pus-filled spots sometimes appear, it is often mistaken for acne—but there are no blackheads or whiteheads. People with rosacea may also get **conjunctivitis** (see page 63).

The cause of rosacea is unknown. It's most common in middle-aged adults, and the rash comes and goes for years. It seems to be made worse by hot or spicy food, alcohol, caffeine, very cold or hot weather, strong sunlight, and rubbing the face.

While rosacea is harmless, it is often unattractive and may get worse over time. If you think you have rosacea, see your doctor; antibiotics can help.

cheek. Try cleaning the receiver often— or buy a headset if you spend long hours on the phone.
➤ Don't pop, pick, scratch, or squeeze your pimples. This may cause scars.

WHEN TO CALL THE DOCTOR

➤ If your acne doesn't get better after 2 to 3 months of over-the-counter treatments. You may need further treatment.
➤ If you have many pimples, if your acne makes you feel shy or ashamed, or if you have signs of scarring. Your physician may give you medication to keep the acne from getting worse.
➤ If you think you may have **rosacea,** a rash around your cheeks and nose (see box, this page).

HOW TO PREVENT IT

Because genetics and hormones are factors in acne, doctors believe you can't prevent it.

FOR MORE HELP

Key Websites: *www.SavonHealth.com*. For more information on acne: *www.SavonAcne.com*.

Organizations: American Academy of Dermatology, Box 4014, Schaumburg, IL 60168-4014. 888-462-3376 or 847-330-0230, M–F 8:30–5 CST; *www.aad.org*. Send a business-size self-addressed stamped envelope for pamphlets on rosacea and acne. Also lists doctors near you.

■ National Institute of Arthritis and Musculoskeletal and Skin Diseases Information Clearinghouse, 877-226-4267, 24-hour recording, or 301-495-4484, M–F 8:30–5 EST; *www.nih.gov/niams/healthinfo/brochpub.htm*. Staff answers questions and sends facts about acne. At Website, click on *Q&A About Acne.*

Books: *Skin Wise: A Guide to Healthy Skin for Women,* by Annette Callan. Facts and advice about acne, skin cancer, and other skin problems. Oxford University Press, 1996, $22.95.

■ *Teenage Health Care,* by Gail B. Slap, M.D., and Martha M. Jablow. Covers teenage growth and a wide range of personal, social, and medical issues. Pocket Books, 1994, $14.

Blisters
www.SavonBlisters.com

SIGNS AND SYMPTOMS

■ Sore, fluid-filled bubbles of skin, sometimes in clusters. They can range in size from a pinpoint to a few inches across.
■ Sometimes itching, redness, and swelling.

Most blisters form because of friction. Simple movements such as rubbing from a shovel handle or a new pair of running shoes can raise one. Insect bites, viruses, certain skin ailments such as **dermatitis** (see page 149), and some drugs and chemicals can also cause them. You can get blisters from **burns** (see page 26), after you've been in the sun, or in extremes of heat or cold.

(see page 26)

WHAT YOU CAN DO NOW

Most of the time no treatment is needed, since new skin forms under the affected area and the fluid is absorbed.

Friction blisters:

➤ Popping a blister makes infection more likely, so it's best to leave a small one alone. To drain a large, painful blister: Clean the area with alcohol. Using a sterile needle, gently pierce one side of the blister. Let it drain. Then apply antibiotic cream and cover it.

➤ Don't pull off or cut away the loose skin from a broken blister. It covers and shields the new skin.

➤ Cover a broken blister to protect it. Use a simple adhesive bandage for a small blister or a gauze pad and adhesive tape for a large one. Change the bandage daily, or more often if it gets wet. Leave the blister uncovered at night to allow it to dry.

Burn blisters:

➤ Flush the affected place right away with lots of cool water or a saline (salt) solution. Don't rub or place ice on burns.

➤ Treat burn blisters like friction blisters.

WHEN TO CALL THE DOCTOR

➤ If a blister has been caused by a burn, covers a large area, and is very painful. Blisters mean a second-degree burn. Some second- and all third-degree burns need a doctor's care.

➤ If the fluid in the blister isn't clear. White, yellow, or green discharge may signal an infection.

➤ If your blisters are the result of a skin ailment or contact with chemicals or other toxic agents.

HOW TO PREVENT IT

➤ Wear gloves for tasks you do only now and then, such as shoveling snow, sweeping, or raking.

➤ Have your feet measured when you buy shoes, and wear only shoes that fit.

➤ Have your shoes repaired often. Worn soles don't protect the feet, and worn linings can chafe the skin.

➤ Keep your feet dry. Wear socks that don't have holes and that soak up moisture. Dust your feet with an antifungal powder if they tend to sweat.

➤ Put petroleum jelly or moleskin pads on areas, such as the heel, where socks are likely to rub. Wear socks that fit well. Socks that bunch up can cause blisters.

FOR MORE HELP

Key Websites: *www.SavonHealth.com*. For more information on blisters: *www.SavonBlisters.com*.

Organizations: American Academy of Orthopaedic Surgeons, 800-824-BONES, 24-hour recording. Ask for brochure titled "If the Shoe Fits, Wear It."

■ American Podiatric Medical Association, 800-366-8227, 24-hour recording that takes requests for free brochures on foot care; *www.apma.org*.

Boils
www.SavonSkinDisorders.com

SIGNS AND SYMPTOMS

■ Redness, swelling, tenderness, pain, or throbbing of a lump under the skin.

■ A red and swollen lump with a white or yellow pus-filled center under the skin (after a number of days).

A boil may look like a bad pimple. But you get a boil when staph bacteria invade a blocked hair follicle (folliculitis) or oil gland. The germs, along with white blood cells and dead skin cells, form pus and cause swelling.

Boils most often appear on the face, neck, scalp, buttocks, armpits, or, sometimes, on a woman's nipple. A cluster of boils is known as a carbuncle—a rarer and more serious form that needs medical help.

Boils are usually not serious. They can be passed from person to person, though this is rare. People with diabetes or immune-system problems and those exposed to some industrial chemicals are the most likely to get them. So are people whose overall health is poor, who wear dirty clothing and don't wash well, whose diet is poor, or who overuse corticosteroids such as cortisone.

Bruises

SIGNS AND SYMPTOMS

- Black and blue or purple skin, turning red or yellow.
- Swelling, or hard lump under the skin.

WHAT YOU CAN DO NOW

➤ Wash the infected area gently with antibacterial soap.

➤ Apply warm compresses (cloths soaked in hot water and wrung out) to help the boil burst and drain.

➤ Put an over-the-counter antibacterial cream on the boil to keep the infection from spreading.

➤ Don't press or prick the boil. This could spread the infection. Most boils will burst on their own after about 10 to 14 days. When one does, hold a warm, clean compress against it to remove all the pus. Next, apply antibacterial cream and cover the boil loosely with a bandage to prevent reinfection.

➤ Since boils can be contagious, wash your hands well and launder towels, clothes, and bed linens in hot water and soap to avoid spreading the infection.

WHEN TO CALL THE DOCTOR

➤ If you have a boil on your face, a cluster of boils, or boils with a fever. You could get a more serious infection.

➤ If the pain is severe. A doctor may lance and drain the boil.

➤ If you get boils often. Your doctor will want to find out what is causing them.

HOW TO PREVENT IT

➤ Shower or bathe often.

➤ If you're prone to getting boils, apply an antibacterial cream after shaving.

➤ Treat minor skin injuries right away.

➤ Don't share towels or clothes. Clean sports gear well—for instance, straps on helmets and gym machines.

➤ Eat balanced meals with lots of fresh fruit and vegetables.

Bruises are a sign of bleeding and damage to tissues just under the skin, most often from a hard blow.

Although the blood under the skin is red, a bruise looks black, blue, or purple because your skin filters out all colors but those. The darker the color, the deeper the bruise. After a few days, it may turn green or yellow as the blood cells begin to break up. This means the bruise is about to fade away.

Most bruises heal on their own, and swift home care can speed the process. But deep bruises, or large ones, may need medical care. They may also be a sign of illness, a blood problem, or a problem with a medication you are taking for another condition.

WHAT YOU CAN DO NOW

➤ Ice packs—wrapped to keep the ice from freezing your skin—and cold compresses used right away can hold down the swelling and damage from most bruises. The cold may also keep the bruise from turning deep purple, and it helps dull pain.

➤ Put a cold compress on the sore place within 15 minutes after an injury. Leave it on for 10 to 20 minutes at a time, then take it off for 30 to 40 minutes. Repeat many times for the next 3 days.

➤ Raise the bruised part above the level of your heart, if you can. This holds down fluid buildup and swelling.

➤ Try not to use the sore area for 1 to 3 days. Use this time to repeat the ice treatment above as often as you can.

➤ Check your medication: Some drugs increase bruising, or your dose may be too high.

➤ Take an over-the-counter painkiller (see **pain relief,** page 315). But avoid aspirin, which can increase bleeding and make the bruise worse. (Never give aspirin to a child or teenager who has chicken pox, a cold, the flu, or any illness you suspect of being caused by a virus; see box on **Reye's syndrome,** page 95.)

WHEN TO CALL THE DOCTOR

➤ If the bruise doesn't fade or go away after 14 days.
➤ If it seems infected: The pain gets worse, it swells more, or you have redness, pus, or a fever.
➤ If you have vision problems with a black eye. The eye may be damaged.
➤ If you bruise often and easily, for no reason. You may have another illness.
➤ If an older person or someone with poor circulation gets a bruise on the lower leg but hasn't bumped or hit the leg. This could be a sign of a blood clot.
➤ If you are taking anticoagulants (they keep the blood from clotting), and you are bruising often or for no reason. Your dose might be too high.

HOW TO PREVENT IT

➤ Eat a balanced diet with plenty of vitamins C and K, which come in many fruits and vegetables (see **the nutrition top ten,** page 298). A lack of C or K can cause bruising.
➤ Accident-proof your house to help avoid falls. Keep clutter off floors and stairs; use night-lights in bathrooms and hallways (see **be careful out there,** page 299).

Corns & Calluses
www.SavonFootProblems.com

SIGNS AND SYMPTOMS

Both corns and calluses are made of thick, hard, dead skin. They differ mainly in where they show up.
Corns:
■ On the tops or sides of toe joints or between the toes.

Calluses:
■ On palms, soles of feet, or any place that rubs a lot against something hard.

Corns and calluses do your body a service, though they can be painful. Both shield the skin from injury. They're common and seldom cause a problem unless they build up or crack open; then they may hurt.

Most corns and calluses on the feet are caused by shoes that don't fit. Open-backed, high-heeled sandals and tapered, narrow-toed shoes cause the most problems.

WHAT YOU CAN DO NOW

➤ Place a corn pad on the toe to help ease the pressure on a corn.
➤ Use a pumice stone or callus file to gently rub dead skin off a callus or hard corn.
➤ Use a small piece of foot plaster, sold in drugstores, to remove the top layer of skin. Leave on as directed. Then rub the corn or callus lightly with a pumice stone and soak in hot, soapy water.
➤ Don't cut or burn off corns or calluses.

WHEN TO CALL THE DOCTOR

➤ If you have constant pain, redness, swelling, or discharge around a corn or callus. You might have an infection.
➤ If you get corns or calluses and you have diabetes or problems with your circulation. You may get an infection. See a doctor before trying home care.
➤ If self-care doesn't work. A foot specialist (podiatrist) may prescribe custom-made shoe inserts (orthotics).

HOW TO PREVENT IT

➤ Buy shoes at the end of the day, when your feet are largest. Wear only shoes that fit properly. The distance between the front of the shoe and your longest toe needs to be half an inch. Make sure toes can wiggle freely, and avoid pointed shoes and high heels.

➤ Keep your shoes in good shape by having them repaired when necessary. Soles shouldn't be so thin that your feet are jarred when you walk. Worn-down heels can't protect the heel bone.

➤ Keep your feet dry, and make sure they don't rub against your shoes. Wearing socks or nylons and using talcum powder will help. Avoid socks made of fibers that don't breathe. Cotton or synthetic fibers designed to wick away moisture are best.

➤ Rub away areas of skin buildup on the feet before they turn into corns or calluses. After bathing, rub the area gently with a pumice stone or callus file, sold in drugstores.

FOR MORE HELP

Key Websites: *www.SavonHealth.com.* For more information on foot problems: *www.SavonFootProblems.com.*

Organizations: American Academy of Orthopaedic Surgeons, 800-824-BONES, 24-hour recording. Ask for brochure titled "If the Shoe Fits, Wear It."

◼ American Podiatric Medical Association, 800-366-8227, 24-hour recording that takes requests for free brochures on foot care; *www.apma.org.*

Website: The Center for Podiatric Information, *www.infowest.com/podiatry/footcare/index.html.* Click on *Corns, Calluses,* or related foot topics.

Dermatitis
www.SavonDermatitis.com

SIGNS AND SYMPTOMS

One or more of these:
◼ Thick, itchy, dry red patches of skin on any part of the body.
◼ A pink or red rash anywhere, caused by something such as a chemical.
◼ Blistered, crusty, or scaly skin in round patches, often on the legs, buttocks, hands, or arms.
◼ Oily yellow scales on or near the face (nose, eyebrows, ears, scalp).
◼ Scaly, reddened skin, sometimes with craterlike sores, on lower legs.

D ermatitis is another name for a skin irritation or rash. There are many types. They vary by the kind of rash and where it is on your body.

Contact dermatitis (red bumps and blisters that often weep and crust over) can appear anywhere on the body. It's most often caused by an irritation or allergy to a skin-care product or a plant such as poison ivy or poison oak (see **poison oak and ivy** box, page 151). You may get this type of dermatitis when your skin reacts to certain soaps (including bubble-bath soap) and detergents, chlorine, and some man-made fibers. Condoms, latex or rubber gloves, and nickel-plated jewelry can cause contact dermatitis. So can leather and new clothing. Be sure to wash new clothes before wearing them for the first time. Perfumes and other items in makeup may also bring it on (see **choosing skin-care products** box, next page).

Another type, **nummular dermatitis,** is marked by round, red, oozing places, most often on the arms and legs. Stress and other skin problems can bring it on. Older people with dry skin or who live in dry climates often get it. It gets worse if you bathe in very hot water. It usually clears up by itself.

Itching

Got an itch? Most of the time, it's nothing to worry about. Often the cause is as simple as an insect bite or dry skin. These minor irritations usually clear up on their own or are easily treated at home with lotion or, in more stubborn cases, with over-the-counter hydrocortisone cream.

Rarely, itching is a sign of a more serious disorder, such as anemia, kidney failure, or skin cancer. If you have itching with a rash, see the **rashes** chart (page 143). If you have an itch that lasts longer than 10 days and you don't know what's causing it, call your doctor for advice and an appointment.

Seborrheic dermatitis appears most of-ten on the scalp (in the form of dandruff) and face. In infants, a yellow, scaly rash is known as cradle cap. Some experts think dandruff comes from a fungus; it may be made worse by plugged oil glands or by stress. People with immune disorders such as AIDS are prone to it.

Stasis dermatitis is a scaly, dry, reddish rash, usually on the lower legs and ankles. Poor circulation can bring it on.

Extreme, constant itchiness anywhere on the body may be **eczema** (see page 152), also known as **atopic dermatitis.**

WHAT YOU CAN DO NOW

➤ For contact dermatitis, seek out the cause and get rid of it. If you find, for example, that nickel-plated jewelry or some type of makeup is the problem, you can simply stop wearing it.

➤ Test yourself if you think your skin reacts to makeup. Apply a small bit of the product to your arm, and cover the spot with a

Choosing Skin-Care Products

If you see a rash on your scalp, neck, or face, something you're using for skin care or makeup could be the culprit. Perfume, makeup, antiperspirant, sunblock, suntan lotion, and shampoo all can upset the skin.

A scent or preservative is most often to blame, but items labeled "unscented" can cause trouble, too. They still may contain irritating fragrances or other chemicals. "Fragrance-free" is a better choice.

Even if a product says it's organic, natural, nonallergenic, or hypoallergenic, your skin may react to it. If you have sensitive skin, choose your skin-care products with caution. Start with a fragrance-free product and apply it to a small area to see how your skin responds. Switch brands until you find one that doesn't cause a rash.

bandage (if you're allergic to these, use gauze and paper tape). If you get a red, itchy rash within 48 hours, the product is the cause, and you'll know to avoid it.

➤ To ease swelling and itching, toss a half-cup of cornstarch or oatmeal bath powder (sold in drugstores) into a warm (not hot) bath. Soak your skin—but only for a half hour so that you don't lose too many of the oils your skin needs. Use a fragrance-free, mild soap or cleanser. Or use the oatmeal as a compress.

➤ For dry or flaky skin, try petroleum jelly or scent-free body lotion. For an oozing rash, use calamine lotion.

➤ Shampoo your hair with a tar shampoo if you have dermatitis on the scalp. Your scalp may sunburn more easily for a few hours after using the shampoo, so stay out of the sun. (Never use this shampoo on children—it's too harsh. Use a baby shampoo instead, and wash your child's hair every day.)

➤ If you have red, oozing sores, apply washcloths that have been soaked in warm, salty water and wrung out. Don't use over-the-counter hydrocortisone cream; it raises your risk of infection.

➤ For stasis dermatitis on the legs and ankles, sit or lie with your legs raised above your hips many times a day. Try wearing support stockings.

➤ Don't scratch. Cut nails short to keep from breaking the skin.

➤ Try hydrocortisone cream on unbroken skin.

WHEN TO CALL THE DOCTOR

➤ If your skin hasn't improved after 2 or 3 weeks of home care, over-the-counter creams, or medicated shampoos.

➤ If you have signs of an infection, such as sores with pus.

HOW TO PREVENT IT

➤ If you've been exposed to a chemical agent, wash your skin with a mild cleanser and water as soon as you can.

➤ To keep the air around you moist, use a humidifier at home and work.

Poison Oak & Ivy

Poison oak, poison ivy, and poison sumac grow as shrubs or vines throughout the United States except in Hawaii, Alaska, and some Nevada deserts. If you're outdoors just about anywhere else, your skin and the clear, oily sap in these plants' leaves, stems, and roots may meet—with nasty results.

The rash you get is a form of contact dermatitis (see **dermatitis,** page 149). Symptoms differ from person to person, but they often include a line or streak on the skin that may look like insect bites within 12 to 48 hours after exposure. Redness and swelling follow, then blisters and severe itching. In a few days, the blisters begin to dry. The rash can take from 10 days to 3 weeks to go away.

You can't pass the rash to another person, or spread the rash to another part of your body. But if the oily poison remains on your clothes or gets in your home and touches your skin, the rash may return.

To prevent exposure:

➤ Learn what poison oak, ivy, and sumac look like in all seasons, and stay away. Be warned, though, that the plants come in many shapes and sizes, and all varieties can get you even when they've lost their leaves. Even in dead plants, the oil can remain active for years.

➤ Cover up as much as possible and use a barrier lotion on exposed skin. These lotions are clay-based compounds that keep the oil from attaching to your skin. Ivy Block was the first of them to be approved as a preventive; other products containing the same active ingredient—5 percent bentoquatam—work as well.

➤ Beware of pets that have run in the woods. The oil can cling to their fur and rub off on you. Hose them down when they return from an adventure.

If you've been exposed:

➤ Clean the oil off exposed skin as soon as you can. If you have rubbing alcohol handy, splash it on, straight from the bottle. It will remove the oil as it runs off. Rinse with plenty of running water. Air dry your skin or pat dry—don't rub—with a towel.

➤ If you don't have alcohol, get to a cold running stream, a lake, or a garden hose quickly. Rinse well. Don't use soap; rubbing the lather can spread the poison.

➤ Or try gently covering exposed skin with sand or even dirt (make sure there aren't any poison oak or ivy leaves in it). This will help absorb the oil. Rinse off with plenty of water.

➤ At the end of a day in the woods, throw your clothes in the washing machine and use a garden hose to rinse your tools, shoes, gear, and pets. Then give yourself a thorough shower.

If you have a rash from poison oak or ivy:

➤ Don't scratch the rash or blisters. To ease itching, calamine lotion is your best bet. Cortisone creams and other over-the-counter anti-itch products are no match for the plants' oils.

➤ Soak often in cool or lukewarm water with a half cup of baking soda or oatmeal bath powder (sold in drugstores).

➤ If your symptoms are severe or if you're getting new outbreaks after 10 days, call your doctor.

➤ If your skin is prone to dermatitis, choose untreated cotton or other natural-fiber fabrics for clothing. Make sure clothing isn't too tight.

➤ Don't wear nickel-plated earrings or other nickel-plated jewelry. Choose surgical stainless steel, sterling silver, or gold jewelry instead.

➤ When washing dishes or handling chemicals, wear cotton-lined rubber gloves to protect your hands.

➤ After washing your hands or bathing, ap-

SKIN, SCALP & NAILS

ply a lotion that has no preservatives or scents while your skin is still damp.

FOR MORE HELP

Key Websites: *www.SavonHealth.com.* For more information on dermatitis: *www.SavonDermatitis.com.*

Organization: American Academy of Dermatology, Box 4014, Schaumburg, IL 60168-4014. 888-462-3376 or 847-330-0230, M–F 8:30–5 CST; *www.aad.org.* Send a business-size self-addressed stamped envelope for a pamphlet on dermatitis. Also lists doctors near you. At Website, click on *Patient Information* and then on *Patient Education,* and choose from listed topics.

Eczema
www.SavonEczema.com

SIGNS AND SYMPTOMS

- Itchy, red, dry, scaly, blistered, or swollen patches of skin, usually on the scalp or face, hands and wrists, and knee and elbow creases.
- Oozing, crusting, thickening, or odd color of the affected skin area (sometimes).

Eczema (atopic dermatitis) tends to run in families and is often related to **allergies** (see page 84), **asthma** (see page 88), and **stress** (see page 218). It can also be triggered by chemical agents, extreme weather, sweating, and infections. Infants are prone to eczema, although many grow out of it before they turn 2. If it lasts after that age, a child is likely to have chronic eczema.

Eczema is usually not a serious health problem, but its symptoms can be stubborn and annoying.

WHAT YOU CAN DO NOW

➤ Don't scratch. Soothe skin and keep it moist by taking warm (not hot) baths daily. Use just a little mild cleanser or

fragrance-free soap, and don't scrub your skin or rub it too hard with the towel. Apply a fragrance-free body lotion after you bathe to restore moisture.

➤ For an older child or an adult, apply over-the-counter hydrocortisone cream. Avoid lotions with scents, oils, or preservatives. These may make your eczema worse.

➤ Try an oral over-the-counter antihistamine to relieve itching. Don't use antihistamine cream or antiseptic sprays.

➤ Wear loose, cool clothing; sweating can make eczema worse. Avoid man-made and wool fabrics, which may irritate the skin.

➤ Wash clothes with mild, fragrance-free laundry soap. Rinse twice. Don't use fabric softener.

➤ Trim nails short. Wear soft cotton gloves or mittens to bed to limit scratching. This is especially helpful for children.

➤ Ease tension with a quick walk or other exercise.

➤ Use a humidifier to keep from breathing dry air (see **hints on humidifiers and vaporizers** box, page 92).

➤ Don't eat foods that seem to make your eczema flare up; some people report problems from cow's milk, eggs, wheat flour, nuts, and citrus juices.

WHEN TO CALL THE DOCTOR

Call for a prompt appointment:
➤ If the affected skin gets a crust, often yellow or brown, or blisters with pus. You may have a bacterial infection that needs antibiotics, or a rare condition—caused by a herpes virus—that may be serious.

Call for advice and an appointment:
➤ If your skin doesn't get better after a week or two of home care, or if the eczema keeps coming back. Your doctor may suggest further treatment.

➤ If you develop an itchy rash that seems to have no cause, and eczema or asthma runs in your family.

HOW TO PREVENT IT

➤ To keep skin from getting dry, take short, warm (not hot) showers or baths, then apply a lotion to put moisture back in your skin right away. Don't use soap every time you bathe.

➤ To keep your hands from getting dry and chapped, wear mittens or gloves in cold weather. Wear cotton gloves under wool or synthetic-fiber gloves to help protect your skin. Use cotton-lined rubber gloves when you are cleaning clothes and dishes.

➤ Avoid skin irritants and allergy-causing agents. These include soaps, detergents, perfumes, dust, pet hair, and tobacco smoke.

➤ Learn to spot stressful times, and do relaxation techniques, such as yoga or meditation (see **relax,** page 303).

FOR MORE HELP

Key Websites: *www.SavonHealth.com.* For more information on eczema: *www.SavonEczema.com.*

Organizations: American Academy of Dermatology, Box 4014, Schaumburg, IL 60168-4014. 888-462-3376 or 847-330-0230, M–F 8:30–5 CST; *www.aad.org.* Send a business-size self-addressed stamped envelope for a pamphlet on eczema. Also provides list of doctors near you. At Website, click on *Patient Information* and then on *Patient Education,* and choose from listed topics.

■ National Eczema Association, 1220 SW Morrison St., Suite 433, Portland, OR 97205. 800-818-SKIN, 24-hour line; *www.eczema-assn.org.* Sends facts about eczema.

Website: Eczema Informant, *www.ei.addr.com.* Covers eczema triggers, treatments, and studies, and lists related links.

Book: *Eczema & Psoriasis: How Your Diet Can Help,* by Stephen Terrass. A guide to nutrition and skin problems. Thorsons, 1995, $9.

Fungal Infections
www.SavonFungalInfections.com

SIGNS AND SYMPTOMS

Athlete's foot:
■ Itching, scaling, and redness that often starts between the toes.
■ Dryness, flaking, or blisters on the toes or soles of the feet.
■ Toenails that thicken and become layered or scaly and yellowish.
■ Odor, in severe cases.

Jock itch:
■ Itchy red bumps in the groin and on the genitals. Rash may extend to the buttocks and inner thigh.

Yeast infection:
■ Thick, white, cheesy discharge from the vagina.
■ Itching, pain, or tenderness around the genitals (men or women). In men, the head of the penis may be inflamed.
■ Pain or soreness during sex.
■ Urge to urinate often. Urine may sting or burn.
■ Creamy yellow or white coating in the mouth or throat or on the tongue that can be easily scraped off and may be painful (thrush).
■ A red, itching rash with flaky white patches on moist skin areas, such as around the genitals, between the buttocks, or under the breasts.

More people get **athlete's foot** (tinea pedis) than any other fungal infection. It can be vexing, but it's easy to control if treated right away.

The fungus that causes athlete's foot is like those that cause jock itch and yeast infections. It breeds in closed, damp places and feeds on dead skin cells. Walking barefoot in the shower at a gym and around pools may increase your chance of getting athlete's foot. Moisture, sweating, and shoes that don't let your feet breathe can make it worse.

Jock itch (tinea cruris) is a fungal infection in the groin that most men get from time to time. Women, on the other hand, may get **yeast infections,** which occur when a fungus that's already in the body displaces the helpful bacteria that keep it under control. The infection begins in the vagina and may spread if left untreated. If you are pregnant or taking oral antibiotics or birth con-

SKIN, SCALP & NAILS

trol pills, you are more likely to get the infection. Men, too, can get yeast infections, which irritate the penis.

Thrush is a yeast infection in the mouth. It makes a white or yellow coating that may look like milk and is easy to scrape away, exposing raw, red skin. Babies frequently get thrush. So do people with AIDS and others with weak immune systems, such as people being treated with chemotherapy for cancer. Taking large doses of antibiotics may bring on thrush. So can the steroid inhalers many people use for asthma.

People who perspire a lot or who are overweight and likely to have folds of skin that rub together also are prone to fungal infections.

Athlete's foot, jock itch, and yeast infections can usually be cured quickly.

WHAT YOU CAN DO NOW

Athlete's foot:
➤ Wash twice a day, and dry well between the toes after showering or swimming.
➤ Apply an over-the-counter antifungal powder or cream to your feet, and sprinkle some powder in your shoes every day.
➤ Wash sports shoes at least once a week.
➤ Wear clean cotton socks, and don't wear the same shoes each day.
➤ Take your shoes and socks off at home to give your feet plenty of air.

Jock itch:
➤ Use an antifungal powder, cream, or spray 2 or 3 times a day until the rash goes away. Keep using the medication for at least a week after that, to make sure the fungus is dead.
➤ Don't wear tight pants or underwear.
➤ Change your underwear and jock strap daily. Wash them in hot water.
➤ Dry your groin well after showering. You can even use a hair dryer set on low.

Yeast infection:
➤ Use condoms or stop having intercourse until you get treatment if you have a yeast infection in the vagina (it can be passed on to others).
➤ If you're sure it's yeast, use an over-the-counter yeast medicine. Read the label and follow the steps.

➤ Wear clean cotton underwear, and avoid panty hose and tight jeans and pants.
➤ Eat plain yogurt containing active cultures if you get a yeast infection after taking antibiotics for another ailment. The bacteria in the yogurt will help control the yeast.
➤ For thrush, try a gentle mouthwash to loosen the white coating.

WHEN TO CALL THE DOCTOR

Athlete's foot:
➤ If your foot has an odor that doesn't go away after treatment at home—a sign that you have a severe case.
➤ If your rash starts to spread or isn't better after 2 weeks of self-care. Once athlete's foot spreads, it is hard to get rid of and often returns.
➤ If the infection has reached your nails. This is hard to clear up. It also makes your nails more prone to bacterial infection because moisture gets trapped in the cracks.

Jock itch:
➤ If over-the-counter treatments fail to work after a couple of weeks.
➤ If you develop an open sore that oozes pus. This is a sign of a secondary infection.
➤ If the rash spreads, gets worse, or keeps coming back.

Yeast infection:
➤ If you suspect you have one and you aren't better after using an over-the-counter medicine. Your doctor can prescribe antifungal suppositories, creams, or tablets for you (and maybe for your sexual partner).
➤ If you see signs of thrush. Your doctor may prescribe antifungal creams, pills, or suppositories.

HOW TO PREVENT IT

➤ Bathe daily and dry your body well.
➤ Avoid tight shoes and underwear, especially in hot weather.

Athlete's foot:
➤ Expose your feet to the air as much as possible. Wear plastic sandals in public dressing rooms and showers.

Jock itch:
➤ Change your clothes as soon as you finish working out, and don't share towels at the

gym. Jock itch is mildly contagious.

Yeast infection:

➤ Don't use feminine hygiene sprays or douches, which may kill the helpful bacteria in the vagina that can ward off a fungus.

➤ Wear underwear and workout clothes made of cotton or another "breathable" fabric. Nylon doesn't let air near the skin and gives fungi a chance to grow.

➤ Wash your workout clothes in hot water after each use.

➤ If you have repeated bouts of the infection and you take the Pill, ask your doctor about trying a different method of birth control.

➤ If you use a steroid inhaler for asthma, rinse your mouth after each use to help prevent thrush (see **asthma,** page 88).

FOR MORE HELP

Key Websites: *www.SavonHealth.com*. For more information on fungal infections: *www.SavonFungalInfections.com*.

Organizations: American Academy of Dermatology, Box 4014, Schaumburg, IL 60168-4014. 888-462-3376 or 847-330-0230, M–F 8:30–5 CST; *www.aad.org*. Send a business-size self-addressed stamped envelope for a pamphlet on athlete's foot. At Website, click on *Patient Information* and then on *Patient Education,* and choose from listed topics.

■ American Podiatric Medical Association 800-366-8227, 24-hour recording that takes request for pamphlets on athlete's foot; *www.apma.org*.

■ National Women's Health Network, 514 Tenth St. NW, Suite 400, Washington, DC 20004. 202-347-1140, M–F 9–5:30 EST; *www.womenshealthnetwork.org*. Call for a brochure on yeast infections.

Hives
www.SavonHives.com

SIGNS AND SYMPTOMS

■ Itchy, raised, red or pink swellings on the skin (called wheals). Each may range in size from smaller than a pea to the size of a dinner plate.

■ Wheals that occur in groups.
■ A wheal with a whitish center, rimmed by a red rash.
■ Wheals that itch or burn and sting. New ones may appear as the old ones fade.
■ Swelling on the lips, tongue, eyelids, or genitals. Swelling may also occur on the backs of the hands and feet.

When an irritant invades your body, your immune system sends chemicals, including histamine, to fight it. This sudden jump in histamine levels can cause an outbreak of hives. Many people—about 1 in 5—get hives at some point.

Milk, eggs, nuts, shellfish, berries, food additives, and medicines such as penicillin and aspirin can all prompt hives in some people. So can insect bites, sunlight, extreme heat or cold, pressure on the skin, and sometimes infections. **Stress** can make hives worse (see page 218).

One form of hives known as angioedema is a deep swelling in skin tissues such as the lips, tongue, eyelids, or genitals. It often lasts 24 hours or more. Most other hives go away on their own within a few days or weeks. If they last longer than 6 weeks, you and your doctor will need to find the cause.

WHAT YOU CAN DO NOW

➤ Take an antihistamine to reduce your body's response and relieve pain.
➤ Soothe your skin with cold compresses or calamine lotion.
➤ Take a cool bath with a few tablespoons of cornstarch (the kind sold in drugstores) added to it.
➤ Relax with a book, some music, or a movie on videotape—tension tends to make hives worse (see **relax,** page 303).

WHEN TO CALL THE DOCTOR

Although usually harmless, hives can signal serious—sometimes fatal—conditions. Call 911 or go to an emergency room **right away:**

SKIN, SCALP & NAILS

➤ If you have hives with hoarseness, wheezing, cold sweats, nausea, dizziness, or trouble breathing after a bee sting, insect bite, eating, or taking a medicine. You may have **shock from allergy** (see page 22). If you have a first-aid kit, give yourself an epinephrine shot. **Caution:** Don't take epinephrine if you're older or if you have heart trouble.

➤ If you have a burning feeling or itchy hives in your throat.

Call for advice:

➤ If you get hives after taking medication. You may be having an allergy attack.

➤ If you have hives that keep coming back for a month or more.

HOW TO PREVENT IT

Find the trigger. If you are reacting to a food, the hives will begin within 2 hours after you start eating. To find the culprit:

➤ For a few days, eat foods that you think won't make you break out. Slowly add other foods back into your diet, watching for a response.

➤ Look for a pattern. Keep a list of what you eat, what you do each day, and the products you use. You'll need this list when you talk with your doctor.

FOR MORE HELP

Key Websites: *www.SavonHealth.com*. For more information on hives: *www.SavonHives.com*.

Organizations: American Academy of Allergy, Asthma and Immunology, 800-822-2762, 24-hour line; *www.aaaai.org*. Ask for brochures on subjects that tie in with allergies and hives, as well as lists of allergists near you.

■ Food Allergy Network, 800-929-4040, M–F 9–5 EST; *www.foodallergy.org*. Provides literature and support.

Ingrown Toenails
www.SavonFootProblems.com

SIGNS AND SYMPTOMS

■ Swelling, pain, and redness at the side of a toenail, most often on the big toe.

Ingrown toenails occur when the sharp corners or sides of the nail push into your skin, mostly because the toenails are cut too short or because tight shoes or stockings press the nail into the flesh. Jamming your toes into the tips of shoes day after day doesn't help matters. Ingrown toenails also seem to run in some families.

Ingrown toenails sometimes become inflamed or infected, but they're easily treated at home. You can treat infections with antibiotics, and badly ingrown nails can be cut away by a doctor using local anesthetic.

WHAT YOU CAN DO NOW

➤ Cut the nail straight across. Push a small wad of sterile cotton between the nail and the skin. Use a new piece of cotton every day until the nail has grown out.

➤ If there's redness, clean the area with hydrogen peroxide, then apply an over-the-counter antibacterial cream. Cover the nail with a bandage.

➤ Soak your foot in warm water or apply a warm compress if your toe aches from the ingrown nail.

➤ If the toe hurts a lot, take an over-the-counter painkiller (see **pain relief** box, page 315).

WHEN TO CALL THE DOCTOR

➤ If redness or swelling around the nail comes with severe pain or discharge.

➤ If you cannot trim the ingrown nail.

➤ If you have diabetes, and an ingrown toenail becomes infected.

HOW TO PREVENT IT

➤ Using nail trimmers, cut straight across, but not too short. Leave some of the white nail at the end. If your nails are very hard, soften them by soaking your feet first.

➤ Wear stockings and shoes that fit well (you should be able to wiggle your toes).

➤ When you buy new shoes, do it at the end of the day, when your feet are at their largest (they tend to swell during the day).

➤ Don't wear pointed shoes.

➤ Don't expect to break in new shoes that pinch. They should feel good when you try them on.

FOR MORE HELP

Key Websites: *www.SavonHealth.com*. For more information on ingrown toenails: *www.SavonFootProblems.com*.

Organizations: American Academy of Orthopaedic Surgeons, 800-824-BONES, 24-hour recording. Ask for brochure titled "If the Shoe Fits, Wear It."

■ American Podiatric Medical Association, 800-366-8227, 24-hour recording that takes requests for free brochures on foot care; *www.apma.org*.

Lice & Scabies
www.SavonLice.com

SIGNS AND SYMPTOMS

Both lice and scabies:
■ Severe itching.
■ Marks and sores on the body from scratching (sometimes).

Head lice:
■ Itchy scalp.
■ Small, grayish white, oval eggs (nits) clinging to hairs close to the scalp.
■ Crusty infection on the scalp.
■ Grayish insects (lice) as long as an eighth of an inch, sometimes visible at the nape of the neck or behind the ears.

Body lice:
■ Raised, red bumps (bites) on the shoulders, trunk, and buttocks.
■ Nits found on clothing, often in the seams of underwear.
■ Headache, fever, and sick feeling with swelling and infected bites

(in severe cases).

Crab lice ("crabs"):
■ Itching around the genitals.
■ Tiny crablike insects (the size of a flake of dandruff or smaller) on the skin in the crotch.
■ Small dark specks (crab feces) on underwear.

Scabies:
■ Itching anywhere that gets worse just after you go to bed.
■ A rough, red, grainy rash with itchy, raised bumps, mainly on the wrists, elbows, breasts, and genitals, on the webs between the fingers and around the waist.
■ Dotted lines or wavy gray ridges like pencil marks on the skin.
■ Large areas of crusty, thick, itchy skin (Norwegian or crusted scabies).
■ In adults, itching from the neck down only. (Babies and young children may have itching on the face.)

As much as they dislike the itching caused by lice and scabies, people are more often upset by the shame they feel at having these tiny pests. But lice and scabies can infest anyone, anywhere. In fact, in recent years there has been a rash of head lice outbreaks in the United States, with 6 to 12 million cases reported yearly.

Lice are wingless insects that feed on human blood. Three types move onto either the scalp, the body, or the pubic region. Lice are found most often from August through November, and they are easily spread by skin-to-skin contact or by sharing clothes, combs, and bedding. Crab lice, the kind that infests your pubic region, are often spread by sex, but you can also get them from a toilet seat because they live away from the body for up to 3 days.

Scabies is an allergic response caused by a burrowing mite that lays eggs in tunnels under the upper layer of human skin. You may not realize you have scabies until you start to itch, and that doesn't happen until about 2 weeks after infestation. Scabies is most often spread through close contact with

SKIN, SCALP & NAILS

other people, including sex, and through sharing clothes and bed linen.

While rapid treatment can get rid of lice and scabies, it doesn't always kill them all on the first try. You may have to reapply treatments a few times, maybe more, before the pests are gone.

WHAT YOU CAN DO NOW

A good way to rid yourself of scabies and lice, many experts say, is to cover the affected part of the body with an over-the-counter shampoo or cream that contains permethrin, pyrethrin, or pyrethrum.

Caution: Because all lice and scabies removers are poisons, you must wait at least 10 days between treatments. Your skin may still itch long after the mites and lice are dead. The chemical lindane, used in some treatments for lice and scabies, is no longer prescribed for children, since it has been known to cause convulsions and other problems. Lindane has shown no such problems in adults, but tell your doctor if you prefer to use a lotion without lindane.

For all lice and scabies:

➤ For itching, try cool soaks, calamine lotion, an oral antihistamine, or pain relievers (see **pain relief,** page 315).

➤ Don't try drastic home care such as scrubbing with harsh soaps or dousing your skin or hair with kerosene.

➤ On the day you start treatment, vacuum your house and car well, and wash sheets, towels, and clothes worn in the last week in hot water and dry them on high heat for at least 30 minutes. Iron or dry-clean clothes that can't be washed. Seal stuffed animals and pillows that can harbor lice in plastic bags, and keep them out of the reach of children for at least 20 days.

Head lice:

➤ Cover the scalp with a shampoo or creme rinse containing 1 percent permethrin, pyrethrin, or pyrethrum. Follow package directions.

➤ None of these products kills the nits (eggs), though. If just a few live through the treatment, they can start a new outbreak. To soften and remove nits, shampoo hair in warm water and comb the nits out with a special fine-tooth comb (sold at drugstores) while the hair is still wet. You may need to use a magnifying glass and pick the nits out by hand.

➤ Boil combs, curlers, and brushes.

➤ If your child has repeated bouts of head lice and you don't want to keep using toxic treatments, some doctors advise this: Mix 50 drops of tea tree oil (sold in health food stores) in 2 ounces of warm olive oil; apply to the hair and scalp. Cover with a shower cap and a hot, moist towel for 2 hours. Then rinse the hair well and comb out the nits with a fine-tooth comb.

Body lice:

➤ Bathe with soap and water.

➤ Apply an antilouse cream to the entire body.

➤ Vacuum floors; wash clothes and linens as directed for all lice and scabies.

Crab lice:

➤ Use an antilouse shampoo. Follow package directions.

➤ Ask your doctor to test you for other sexually transmitted diseases.

➤ Be sure your sexual partner is treated.

Scabies:

➤ Call your doctor for a prompt appointment. The most effective treatment (a lotion containing 5 percent permethrin or pyrethrin) is given only by prescription.

➤ Wash clothes and linens as directed for all lice and scabies.

➤ Be sure all family members and people with whom you've been in close contact are treated at the same time.

➤ Try an over-the-counter antihistamine for relief from itching.

WHEN TO CALL THE DOCTOR

Call for advice and an appointment:

➤ If you suspect you have scabies.

➤ If you are unsure of the cause of your itching. Other rashes and problems can mimic the signs of scabies.

➤ If the pests come back after treatment.

➤ If your sores become infected and ooze.

➤ If you have lice on your eyelashes. Your doctor may need to remove the pests.

➤ If a baby or young child is infested.

➤ If the itching is driving you crazy.
➤ If you develop a rash or have a seizure after using a medicated lice or scabies treatment.

HOW TO PREVENT IT

Head lice:
➤ Use a flashlight to check your children for lice, especially from August through November, if you see a child scratching or your school warns you of an outbreak. Look for bites, nits, or lice at the nape of the neck and behind the ears.

All infestations:
➤ Wash clothes after 1 or 2 wearings.
➤ Wash towels and linens often.
➤ Bathe or shower daily.
➤ Don't share hats, combs, headphones, and other such items.
➤ If you have a new sexual partner, trade news about any lice or scabies either of you has had.

FOR MORE HELP

Key Websites: *www.SavonHealth.com*. For more information on lice and scabbies: *www.SavonLice.com*.

Organizations: American Academy of Dermatology, Box 4014, Schaumburg, IL 60168-4014. 888-462-3376 or 847-330-0230, M–F 8:30–5 CST; *www.aad.org*. Send a business-size self-addressed stamped envelope for a pamphlet on scabies and a list of doctors near you. At Website, click on *Patient Information* and then on *Patient Education,* and choose from listed topics.

■ National Pediculosis Association, Box 610189, Newton, MA 02461. 800-446-4672, M–F 9–4 EST; *www.headlice.org*. Ask for information on screening programs, educational materials, and the latest lice and scabies treatments.

Website: North Carolina State University, Department of Entomology, *www.ces.ncsu.edu/depts/ent/notes/Urban/lice.htm*. Offers a survey of head, body, and pubic lice and discusses treatment.

Psoriasis
www.SavonPsoriasis.com

SIGNS AND SYMPTOMS

■ Pink, raised skin flaked with white scales. Sometimes itchy or painful. Can appear anywhere, but most often on scalp, knees, and elbows; less frequently in armpits, under breasts, on genitals, and around the anus.
■ Rough, pitted fingernails that may crumble or come off.
■ Raised areas on the hands and feet that may crack or form blisters filled with pus.
■ Stiffness and inflamed flesh in fingers and toes—a form of arthritis found in 10 percent of cases.
■ Small, scaly patches along with a sore throat and strep infection (mostly in teens and young adults).

The scales of psoriasis are dense piles of dead skin formed when cells in the outer layer (the epidermis) grow faster than they can be worn away. Psoriasis, which shows up most often in people between the ages of 10 and 30, may run in families. The disorder is not contagious.

Skin injuries, strep infection, and heavy alcohol use may be causes. Stress may also be a culprit, though some experts say it isn't. Often, the ailment itself brings on feelings of low self-esteem and depression—so dealing with the accompanying emotions is a vital part of the treatment.

Some people keep psoriasis in check by using moisturizers. Others, especially those who have it on the hands and feet or on more than 30 percent of the body, may need to use stronger measures.

Psoriasis can't be cured, but home care combined with medical help often keeps it under control. Some common medical treatments include steroid creams, ultraviolet light, and oral medications, including methotrexate, an anticancer drug.

SKIN, SCALP & NAILS

WHAT YOU CAN DO NOW

➤ Follow your doctor's advice on caring for your skin, even if it takes a lot of time.

➤ Don't pick at scales. New ones may form.

➤ Use warm (not hot) water to soak the scaly spots. When the scales are plumped up with water, gently remove whatever will come away easily with a loofah sponge or pumice stone.

➤ Shampoos and lotions made with tar may help psoriasis or even get rid of it for up to 2 years. If your psoriasis is on your scalp, a dandruff shampoo may help.

➤ Use lotions to keep your skin moist. Petroleum jelly and cooking oil don't cost much and they will do the job.

➤ Sunlight helps clear up the skin. The trick is to stay in the sun until just before you burn. Talk with your doctor about finding the right balance. Use a sunscreen on skin without psoriasis. If you're using tar products, your skin may be less able to handle the sun.

➤ If you suspect your flare-ups are triggered by stress, learn to reduce it. Techniques such as yoga or meditation may help (see **relax,** page 303).

WHEN TO CALL THE DOCTOR

Call for a prompt appointment:

➤ If you get pus-filled blisters or your whole body is red and scaly; you may need treatment right away.

Call for advice:

➤ If psoriasis flares up whenever you have a sore throat; ask your doctor for medication to combat a sore throat at the first sign of illness.

➤ If home care doesn't improve or control your psoriasis.

HOW TO PREVENT IT

There is no known way to prevent psoriasis.

FOR MORE HELP

Key Websites: *www.SavonHealth.com*. For more information on psoriasis: *www.SavonPsoriasis.com*.

Organizations: American Academy of Dermatology, Box 4014, Schaumburg, IL 60168-4014. 888-462-3376 or 847-330-0230, M–F 8:30–5 CST; *www.aad.org/pamphlets/Psoriasis.html*. Explores causes and treatments.

■ National Institute of Arthritis and Musculoskeletal and Skin Diseases Information Clearinghouse, 877-226-4267, 24-hour recording, or 301-495-4484, M–F 8:30–5 EST; *www.nih.gov/niams*. Request a packet of recent articles on psoriasis.

■ National Psoriasis Foundation, 800-723-9166, M–F 8–5 PST; *www.psoriasis.org*. Staff answers questions about causes and treatments, gives names of doctors near you, and sends pamphlets and a newsletter.

Book: *Eczema & Psoriasis: How Your Diet Can Help,* by Stephen Terrass. A guide to nutrition and skin problems. HarperCollins, 1995, $9.

Shingles
www.SavonVaricella-Zoster.com

SIGNS AND SYMPTOMS

The first symptoms of shingles vary widely from person to person and can mimic other sources of pain, including muscle strain or a heart attack. Watch for:

■ Puzzling pain (sometimes pulsing or unbearable) and tingling, itching, or extreme tenderness in an area of skin on only one side of the body or face.

■ Fever and headache.

■ A red, blistering rash in a band on one side of the body. This rash may show up 1 to 3 days after the first symptoms. If confined to one side of the body, it almost always means shingles. In rare cases, the rash may appear on both sides.

■ Fluid-filled blisters that scab over, most often in 2 to 3 weeks.

■ Pain and tenderness that may last longer than the blisters.

(continued on page 177)

The Body
Illustrated

Each part of the human body works with other parts to keep the whole system in good repair—most of the time. Sometimes, as you can see in the striking illustrations on the next 16 pages, something breaks down: Thinning cartilage in a joint can lead to arthritis, for example; thickening artery walls to a heart attack; or (below) aging of the eye's lens to cataracts.

A new lens for cataracts

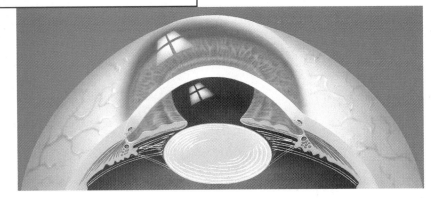

THE HEALTHY EYE ACTS LIKE A CAMERA. The clear cornea and the saucer-shaped lens focus light on the retina; from there, signals travel through the optic nerve to the brain, where they are turned into images. A cataract—clouding of the lens—distorts the focus, blurs vision, and can cause blindness.

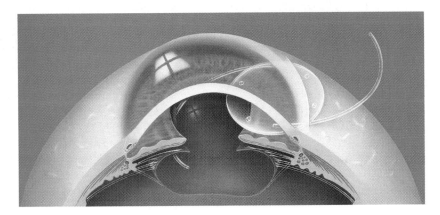

WHEN A CATARACT BECOMES SEVERE enough that a change in your eye-glass prescription no longer helps, surgeons can repair it by making a small cut in the side of the cornea, popping out the cloudy lens, and slipping a clear plastic lens in to replace it. You can go home the same day. Stitches, if you have any, rarely need to be removed; they usually dissolve naturally.

Vision problems

If you are nearsighted or farsighted, you see everything out of focus. Other vision problems have their own distinct signatures: Each has its own way of distorting or blocking the images you see.

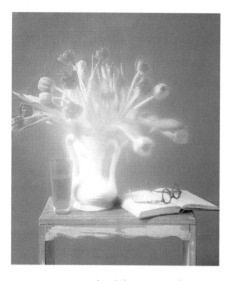

CATARACTS can cloud the center of your visual field more than the edges. Also, they can make your eyes more sensitive to glare (especially at night or in bright sunlight), cause "ghost" images, and increase nearsightedness.

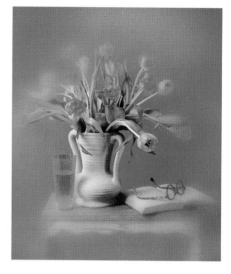

GLAUCOMA, unlike cataracts, blurs peripheral vision—the outer rim—before it affects the center. It can creep up so gradually, with so few other symptoms, that you don't notice it until your optic nerve is badly damaged.

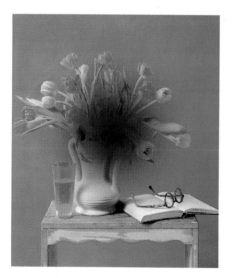

MACULAR DEGENERATION blocks the center of what you see, but it doesn't destroy peripheral vision. If it affects both eyes, you may see an empty or dark area, as above, or distorted straight lines, or blurred words on a page.

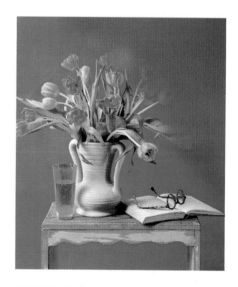

RETINAL DETACHMENT, a bubble or a rip in the retina, can suddenly black out part of your vision. This is one possible symptom; others are flashing-light sensations and dark "floaters" that look like spots or stringy shapes.

Upper respiratory

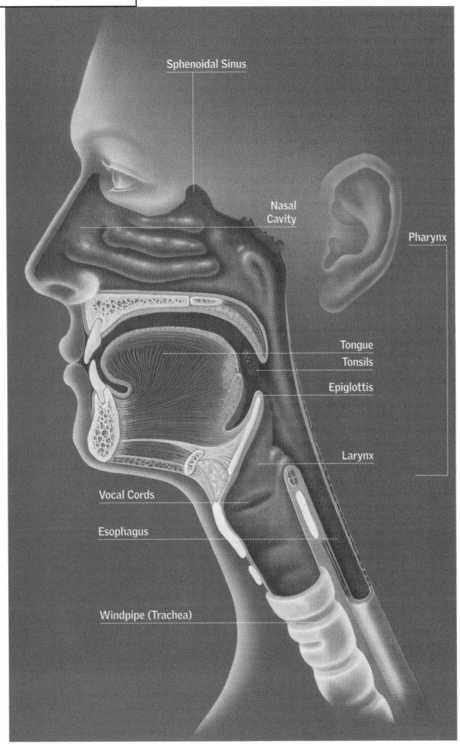

Sphenoidal Sinus

Nasal Cavity

Pharynx

Tongue

Tonsils

Epiglottis

Larynx

Vocal Cords

Esophagus

Windpipe (Trachea)

THE BODY ILLUSTRATED

Asthma

Most of the 16 million people in the United States who have asthma feel as if they can't get enough air into their lungs during an attack. But that isn't because they can't breathe in; when their airways narrow and clog, they can't breathe out.

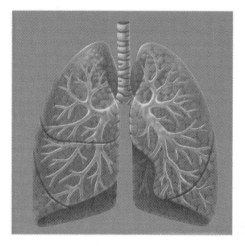
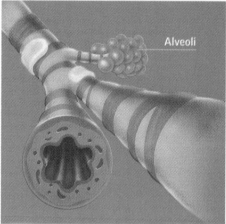

WHEN YOU BREATHE IN, muscles around your lungs expand your chest, allowing the lungs to stretch and pull in air. The air travels through bronchial tubes that branch like tree limbs into smaller and smaller passages (above, left). Eventually it reaches the alveoli, grapelike clusters of cells that pass oxygen into the bloodstream. The muscles are strong enough to pull air in, even when airways are narrowed. But they're not so good at pushing air out. In an asthma attack, stale air stays trapped in the lungs, so fresh air can't enter.

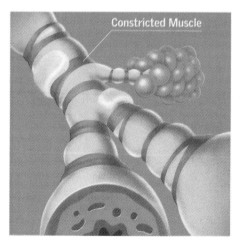
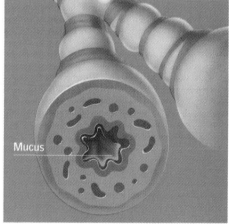

WHEN YOU HAVE ASTHMA and you inhale dust, pollen, or any other allergy-causing substance, the lining of your bronchial tubes swells (above, left). You may wheeze when you breathe. Also, muscles around your bronchial tubes can tighten, making breathing even harder. People with asthma use up to 25 times more effort to take a breath than people without it. In a severe attack, the lining of the tubes produces too much of the mucus that normally helps keep the lungs free of dust and other debris, so there is even less room for air.

Osteoarthritis

Arthritis is a name for many kinds of swelling, stiffness, and pain in the joints. Osteoarthritis, the wear-and-tear type, is the most common. More than half of all people over 65 have it in varying degrees, from mild to disabling.

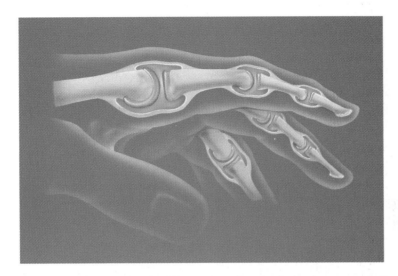

HIGHLY MOBILE JOINTS, such as those in the hands, are usually the first to feel stiff and painful. Other common sites are in the knees, hips, and spine. Here's how osteoarthritis comes on: In a young joint, a layer of smooth cartilage cushions the place where the 2 bones meet. The joint itself is sealed in a capsule filled with synovial fluid—a thick lubricant that looks like egg white.

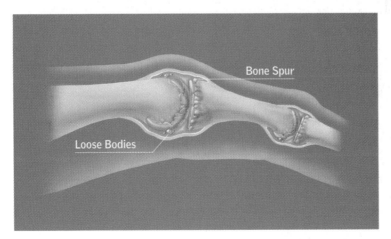

Bone Spur

Loose Bodies

WITH AGE, THE CARTILAGE becomes pitted and frayed. As the ends of the bones become more and more exposed, they roughen and rub against each other. They may also grow small bumps—spurs—that cause pain. Bits of bone and cartilage, called loose bodies, may break free and float in the joint space, causing more pain and making it even more difficult for the joint to move.

THE BODY ILLUSTRATED

Low back pain

Every year, half of all the adults in the United States have back pain, most often in the lower back—the lumbar region—which supports 70 percent of the body's weight. Even sitting at a desk can lead to low back pain.

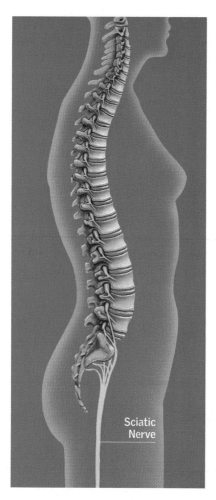

Sciatic Nerve

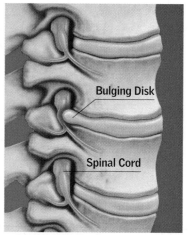

Bulging Disk

Spinal Cord

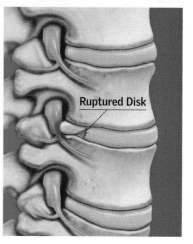

Ruptured Disk

THE SPINE IS A COLUMN OF 26 BONES, the vertebrae. It supports the head, allows human beings to stand upright, anchors the ribs and back muscles, and protects the spinal cord, a thick cable of nerves that runs from the brain down through a channel in the vertebral column.

Disks between the vertebrae allow the vertebral column to move. They also absorb shock and cushion the impact of walking and other motion. Their tough outside shell protects a soft, gel-like center. Aging and stress on the spine can cause the shell of a disk to bulge—this is what's known as a herniated, or slipped, disk—and even to rupture and leak some of its contents.

The bulging disk may press on a nerve and cause pain, sometimes a lot of it. When that happens to the sciatic nerve (left, descending from the base of the spine), you may feel burning pain or sometimes tingling or numbness far from your back, in your legs. That is because the sciatic nerve carries nerve impulses all the way down the legs to your feet.

Osteoporosis

Though it looks solid, bone is built around a spongy core that helps make it both light and strong. A breakdown of the core results in osteoporosis ("porous bone"), the main cause of bone fractures among Americans over 45.

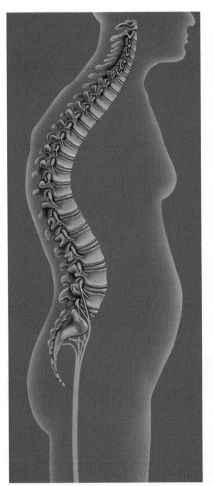

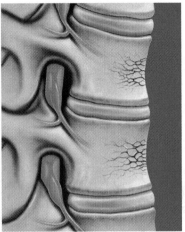

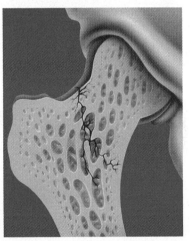

BONE IS LIVING TISSUE that renews and repairs itself. It can be as tough as steel, yet is far lighter and more flexible, because it is built in 2 layers. Its spongelike core consists of many spaces connected by bony bridges. A hard, dense outer layer protects the core. In both, special cells constantly tear down old bone and build new bone with calcium and other minerals.

After middle age, bones tend to lose minerals faster than they can be replaced. More bone is torn down than rebuilt. If you don't halt this loss, the bridges in the core become thin and brittle: Osteoporosis sets in. When osteoporosis weakens bones in the spine, even the normal pressure of body weight can cause tiny cracks called crush fractures (upper right). Over time, these cracks can lead to chronic back pain, loss of height, and the curving upper spine known as dowager's hump (left). The first symptom of osteoporosis may be a bone that breaks for no clear reason. Bones with large spongy areas, like those of the hip joint (lower right), are the most subject to fractures.

The heart

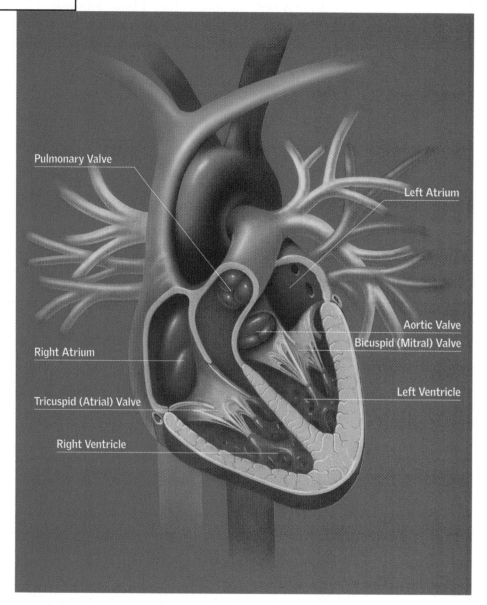

Pulmonary Valve

Left Atrium

Right Atrium

Aortic Valve

Bicuspid (Mitral) Valve

Tricuspid (Atrial) Valve

Left Ventricle

Right Ventricle

YOUR HARDEST-WORKING MUSCLE is your heart. Every day it beats about 100,000 times, pumping more than 1,900 gallons of blood. It is as durable as it is complex; usually it works without complaint. And if something does go wrong with one of its parts, the defect can very often be repaired.

The right side of the heart pumps "spent" blood to the lungs for a fresh supply of oxygen. Then the left side pumps oxygen-rich blood to the rest of the body. Four valves keep blood from leaking backward as it moves through the chambers of the heart. A murmur may be a sign of something disrupting blood flow—a narrowed valve, perhaps, or one that doesn't close tightly. In mitral valve prolapse, for instance, part of the valve flops back too far, allowing backflow. For most people this is not a serious problem, but some need medication to prevent infection of the valve, and some may even need surgery.

Atherosclerosis

In atherosclerosis, the arteries slowly grow thicker and harder. The process can start as early as childhood, and it can go on without symptoms for decades until the buildup causes a heart attack or a stroke.

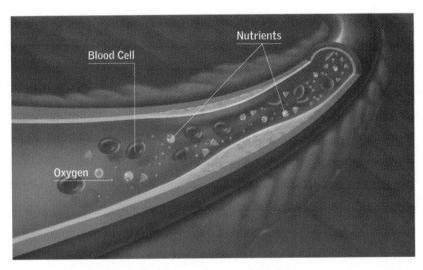

THE ARTERIES CARRY BLOOD rich in nutrients, oxygen, and other vital substances, including cholesterol, from the heart and lungs to the body.

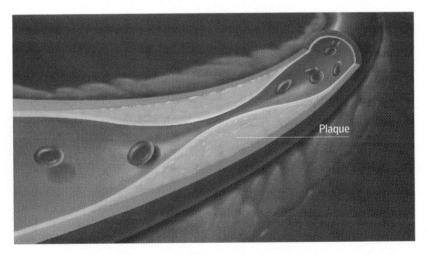

THE WALLS OF AN ARTERY, over time, may collect dense streaks of minerals and fats. These streaks, which bulge from the wall, are called plaque.

As plaque builds up and narrows an artery, it restricts the amount of blood that can flow through. The bulges and rough spots on its surface allow clots to form easily. A clot that wedges in a narrowed spot and blocks the flow of blood can cause a heart attack or a stroke.

THE BODY ILLUSTRATED

Bones

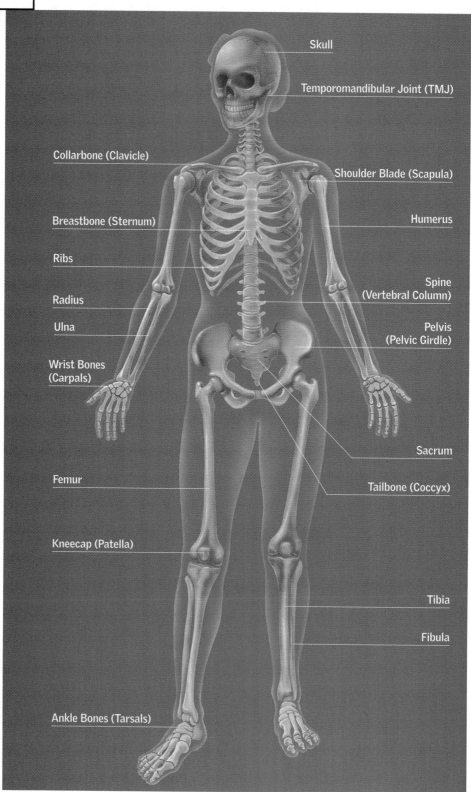

Skull

Temporomandibular Joint (TMJ)

Collarbone (Clavicle)

Shoulder Blade (Scapula)

Breastbone (Sternum)

Humerus

Ribs

Spine
(Vertebral Column)

Radius

Ulna

Pelvis
(Pelvic Girdle)

Wrist Bones
(Carpals)

Sacrum

Femur

Tailbone (Coccyx)

Kneecap (Patella)

Tibia

Fibula

Ankle Bones (Tarsals)

Muscles

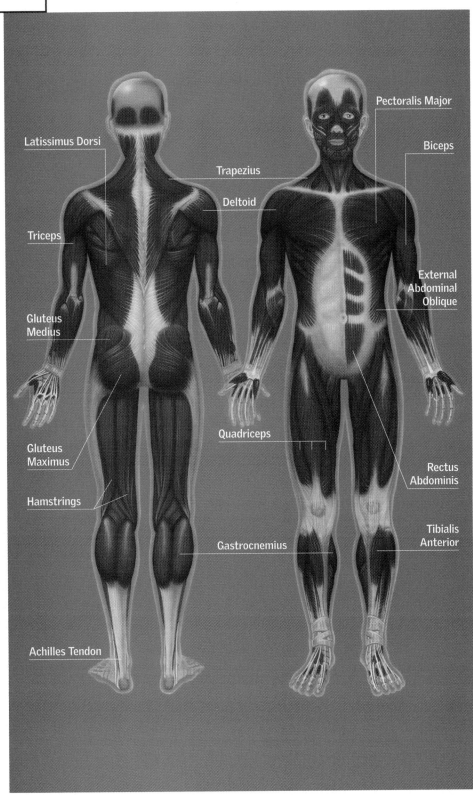

Latissimus Dorsi

Trapezius

Deltoid

Triceps

Gluteus
Medius

Gluteus
Maximus

Hamstrings

Quadriceps

Gastrocnemius

Achilles Tendon

Pectoralis Major

Biceps

External
Abdominal
Oblique

Rectus
Abdominis

Tibialis
Anterior

THE BODY ILLUSTRATED

Skin cancer

Most skin cancers are caused by ultraviolet (UV) rays from the sun. Basal and squamous cell cancers are common but seldom fatal; melanoma is rare but often deadly. You can reduce skin damage by covering up and using sunscreen.

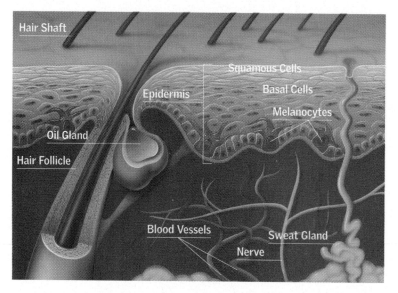

THE TOP LAYER OF THE SKIN (the epidermis) is made of 3 kinds of cells: squamous cells, basal cells, and melanocytes. Cancer occurs when skin cells begin to grow out of control, forming tumors.

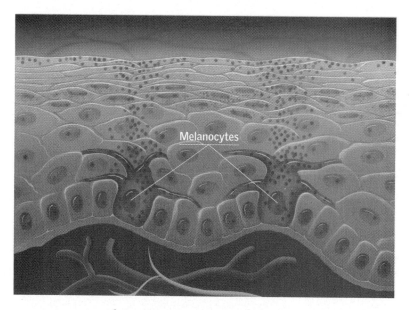

A TAN IS THE SKIN'S EMERGENCY RESPONSE to UV rays from the sun. When UV light hits, melanocytes try to repair the damage it does by putting out more melanin, a dark pigment, and multiplying faster than usual. Over time, UV rays make stretchy tissues in the lower layer of cells begin to sag.

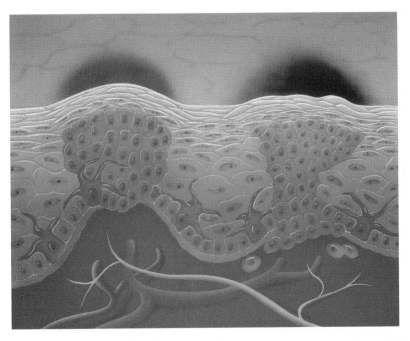

A MOLE FORMS when a cluster of melanocytes pushes to the surface of the skin, forming a dark and compact, but harmless, growth.

Sun exposure can push melanocytes to grow wildly into a cancerous tumor known as a malignant melanoma. Sometimes cells from a melanoma break away and form cancerous tumors in other parts of the body.

THESE SIGNS HELP you tell a melanoma from a normal mole:

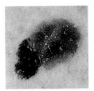 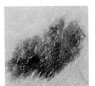 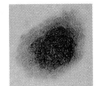 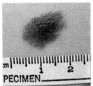

Asymmetrical shape.   **B**orders are blurry.   **C**olor varies within mole.   **D**iameter larger than a pencil eraser.

Internal organs

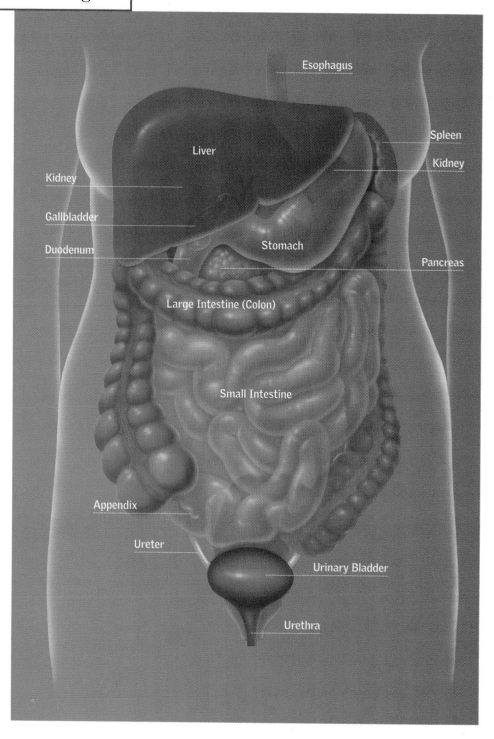

Esophagus

Spleen

Kidney

Liver

Kidney

Gallbladder

Duodenum

Stomach

Pancreas

Large Intestine (Colon)

Small Intestine

Appendix

Ureter

Urinary Bladder

Urethra

Reproduction

The female and male reproductive systems produce and store the cells that combine and become new human beings. When a woman's egg and a man's sperm cell join, the fertilized egg is a tiny speck weighing less than one-twentieth of a millionth of an ounce.

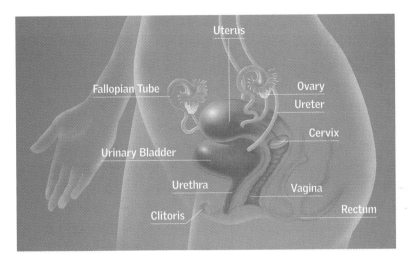

A GIRL'S OVARIES contain all the eggs she'll ever have—200,000 of them—6 months before she is born. As she reaches her teens, her ovaries begin to release one or more of the eggs every month into the fallopian tubes, which carry them to the uterus. If an egg is not fertilized, the lining of the uterus (the endometrium) will shed during menstruation. Sometimes fragments of endometrial tissue grow outside the uterus (the problem is called endometriosis) and cause painful menstruation.

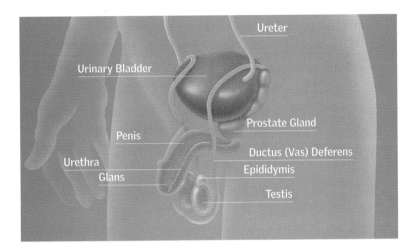

A MAN'S TESTES produce spermatozoa that move on to the epididymis, where they mature. When a man ejaculates, he releases 300 to 500 million sperm cells. The prostate gland, which produces fluid that nourishes sperm and makes them more active, often becomes enlarged as a man grows older. The enlarged gland may squeeze the urethra and make urination difficult.

Referred pain

Have you ever wondered why a person having a heart attack might feel pain not in the heart but in the shoulder, chest, or left arm? The answer is referred pain. Sensations from an internal organ are sometimes referred to—felt in—other places served by nerves from the same part of the spinal cord as that organ.

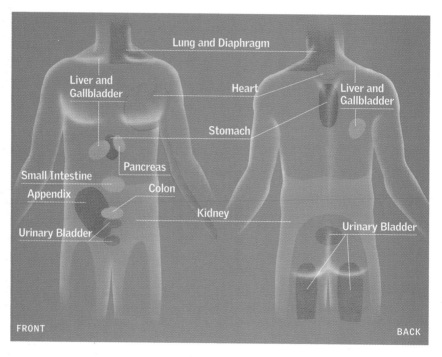

Lung and Diaphragm

Liver and Gallbladder

Heart

Liver and Gallbladder

Stomach

Pancreas

Small Intestine

Colon

Appendix

Kidney

Urinary Bladder

Urinary Bladder

FRONT

BACK

PAIN FROM AN INTERNAL ORGAN often shows up on the skin or just under it. It can occur close to the organ or sometimes far from it. For example, pain from liver and gallbladder trouble (green) may be felt in the right side of the neck, the front of the chest, or the right shoulder blade, and pain from the stomach (red) may appear high in the abdomen and between the shoulders.

PAIN IN THE FACE (the shaded areas) is often a sign of a deeper problem.

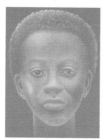
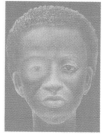
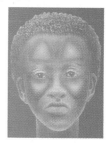
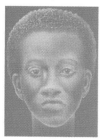

If pain gets worse when you bend your head forward, you may have a sinus infection.

If a throbbing pain gets worse at night, you may have a tooth abscess.

If your nose and one eye are runny and you have a headache, you may have a migraine.

If you have a blood-shot eye, blurry vision, and intense pain, you may have acute glaucoma.

(continued from page 160)

Thought chicken pox was behind you? Think again. Anyone who has had chicken pox has a chance of getting shingles as an adult. That's because chicken pox and the painful blisters of shingles are caused by the same herpes virus. Instead of going away when the chicken pox sores dry up, the virus hides in the nerve cells near the spine, sometimes for decades. Later, perhaps because the immune system is weakened or stressed, the virus comes back in its new form, inflaming certain nerve pathways.

Shingles is most common in adults over 50, and half of people over 85 have had it. People with immune systems weakened by AIDS, Hodgkin's disease, leukemia, or some kinds of drugs also are more likely to get this disorder.

You can't catch shingles. But if you've never had chicken pox, there's a small chance that you'll get chicken pox if you come into contact with fluid from the broken blisters of someone with shingles. That risk is highest for newborns.

In its worst form, which happens in 10 to 15 percent of cases, the ailment can cause intense shooting, burning pain (post-herpetic neuralgia) for a month or more after the blisters are gone. But antiviral drugs can halt the disease. Prompt treatment reduces the chances of having this type of pain.

Shingles may also involve the nerves to the iris of the eye. This can lead to glaucoma and even blindness. Watch for blisters on the nose—they're the first sign the eyes may be affected. In those with other diseases, shingles may affect skin all over the body, and even the internal organs.

Most people who get shingles get over it in a few weeks, and the disease rarely recurs.

WHAT YOU CAN DO NOW

Call your doctor for advice if you notice the first signs of shingles. There are medicines that fight the virus. In mild cases, you may not need drugs—but if you do, the sooner you take them, the better your chance of avoiding the pain of shingles.

➤ Soothe the pain with cool compresses or ice packs.

➤ Take an over-the-counter painkiller (see **pain relief,** page 315).

➤ Relieve the itching with calamine lotion.

➤ Ask your doctor about using over-the-counter capsaicin cream, made from the fiery substance in chili peppers, to help reduce the severe pain of post-herpetic neuralgia. Use it only after the blisters are healed.

➤ Put a few tablespoons of cornstarch or oatmeal bath powder (the kind sold in drugstores) in your bathwater.

➤ Cut nails short. Do not scratch. The blisters can become infected or leave scars.

➤ Wear gloves at night so you won't scratch in your sleep.

➤ If you have severe pain that won't go away, join a chronic pain support group.

WHEN TO CALL THE DOCTOR

Call your doctor for emergency advice (if you can't get any, call 911 or go to an emergency room):

➤ If you have eye pain or a fluid-filled blister on your face. You may be at risk of getting herpes in your eye, which can lead to blindness.

Call for a prompt appointment:

➤ If you have a fever over 101 degrees or swelling, redness, and pus. This can signal a systemwide infection or a bacterial infection in the blisters.

Call for advice:

➤ If you have symptoms of shingles.

HOW TO PREVENT IT

There is no known way to prevent shingles. A vaccine for chicken pox is now in use, but its effects on shingles are unknown.

FOR MORE HELP

Key Websites: *www.SavonHealth.com*. For more information on shingles: *www.SavonVaricella-Zoster.com*.

Organizations: American Chronic Pain Association, Box 850, Rocklin, CA 95677. 916-632-0922, 24-hour line. Ask for facts about shingles and advice on support groups for those with chronic pain.

SKIN, SCALP & NAILS

■ National Institute of Neurological Disorders and Stroke, 800-352-9424, M–F 8:30–5 EST; *www.ninds.nih.gov.* Ask for facts about shingles and post-herpetic neuralgia.

Sunburn
www.SavonSunburn.com

SIGNS AND SYMPTOMS

■ Red, "burned" skin (even in dark-skinned people).
■ Pain and (sometimes) blisters.

Not too long ago, a suntan—or even a slight burn—was considered a sign of good health. Now we know it's the body's attempt to protect itself from the sun, and a sign of skin damage.

That's because some rays of sun—called ultraviolet A and B (UVA and UVB)—damage skin cells. If you're out in the sun year after year, even if you never burn, the result is wrinkles and perhaps **skin cancer** (see facing page and illustrations, pages 172 and 173).

A sunburn raises the risks. People of all skin colors can get a sunburn, but those with fair skin are the most likely to get long-term skin damage or skin cancer from it.

WHAT YOU CAN DO NOW

➤ Soothe the burned skin with a cool bath or a compress.
➤ Try ice for pain. Take one cube and melt it slightly so that it has no rough edges. Glide it over the burn until it melts, keeping it moving to avoid skin damage. Repeat every hour as needed for pain.
➤ Try lotions or gels with aloe vera to soothe pain and speed healing.
➤ Use an over-the-counter painkiller (see **pain relief,** page 315). Aspirin works best because it blocks a chemical the body makes in response to burns. (Never give aspirin to a child or teenager who has chicken pox, a cold, the flu, or any other illness you suspect of being caused by a virus; see box on **Reye's syndrome,** page 95.)

➤ Consider a lotion or spray that contains benzocaine for pain relief. **Caution:** It may cause an allergic response. Don't use it if you have skin allergies or if allergies run in your family.
➤ Watch for signs of dehydration—dry mouth, sticky saliva, dizziness or weakness, and dark yellow urine—especially if the sunburned person is a child. Give water or a **rehydration** drink (see box on page 120).
➤ Watch out for **heatstroke** and **heat exhaustion** (see page 38). **Caution:** If you suspect heatstroke, don't give the person anything to drink.

Later:
➤ If skin peels, use a lotion to add moisture and ease itching. Lotions with aloe vera are soothing at any point.
➤ If you must go back into the sun, keep the burn from getting worse by covering up and using sunscreen with an SPF (sun protection factor) of at least 15.

WHEN TO CALL THE DOCTOR

➤ Call 911 or go to an emergency room **right away** if you see signs of heat stroke.
➤ Call for advice if the skin blisters. Don't cover the blisters.

Simple Steps to Save Your Skin

➤ Standing in front of a mirror, look at your front and, using a hand mirror, at your back. Look for any strange lumps or new growths.
➤ Raise your arms and turn to the right and left as you examine your sides and underarms.
➤ Bend your arms and inspect them from fingertips to shoulders, including the undersides.
➤ Sit down and use a hand mirror to look at the backs of your legs; also examine the tops of your feet and the spaces between your toes.
➤ Use the hand mirror to look at the back of your neck and your scalp, or ask someone to check these areas for you.

Skin Cancer

In the United States, 1 person in 5 will have skin cancer during her or his lifetime. The good news is that it can nearly always be cured if caught in time. And because sunlight is the major cause, most skin cancer can be prevented.

The 3 main kinds of skin cancer are:

Basal cell carcinoma. This is the most common type. Often found on the face, it develops slowly and, most of the time, doesn't send cancer cells to other parts of the body. The symptoms are:

- A pearly or shiny skin growth, often with a dent in the center and raised edges, that expands over time.
- A patch of skin that itches, bleeds, hurts, or forms a scab.
- An open sore that fails to heal in a month, or one that closes and then reopens.

Squamous cell carcinoma. This usually appears on the face, lips, or rim of the ear. It grows quickly and can form large masses. If ignored, it can spread to other parts of the body. The symptoms are:

- Reddish or brownish rough, scaly patches on skin that has been exposed to sunlight.
- A stubborn, scaly patch that sometimes crusts or bleeds.
- A raised growth that looks like a wart and sometimes bleeds.
- A firm, fleshy lump that grows bigger and bigger.

Malignant melanoma. This is the most harmful type of skin cancer. A cancer of the cells that produce melanin, it often spreads to other parts of the body and can be fatal. The symptoms are:

- A mole that changes the way it looks. It may become scaly or ooze, bleed, or enlarge.
- A dark area of the skin that feels itchy, or the sudden growth of a "bubbly" mole.
- Dark spots or moles that have these "ABCD" traits: Asymmetrical, Border blurry, Color uneven, Diameter larger than a pencil eraser.

See a doctor promptly if you have any of the symptoms of skin cancer. The earlier skin cancer is detected, the better your chances that treatment will cure it.

Call for a prompt appointment if you have an itchy mole or a dark spot or bump that changes color, bleeds, or oozes. Call for advice if you see any of the signs of skin cancer; if what looks like a pimple crusts over, doesn't go away, and gets bigger; or if you develop a lump on or beneath an area of your skin that is often exposed to the sun and doesn't go away after 2 weeks of home treatment with warm compresses.

For more information, contact:

- The American Academy of Dermatology, Box 4014, Schaumburg, IL 60168-4014. 888-462-3376 or 847-330-0230, M–F 8:30–5 CST; *www.aad.org*. Send a business-size self-addressed stamped envelope for a pamphlet on skin cancer. At Website, click on *Patient Information,* then *Patient Education,* then *Skin Cancer* for facts about skin cancer.
- American Cancer Society, 800-227-2345, staff is available to speak with you 24 hours a day; *www.cancer.org*. Provides referrals; information about support groups, treatment options, and events; and a list of American Cancer Society offices near you.
- National Cancer Institute's Cancer Information Service, 800-4-CANCER, M–F 9–4:30 your time, *www.cis.nci.nih.gov*. In English and Spanish. Provides brochures, information on standard treatment options, access to a database of clinical trials, and names of cancer-related resources near you.

SKIN, SCALP & NAILS

➤ Apply a sunscreen of SPF 15 or higher 30 minutes before you go outside (to give it time to bond to the skin). You need protection whenever you plan to be out more than a few minutes, even in winter or when it's overcast.

➤ Reapply sunscreen every 2 hours, even if it's waterproof (no matter what their SPF, waterproof sunscreens by current law have to protect for just 80 minutes when wet, and they're not necessarily sweatproof). **Caution:** If you have allergies or tender skin, test the sunscreen on a small spot to see if you react. You might want to avoid sunscreens with PABA, or try a product with titanium dioxide. Don't put sunscreen on the faces of babies younger than 6 months—it can get in their eyes or mouth. Keep infants out of the sun.

➤ When possible, avoid being outdoors between 10 AM and 2 PM, when the sun's rays are most intense.

➤ Wear protective clothing and a hat with a wide brim. But remember, you can get a sunburn through most clothes. The average white T-shirt has an SPF of 9 at most, and that drops to 3 if the shirt is wet. A few companies manufacture special clothing that blocks UV rays.

➤ Don't go to tanning salons; they use harmful ultraviolet light.

➤ Don't use suntan oil; it doesn't protect your skin.

➤ Do a skin self-exam every month (see **simple steps to save your skin** box, page 178). If you are light-skinned, have freckles, burn without tanning, or have a family history of skin cancer, see your doctor for a checkup and to learn the danger signs (see box on **skin cancer,** page 179).

Which SPF Is Best for You?

With stores swimming in lotions with SPF 30, 45, and even 60, it's useful to know what SPF means. The term—which refers to "sun protection factor"—is meant to help you figure out how long a product will let you stay in the sun before you burn. An SPF 15 lets you linger 15 times longer than if your skin were unprotected; an SPF 8 sunscreen, 8 times longer. The key is your coloring. If you're very fair and burn after 10 minutes of sun, SPF 15 gives you about 150 minutes of protection; if you take 20 minutes to redden, it protects you for 300 minutes. Reapplying doesn't increase the total amount of time you can be in the sun before burning.

The Food and Drug Administration has moved to bring order to the world of sunscreen labels. By May 2001, products that claim to fight off the sun's wrinkle- and cancer-inducing rays will be ranked "minimum" if they have an SPF of 2 to 11, "moderate" (12 to 20), or "high" (30 or above). Terms like "sunblock," "all-day protection," and "waterproof" will have vanished. Instead, you'll read "water resistant" if a product continues protecting for 40 minutes after exposure to moisture (including sweat) and "very water resistant" if it works for 80 minutes. The FDA may do some tinkering before the changes are final.

Key Websites: *www.SavonHealth.com*. For more information on sunburn: *www.SavonSunburn.com*.

Organizations: American Academy of Dermatology, Box 4014, Schaumburg, IL 60168-4014. 888-462-3376 or 847-330-0230, M–F 8:30–5 CST; *www.aad.org*. Send a business-size self-addressed stamped envelope for the pamphlets on skin cancer. At Website, click on *Patient Information* and then on *Skin Savvy*.

■ National Institute of Arthritis and Musculoskeletal and Skin Diseases Information Clearinghouse, 877-226-4267, 24-hour recording, or 301-495-4484 M–F 8:30–5 EST; *www.nih.gov/niams*. Request the "Sun and Skin" packet.

Warts

www.SavonWarts.com

SIGNS AND SYMPTOMS

Common warts:
- Small, hard, rough, raised growths that most often appear on the skin of the hands and fingers.

Plantar warts:
- Same hard growths as common warts but on the soles of the feet, sometimes making walking painful.

Flat warts:
- Small, flat growths, clustered in groups of many hundreds. Often found on the hands, wrists, forearms, knees, face, neck, and chest.

Filiform warts:
- Slim, stringlike growths that take root on the face or neck.

Genital warts:
- Itchy, small bumps, round or flat, sometimes in groups, that appear on or near the genitals. Can be passed from person to person.

The source of warts is any one of about 70 types of the human papilloma virus.

You pick up the virus by coming into contact with skin shed from a wart (either your own or someone else's). The virus enters through a cut or nick in the skin, causing skin cells to grow quickly, creating a new wart. This doesn't happen easily, except in the case of genital warts.

Children, young adults, and people with weakened immune systems are most likely to get warts. Children's warts nearly always go away within a year or so, but in adults they may take longer, or may need to be removed.

WHAT YOU CAN DO NOW

Warts are harmless, and can go away by themselves. You can often remove them at home. If you're over 45 and a new wart appears, check with a doctor before trying home care.

- If you have genital warts, see your doctor.
- You can remove warts, when they are not on the face or the genitals, with an over-the-counter product that contains salicylic acid. It gently peels the surface of the wart away. You may need to apply the acid many times.
- Don't cut or burn a wart.
- Plantar warts often extend below the surface of the skin. You may need the help of a skin doctor to remove them. Padded insoles in your shoes may reduce pain.
- Some experts believe you can think your warts away. Sit quietly, close your eyes, and create an image of the wart shrinking and vanishing. Do it for 5 or 10 minutes 2 or 3 times a day for several days.

WHEN TO CALL THE DOCTOR

- If you or your partner has genital warts, which can be passed on to others and also may be related to cervical cancer in women (see **sexually transmitted diseases** chart, page 221).
- If you are over 45 and you find a new wart. Your doctor will want to check it to make sure it's not **skin cancer** (see page 179; see also color illustration, page 172).
- If you want a wart on your face removed.
- If you have a wart that does not respond to home treatment, especially if it bleeds, changes color, or looks infected.

HOW TO PREVENT IT

- Don't scratch warts.
- When shaving, use an electric razor to avoid the small nicks and scratches that may allow viruses to enter.
- Don't touch other people's warts.
- When using public showers, wear footwear.

FOR MORE HELP

Key Websites: *www.SavonHealth.com*. For more information on warts: *www.SavonWarts.com*.

Organization: American Academy of Dermatology, Box 4014, Schaumburg, IL 60168-4014. 888-462-3376 or 847-330-0230, M–F 8:30–5 CST; *www.aad.org*. Send a business-size self-addressed stamped envelope for a pamphlet on warts. At Website, click on *Patient Information* and then on *Patient Education*, then choose from listed topics.

SKIN, SCALP & NAILS

Muscles, Bones & Joints

Arthritis

www.SavonArthritis.com

SIGNS AND SYMPTOMS

Osteoarthritis:
- Joint pain that is made worse by movement.
- Stiffness in the morning.
- Knobby growths on finger joints.

Rheumatoid arthritis:
- Painful, swollen joints that may feel warm.
- Low fever, loss of weight and appetite, feeling "sick all over."
- Morning stiffness.
- Skin lumps, often on the elbows, fingers, or buttocks.
- Dry, itching eyes and dry mouth.

Gout:
- Severe, sudden pain in a joint, often the wrist, big toe, or knee.
- Redness, swelling around joint.
- Fever.

Arthritis is a name given to more than 100 kinds of mild to crippling joint problems that cause swelling, pain, and stiffness. Three types are most common:

Osteoarthritis is caused by chips and cracks in the smooth cartilage that cushions the joints (see color illustrations, page 165). When bone surfaces have too little cushioning, they rub together and may grow bumps, called spurs, that irritate nearby tissue. Osteoarthritis is the most common form of arthritis, affecting more than 23 million Americans. More than half of those older than 65 have osteoarthritis. It most often occurs in the hands or in weight-bearing joints such as the knee and hip.

Rheumatoid arthritis results when the lining of the capsule around a joint becomes inflamed and thickened, causing swelling, pain, and stiffness. Rheumatoid arthritis can also inflame the eyes and lungs. Some experts think it's the result of a problem with the body's immune system—the body attacking its own tissues as if they were foreign invaders. It may also be hereditary. Rheumatoid arthritis most often affects people between 20 and 50, and more women than men, some 2.5 million Americans.

Gout usually affects men over 40 and is caused by high blood levels of uric acid, one of the body's waste products, which forms crystals in the joints. The immune system tries to defend the body against these crystals, and the joint becomes inflamed and painful. Symptoms of each attack go away in about a week.

Treatment of arthritis depends on the type and how bad it is. Most can be treated with gentle exercise to keep the bones and muscles strong and supple. Drugs also reduce pain, swelling, and stiffness. New painkillers called COX-2 inhibitors offer relief with less risk of the stomach ulcers and bleeding caused by common arthritis drugs. For rheumatoid arthritis, two new types of drugs help ease pain by actually slowing the disease's progression; there's even a new device that filters inflammation-causing antibodies from the blood in advanced cases. Gout can be treated with drugs to reduce uric acid in the blood. And in some severe cases of osteoarthritis and rheumatoid arthritis, surgery may be used to smooth rough joint surfaces or replace a damaged joint.

Neck Pain

Neck pain is most often a sign of simple muscle strain that you can take care of at home, but it can be a symptom of more serious problems.

SYMPTOMS	WHAT IT MIGHT BE	WHAT YOU CAN DO
Severe headache, then neck pain and stiffness; sometimes with nausea, drowsiness, or trouble seeing in bright light.	Meningitis—infection of tissue around brain (see page 55).	Call 911 or go to emergency room **right away.**
Severe pain and/or swelling in neck after injury; numbness, weakness, or paralysis below injured spot; lack of bladder or bowel control; shock.	Spinal cord injury (see head, neck, and back injuries, page 36).	Call 911 **right away.** Never attempt to move someone who may have a spinal cord injury.
Bad neck pain, worse when moving head; or tingling, numbness, pain, or weakness in shoulder, arm, or hand.	Protruded disk pressing on a nerve (see low back pain, page 190).	With sudden numbness or weakness, call doctor for advice and appointment **right away;** if you can't get one, call 911 or go to emergency room. Take painkillers (see box, page 315), and rest.
Pain and stiffness that begin in neck and move to shoulders, upper arms, hands, or back of head; numbness or tingling in arms, head, and fingers; weakness in arms and legs.	Cervical spondylosis—breakdown of joints in neck that may cause them to press on nerves and muscles.	With numbness and tingling, call doctor for prompt appointment. Otherwise, call for advice. Apply moist heat. Sleep with thin pillow under head and thin, rolled-up towel under neck.
Pain and soreness in front of neck, fever, swelling.	Thyroiditis (see thyroid problems, page 288).	Call doctor for prompt appointment.
Stiff neck that may come with pain or swelling in other joints.	Arthritis.	See arthritis, facing page.
Pain with swelling on back or side of neck.	Swollen lymph nodes from infection.	See infections, page 281.

(continued)

MUSCLES, BONES & JOINTS

Neck Pain (continued)

SYMPTOMS	WHAT IT MIGHT BE	WHAT YOU CAN DO
Neck pain or stiffness that starts within 24 hours of a jolt (such as a car stopping suddenly); sometimes with dizziness, headache, vomiting, or trouble walking.	Whiplash—also known as cervical acceleration/deceleration injury.	Call doctor for prompt appointment. Wear soft, padded collar to hold neck still. Sleep with thin pillow under head and thin, rolled-up towel under neck. Apply ice pack, and take pain-killers (see box, page 315).
Stiff neck or pain on waking, or when sitting or standing.	Strained neck muscles or ligaments from sleeping or sitting in awkward way.	Sleep with thin pillow under head and thin, rolled-up towel under neck. If stiffness or pain lasts more than 24 hours, call doctor for advice and appointment.

WHAT YOU CAN DO NOW

➤ For rheumatoid arthritis, take aspirin or the anti-inflammatory painkiller recommended by your doctor. If these upset your stomach, try an "enteric-coated" brand that delays release of the drug until it has passed through your stomach. Or ask your doctor about other drugs aimed at reducing the risk of ulcers.

➤ For osteoarthritis, use acetaminophen. If you have gout, don't take aspirin, which inhibits the body's ability to excrete uric acid. Take aspirin, ibuprofen, or naproxen separately; never combine them (see **pain relief** box, page 315).

➤ Apply cold packs to swollen, painful joints, or warm packs for stiffness without other symptoms, for 10 minutes every hour.

➤ For pain relief, apply over-the-counter creams that contain methyl salicylate or capsaicin, a substance in hot peppers.

➤ Twice a day, put each joint gently through a full range of motion to prevent stiffness.

➤ Take a warm shower or bath in the morning to relieve stiffness.

➤ Enroll in an arthritis self-help program or join a support group with other people going through the same things you are.

➤ To ease the strain on painful hand joints, use electric can openers and large rubber grips for pens or tools.

➤ Don't grip objects tightly for a long time.

➤ Eat more than 2 servings a week of fish rich in omega-3 polyunsaturated fatty acids (salmon, mackerel, or sardines) or take omega-3 in capsule form to help reduce inflammation.

➤ Get lots of rest.

WHEN TO CALL THE DOCTOR

➤ If you have joint pain or stiffness that gets in the way of normal activities.

➤ If you have fever or chills along with other arthritis symptoms. You may have infectious arthritis, caused by bacteria, which can be treated with antibiotics.

➤ If you get the painful symptoms of gout.

➤ If your arthritis doesn't get better.

HOW TO PREVENT IT

Osteoarthritis:

➤ Exercise gently and often to keep your bones and muscles strong. Swimming, biking, yoga, and low-impact or water aerobics are ideal.

➤ If you weigh more than you should, lose those extra pounds. Too much weight puts added pressure on the joints.

➤ Try not to do the same movements over and over—for instance, typing.

➤ Stand up straight to ease strain on joints.

Rheumatoid arthritis:

There's no known way to prevent rheumatoid arthritis.

Gout:

➤ Control your weight, but don't fast; fasting can raise levels of uric acid.

➤ If you drink, drink moderately—no more than 2 drinks a day if you're a man, 1 if you're a woman. A drink is a 1.5-ounce shot of hard liquor, a 5-ounce glass of wine, or a 12-ounce beer.

➤ Avoid protein-rich foods such as organ meats, shellfish, and beans.

➤ Drink plenty of water—at least 10 big glasses a day to help flush out uric acid.

COMPLEMENTARY CHOICES

➤ Acupuncture may help. Studies by the National Institutes of Health and others have found it relieves chronic arthritis pain. (See page 310 for tips on finding a reliable acupuncturist.)

➤ Some people with arthritis find that stress reduction such as yoga or meditation eases their pain (see **relax,** page 303). Massage also may help.

➤ Supplements of two natural substances, glucosamine and chondroitin, appear to help maintain cartilage and even repair damage from arthritis.

FOR MORE HELP

Key Websites: *www.SavonHealth.com.* For more information on arthritis: *www.SavonArthritis.com.*

Organizations: Arthritis Foundation, 1330 W. Peachtree St., Atlanta, GA 30309. 800-283-7800, 24-hour recording, or 404- 872-7100, M–F 9–5 EST; *www.arthritis.org.* Provides tips on exercise and pain control, and lists support groups near you. Membership, starting at $20, includes a subscription to *Arthritis Today* magazine.

■ National Institute of Arthritis and Musculoskeletal and Skin Diseases Information Clearinghouse, 1 AMS Circle, Bethesda, MD 20892-3675. 877-226-4267, M–F 8:30–5 EST; *www.nih.gov/niams.* Click on *Health Information* and then on *NIAMS Brochures and Other Publications.*

Website: Johns Hopkins Health Information, *www.intelihealth.com.* Click on *Arthritis* for facts and articles on the disorder.

Books: *The Arthritis Foundation's Guide to Alternative Therapies,* by Judith Horstman. Advice on nontraditional arthritis treatment. Longstreet Press, 1999, $24.95.

■ *250 Tips for Making Life With Arthritis Easier,* by Shelley Peterman Schwartz. Longstreet Press, 1997, $9.95.

Bunions & Hammertoes
www.SavonFootProblems.com

SIGNS AND SYMPTOMS

Bunion:

■ A lump on the side of the joint that connects the big toe to the foot.

■ A big toe that points in or out.

■ Pain, swelling, or stiffness in the joint.

Hammertoe:

■ A toe (often the second one) bent downward in a clawlike position.

■ A corn at the top of the toe.

■ Pain in the toe.

One in 6 people in the United States has a foot problem. Among the most common complaints are bunions and hammertoes. Both conditions tend to run in families, but ill-fitting shoes can cause them or make them worse.

Bunions are most often harmless, but they can hurt. A bunion may become inflamed when a tight shoe rubs against it. Long-term pressure can cause **bursitis** (see page 187).

A hammertoe occurs when the tendons in the toe tighten and bend it down so it can't straighten. Where the toe rubs against shoes, a painful **corn** (see page 148) can develop. For some people, the pain may interfere with walking and standing.

These problems can be prevented or helped with shoes that fit well (you should be able to wiggle your toes in them). Severe cases can be fixed with surgery.

MUSCLES, BONES & JOINTS

Shoulder Pain

Most shoulder pain results from injury or overuse. Rest and self-care are often all that's needed.

SYMPTOMS	WHAT IT MIGHT BE	WHAT YOU CAN DO
After injury, severe pain and tenderness, worse when moving; numbness, tingling in arm; joint may be misshapen.	Shoulder dislocation or fracture of collarbone (see fractures and dislocations, page 35).	Call doctor for advice right away. If you can't get one, call 911 or go to emergency room.
Sudden joint pain with flu or other infection.	Side effect of infection.	Take over-the-counter painkillers (see box, page 315). If temperature is over 101, call doctor for prompt appointment.
Pain and swelling around shoulder, painful movement, fever (sometimes).	Bursitis (see facing page).	If temperature is over 101, call doctor for prompt appointment; bursa may be infected.
Pain and stiffness that begin in neck and move to shoulders; numbness or tingling in arms, hands, and fingers; weakness in arms and legs.	Cervical spondylosis—a breakdown of joints in neck that may put pressure on nerves and muscles.	With numbness and tingling, call doctor for prompt appointment. Otherwise, call for advice. Apply moist heat. Sleep with thin pillow under head and thin, rolled-up towel under neck.
Severe pain during movement, trouble moving arm, ache when not being used.	Frozen shoulder—inflamed shoulder joint from lack of use (often because of injury).	Call doctor for advice and appointment. Use RICE treatment (see box, page 198).
Pain or dull ache in shoulder, trouble raising or lowering arm, weakness in shoulder.	Rotator cuff injury—inflammation of tendons that hold shoulder in place.	Call doctor for advice and appointment.
Pain and stiffness in shoulders (or other joints).	Arthritis.	See arthritis, page 182.
Pain in distinct spot, worse when moving or after injury, exertion, or heavy lifting.	Strained or torn tendon, ligament, or muscle.	See sprains and strains, page 44.
Pain and tenderness, often worse at night; muscle spasms.	Tendinitis.	See tendinitis, page 202.

WHAT YOU CAN DO NOW

Self-care won't get rid of a hammertoe or bunion, but it can ease the pain.

➤ Wear shoes that are wide enough to relieve pressure on the foot.

➤ For relief around the house, wear old shoes with a hole cut out for the bunion.

➤ To relieve the pain of a hammertoe, buy toe caps (padded sleeves that go around the top of a toe).

➤ Try a "contrast soak"—soak your foot in cold water for 1 minute, then warm water for 5 minutes, then another minute in cold water. Repeat 3 or 4 times. Ice packs and heating pads also work well.

➤ Put a small sponge or pad between your big toe and second toe to help align them with the other toes.

➤ Cushion the sore area with moleskin or foot pads to prevent rubbing.

➤ Take an over-the-counter painkiller (see **pain relief** box, page 315).

WHEN TO CALL THE DOCTOR

➤ If redness, pain, or swelling lasts long.

➤ If your feet hurt so much that you find it hard to walk, wear shoes, or go about your normal activities.

➤ If you have diabetes or poor blood flow in your limbs and notice irritated skin over a bunion or hammertoe; it can become infected and lead to problems such as gangrene (tissue death).

HOW TO PREVENT IT

➤ Wear roomy, low-heeled shoes that don't pinch your toes.

➤ Fit new shoes to your larger foot. Most people's feet are not exactly the same size.

➤ Feet tend to swell during the day, so shop for new shoes at the end of the day, when your feet are largest.

➤ If you have early signs of a bunion or hammertoe, ask your doctor or podiatrist about orthotics, custom-made shoe inserts that can reduce the risk of foot problems.

FOR MORE HELP

Key Websites: *www.SavonHealth.com*. For more information on bunions or hammertoes: *www.SavonFootProblems.com*.

Organizations: American Academy of Orthopaedic Surgeons, 800-824-BONE, 24-hour recording. Request free brochures on how to choose shoes and how to exercise without injury.

■ American Podiatric Medical Association, 800-366-8227, 24-hour recording that takes requests for free brochures on topics about feet; *www.apma.org*.

Bursitis
www.SavonBursitis.com

SIGNS AND SYMPTOMS

■ Pain and swelling in or near a joint.

■ In bursitis of the shoulder, pain moving into the neck, arms, or fingers.

■ Fever, if infection is present.

Where your bones, tendons, and ligaments move against each other, they are cushioned by small fluid-filled sacs called bursae. These sacs help joints move smoothly. Bursitis occurs when a bursa becomes inflamed—often from too much pressure, overuse, infection, or injury.

Athletes and people who do heavy lifting or the same motions again and again, such as hammering, tend to get bursitis. Working for a long time in an odd posture also can bring it on. Calcium deposits near the bursae closest to joints can make it worse. Bursitis can also be an early sign of arthritis.

Bursitis is seldom serious and often gets better in 1 to 2 weeks, as long as you take a break from whatever caused the problem. Bursitis may come back, though, and can become chronic—meaning it may last a long time, with symptoms that come and go.

Bursitis responds well to rest, self-care, and gentle exercise that helps restore normal movement and prevent stiffness. In the worst cases, a doctor may need to drain fluid from the bursa, inject drugs to reduce pain and swelling, or surgically remove the bursa.

WHAT YOU CAN DO NOW

➤ Rest the sore joint.

➤ Change movements that cause pain.

➤ Take aspirin, ibuprofen, or naproxen to ease pain and reduce swelling (see **pain relief** box, page 315).

➤ Hold an ice pack on the sore joint for 20 minutes at a time 3 or 4 times a day for 2 days to reduce pain and swelling. A bag of frozen peas wrapped in a washcloth works well. After 2 days, if pain returns, apply warmth for 15 to 20 minutes 3 or 4 times a day. Use a washcloth soaked in warm water and wrung out.

➤ Exercise the tender joint twice a day: Move the joint gently as far as you can through its range of motion. Let pain be your guide; stop when it hurts.

➤ As you get better, begin to add gentle strength training to build muscle around the joint. This will help protect the joint and prevent future problems.

WHEN TO CALL THE DOCTOR

Call for a prompt appointment:

➤ If your temperature is over 101 or if the skin around the joint turns red and swollen; you may have an infected bursa.

Call for advice and an appointment:

➤ If pain or swelling lasts for more than 2 weeks despite rest and home care; you may have chronic bursitis or early arthritis.

HOW TO PREVENT IT

➤ Warm up before exercise; cool down afterward (see **overuse injuries,** page 198).

➤ Wear padding to play contact sports.

➤ Avoid repetitive movement, such as hammering or kneeling on a hard surface.

➤ If you can't avoid such things, change your position often and take 5-to-10-minute breaks every hour.

➤ To prevent bursitis in the feet, don't wear high heels or badly worn running or walking shoes.

➤ To avoid bursitis in the hip, sit on cushioned chairs. Get up often.

➤ Stretching or yoga can help.

FOR MORE HELP

Key Websites: *www.SavonHealth.com*. For more information on bursitis: *www.SavonBursitis.com*.

Organizations: American Chronic Pain Association, Box 850, Rocklin, CA 95677. 916-632-0922, 24-hour line; *www.theacpa.org*.

■ Arthritis Foundation, 1330 W. Peachtree St., Atlanta, GA 30309. 800-283-7800, 24-hour recording, or 404-872-7100, M–F 9–5 EST; *www.arthritis.org*.

Website: American College of Rheumatology, *www.rheumatology.org/patients/factsheets.html*. Covers bursitis and lists doctors.

Carpal Tunnel Syndrome
www.SavonCarpalTunnel.com

SIGNS AND SYMPTOMS

■ Numbness and tingling in the first 3 fingers.

■ Shooting pain in the hand, wrist, and sometimes forearm.

■ Pain that may be worse at night, causing trouble sleeping.

■ Weakness in the hands and fingers (in severe cases).

The pain and numbness of carpal tunnel syndrome (CTS) come from repeated use of the wrists in the workplace, often for typing, or in sports. Also known as a repetitive strain injury (RSI), it happens when a nerve that runs through a narrow channel covered by ligaments below the surface of the wrist is squeezed by fluid or inflamed tissue in the carpal (wrist) tunnel.

CTS is also common in women when pregnancy or menopause causes fluid build-up. **Arthritis** (see page 182), **diabetes** (see page 277), and hypothyroidism (see **thyroid problems,** page 288) may also cause it.

CTS is easy to treat if it's caught early; left untreated, it can damage nerves and muscles. Injections in the wrist may help reduce the worst pain and swelling. As a last resort,

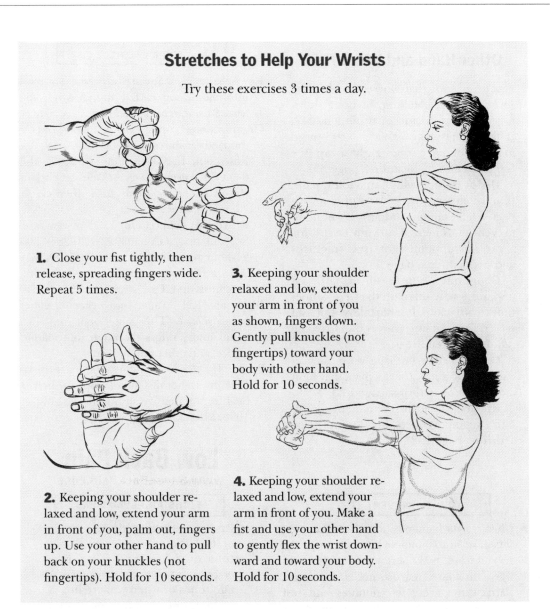

Stretches to Help Your Wrists

Try these exercises 3 times a day.

1. Close your fist tightly, then release, spreading fingers wide. Repeat 5 times.

2. Keeping your shoulder relaxed and low, extend your arm in front of you, palm out, fingers up. Use your other hand to pull back on your knuckles (not fingertips). Hold for 10 seconds.

3. Keeping your shoulder relaxed and low, extend your arm in front of you as shown, fingers down. Gently pull knuckles (not fingertips) toward your body with other hand. Hold for 10 seconds.

4. Keeping your shoulder relaxed and low, extend your arm in front of you. Make a fist and use your other hand to gently flex the wrist downward and toward your body. Hold for 10 seconds.

MUSCLES, BONES & JOINTS

pressure on the nerve can sometimes be eased by surgery in the doctor's office.

WHAT YOU CAN DO NOW

➤ Stretch and exercise your wrists every day (see box, above).

➤ Rest the hand and wrist when possible.

➤ If you have trouble sleeping, wear a wrist splint at night to reduce pressure on the nerve. Most drugstores carry splints.

➤ At work, wear a wrist splint if it helps, and change movements that cause pain.

➤ If you do much typing, try using a variable-position keyboard. Also put a pad in front of the keyboard to support your wrists.

➤ Cut salt from your diet; this may help reduce swelling.

➤ Drink plenty of water—at least 8 large glasses a day.

➤ Take ibuprofen, naproxen, or aspirin to reduce pain and swelling (see **pain relief** box, page 315).

➤ Apply a cold pack, 10 minutes on, 10 minutes off, for an hour. A bag of frozen peas wrapped in a washcloth works well.

WHEN TO CALL THE DOCTOR

➤ If pain and other symptoms persist or get worse despite a month of home care.

Other Hand and Wrist Pain

Fracture: pain that worsens with pressure; swelling, bleeding, or bone showing. Call your doctor for prompt advice. If he or she isn't available, call 911 or go to an emergency room **right away** (see **fractures and dislocations,** page 35).

Dislocation: swelling in a joint, pain, trouble moving the joint. Apply an ice pack for swelling, and use a splint to prevent movement. Call your doctor for a prompt appointment (see **fractures and dislocations,** page 35).

Ganglion: a round, soft or hard cyst under the skin, often on the wrist, sometimes with pain. It's harmless, but call your doctor if it hurts or swells. He or she can drain or remove it.

Osteoarthritis: cartilage worn away in one or more joints. Causes pain, may limit movement (see **arthritis,** page 182).

Rheumatoid arthritis: pain in a joint, with swelling, redness, and stiffness (see **arthritis,** page 182).

HOW TO PREVENT IT

➤ Change your hand position often when typing. Take 5-to-10-minute breaks hourly.
➤ As you work, make sure your hands are in line with your forearms, not cocked backward. Pause every few minutes and rest your wrist on a pad; office supply stores carry them.
➤ Some people find that vitamin B6 helps. Take no more than the recommended daily amount; high doses can be harmful.
➤ Ask your employer to check with an expert in workplace design about ways to ease wrist strain on the job.

COMPLEMENTARY CHOICES

➤ Seek some kind of physical therapy such as massage, hydrotherapy, low-level electrical stimulation, or ultrasound to reduce inflammation and swelling.
➤ A soothing compress made with grated ginger and hot water may offer relief.

FOR MORE HELP

Key Website: *www.SavonHealth.com*. For more information on carpal tunnel syndrome: *www.SavonCarpalTunnel.com*.

Organizations: American Academy of Orthopaedic Surgeons, 6300 N. River Rd., Rosemont, IL 60018. 800-346-2267, M–F 8–5 CST; *www.aaos.org*. At Website, click on *Patient Education,* then *Hand,* then *Carpal Tunnel Syndrome.*

■ Arthritis Foundation, 1330 W. Peachtree St., Atlanta, GA 30309. 800-283-7800, 24-hour recording, or 404-872-7100, M–F 9–5 EST; *www.arthritis.org*. Sends free brochures on CTS.

Website: RSI Page, *www.engr.unl.edu/ee/eeshop/rsi.html*. This site about repetitive strain injury offers thorough information, advice, and other online help.

Book: *The Repetitive Strain Injury Recovery Book,* by Deborah Quilter. Tips on how to heal from repetitive strain injuries. Walker, 1998, $15.95.

Low Back Pain
www.SavonBackPain.com

SIGNS AND SYMPTOMS

■ Pain in the lumbar (lower) region of the back; may be severe. It can come on quickly or slowly; it may be constant or occur only at certain times or when you are in a certain posture; it may be confined to one place or move to other parts of your back.
■ Numbness, tingling, or a shooting pain in your legs or buttocks, often on one side only.
■ Pain made worse by coughing, sneezing, or twisting.
■ Stiffness.

Call a doctor **right away** if you also have these symptoms of nerve damage:

■ Numbness or weakness, especially numbness around your groin or rectal area.
■ Bladder or bowel control trouble.
■ Weakness in one or both legs.

Most of us get a bit of back pain now and then, frequently in the lower back. In fact, every year half of the working people in the United States are bothered by low back pain at some time.

The spinal column, also called the backbone, is a series of bones (vertebrae) cushioned by small shock absorbers (disks) and held up by muscles and ligaments (see color illustration, page 166). Most low back pain comes from muscle or ligament strain, disk problems, stress, or sometimes all of these. The pain often goes away on its own, but it may return later.

Disks break down somewhat with age or from a lot of bending and twisting. In some cases, a swollen disk may press on a nerve in the lower back and send pain down the buttocks or legs. Most disk problems will clear up with the proper care. In severe cases, surgery to remove the disk or part of it may help stem the pain and allow the back to be more functional.

WHAT YOU CAN DO NOW

➤ When your back starts hurting, apply an ice pack to reduce pain and swelling. Leave it there 10 to 15 minutes every hour. After 2 days, apply a heating pad or hot towel, or take hot showers. The heat will increase blood flow, bringing healing white cells to the sore spot.

➤ When pain is bad, lie flat on the floor with your knees bent and your lower legs on a chair or pile of pillows. This helps flatten the lower back and ease the strain.

➤ Sitting may be hard on a sore back. Stay away from soft chairs. Instead, try a straight-backed chair and don't sit down for a long time. Don't sit up in bed.

➤ Walk as much as you can, but only if it doesn't make your pain worse.

➤ If pain disturbs your sleep, put pillows under your knees when lying on your back.

➤ If you sleep on your side, bend your knees and put a pillow between them. Don't lie on your stomach.

➤ Take acetaminophen, aspirin, or ibuprofen for the pain (see **pain relief** box, page 315). Don't bother with prescription drugs for relaxing muscles; they work no better and often have side effects.

The Spine

The curves of the spine give it strength and allow humans to walk upright.

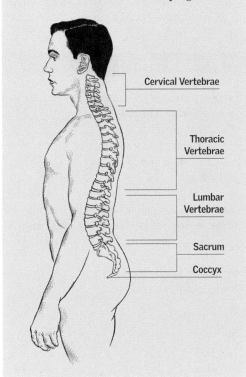

Cervical Vertebrae

Thoracic Vertebrae

Lumbar Vertebrae

Sacrum

Coccyx

WHEN TO CALL THE DOCTOR

Call for advice **right away** (if your doctor is not in, call 911 or go to an emergency room):

➤ If you have back pain with symptoms of nerve damage, especially loss of bladder or bowel control.

Call for advice and an appointment:

➤ If back pain is severe or disrupts your normal activities.

➤ If the pain doesn't go away within a few days or keeps coming back.

HOW TO PREVENT IT

➤ Exercise as often as you can. Avoid twisting or wrenching your body, or doing anything that seems to make your back pain worse. Walking, swimming, and even walking in a swimming pool are ideal.

➤ Do exercises to strengthen the abdominal muscles (always do abdominal crunches with

MUSCLES, BONES & JOINTS

Back Pain

Most backaches have no clear cause. Many come from simple strain, because the stacked bones and disks of the spine are not well suited to our upright posture, and gravity takes its toll. Sometimes, though, the pain signals a problem you can trace to another source.

SYMPTOMS	WHAT IT MIGHT BE	WHAT YOU CAN DO
Stubborn pain, often worse at night; numbness, tingling, and weakness that gets worse; in some cases, loss of bladder or bowel control.	Spinal tumor.	With loss of bladder or bowel control, call doctor for advice and appointment **right away;** if you can't reach one, call 911 or go to emergency room.
Severe low back pain made worse by twisting, bending, coughing, or lifting (pain may shoot down one leg); in the worst cases, loss of bladder or bowel control.	Bulging disk pressing on a nerve (see low back pain, page 190).	With loss of bladder or bowel control, call doctor for advice right away; if you can't get one, call 911 or go to emergency room. Otherwise, call doctor for an appointment, take painkillers (see box, page 315), and rest.
Low back pain that comes and goes (may be worse at night); back or hip stiffness in morning that improves with activity; pain and stiffness in rib area; neck or chest pain; fatigue, weight loss, and poor appetite; fever; eye pain; blurred vision.	Ankylosing spondylitis—a rare form of arthritis that chiefly affects spinal column, usually in men under 40.	Call doctor for advice and appointment. Physical therapy, strength training, massage, and over-the-counter painkillers (see box, page 315) may help.
Numbness, weakness, and/or mild pain in back and legs; worse when walking, eases when sitting.	Spinal stenosis—narrowed spinal canal due to arthritis, thickened ligaments, or bulging disks.	Call doctor for advice and appointment. Weight loss and abdominal strengthening exercises may help.
Stiffness and pain in back, buttocks, and thighs; trouble moving or bending.	Arthritis.	See arthritis, page 182.
Low back pain in women more than 4 months pregnant.	Stress on back from extra weight. ■ Sign of early labor.	See pregnancy, page 238.

Back Pain

SYMPTOMS	WHAT IT MIGHT BE	WHAT YOU CAN DO
Stiffness and soreness after exertion or injury, or soreness that develops slowly during night; may spread to buttocks and thighs.	Back sprain or strain (see low back pain, page 190).	Rest for a few days; take over-the-counter painkillers (see box, page 315); return to normal activities when comfortable.
Aching, pain, and stiffness in back muscles (also pain elsewhere); points on body feel sore when pressed; fatigue, headaches, and trouble sleeping.	Fibromyalgia.	See box on fibromyalgia, page 276.
Backache; easily broken bones, especially in spine, wrists, and hips; stooped or hunched posture.	Osteoporosis.	See osteoporosis, page 196.

your knees bent). Also, stretch the muscles that run parallel to your spine (lie flat on your back; pull one knee, then the other, toward your chest until both knees are tucked).

➤ Try yoga. Doctors and people with back pain like it for building strength and flexibility. It also helps you relax.

➤ Wear comfortable, low-heeled shoes.

➤ If you sit for long periods, make sure your work surface is at the right height for comfort and that your chair provides good lower back support. Walk around for a few minutes every half hour or so. If sitting is painful, try changing your work space so that you can stand with one foot on a low block.

➤ Don't lift and twist at the same time. Lift by bending your legs, not your back, and lift as little weight each time as possible.

➤ Lose weight if you need to. A big belly puts strain on the lower spine.

COMPLEMENTARY CHOICES

➤ Studies by the National Institutes of Health and others have found that acupuncture can be used to relieve pain from many conditions, including migraines, bladder infections, and chronic musculoskeletal problems (see **how to choose a natural healer,** page 310.)

➤ Chiropractic or osteopathic treatment may help. Some back pain is caused by misaligned spinal vertebrae, which affect surrounding muscles and may pinch nerves. Realignment of the spine through chiropractic, or gentle manipulation of other areas of the body through osteopathy, often relieves pain.

➤ Massage can loosen tight, painful muscles. Swedish massage, shiatsu, and rolfing are common types. Techniques vary, so you may need to try several to find a type that works for you.

➤ If you think stress could be the cause, learn to spot—and avoid—situations that make you tense. Many people don't realize that stress is making them tighten their back muscles (see **stress,** page 218).

➤ Learning some relaxation methods may help ease the pain. Practice deep breathing or meditation (see **relax,** page 303).

➤ Biofeedback—using electronic devices to monitor and control signals from your body—can help relieve pain. Biofeedback also helps reduce stress.

MUSCLES, BONES & JOINTS

Leg Pain

Most leg pain comes from an injury or overuse. But sometimes it can signal a more serious problem in the blood vessels. If you have leg pain that isn't from an injury or other cause you know of, be sure to talk with your doctor about it.

SYMPTOMS	WHAT IT MIGHT BE	WHAT YOU CAN DO
Severe leg pain, swelling, and tenderness after an injury; you can't move leg.	Bone fracture (see fractures and dislocations, page 35).	Call 911 or go to emergency room **right away.**
Leg pain after injury, but you can move leg.	Strained, inflamed, or torn tendon, ligament, or muscle (see sprains and strains, page 44).	Call doctor for prompt appointment.
Pain and fatigue in muscles of thighs, calves, feet, or hips when active; stops with rest; mostly in older adults.	Peripheral vascular disease (see artery disease, page 104).	Call doctor for prompt appointment.
Pain and burning with redness, tenderness, and itching; hard, cordlike swelling beneath skin along length of a vein in leg (in phlebitis). Swelling, warmth, and redness throughout leg; bluish color in toes (in deep-vein thrombosis).	Phlebitis (also known as thrombophlebitis)—inflamed vein near surface of skin, most often from infection or injury, causing clotting. ■ Deep-vein thrombosis—blood clots in deep veins.	Call doctor for prompt appointment. Phlebitis is rarely harmful, but deep-vein thrombosis can cause clots that break off and travel to lungs. Varicose veins (see page 115) may increase risk of both ailments.
In children: pain that comes and goes in leg muscles, most often at night; goes away by morning.	Growing pains—common in children 3 to 12.	Gently massage area. For pain, give acetaminophen with food at bedtime (never aspirin; see Reye's syndrome box, page 95). Call doctor for advice if pain persists.
Pain in front or side of lower leg that begins during or just after exercise.	Shinsplints—inflamed bone, tendon, or muscle in calf or shin.	Rest. Use ice for pain and swelling. Switch from high-impact sports, such as running, to gentler ones such as swimming or bicycling. Call doctor if pain persists.
Leg muscles tighten for a few minutes, then return to normal.	Leg cramps.	See muscle cramps, facing page.

Leg Pain

SYMPTOMS	WHAT IT MIGHT BE	WHAT YOU CAN DO
Pain and sometimes swelling after physical activity.	Overuse injury.	See overuse injuries, page 198.
Numbness, tingling, or pain in buttocks or back of one leg.	Disk in spine pressing on sciatic nerve in leg. ■ Other sciatic nerve injury.	See low back pain, page 190.
Aching or itching in legs, with blue or purple veins; sometimes swelling in feet or ankles.	Varicose veins.	See varicose veins, page 115.

FOR MORE HELP

Key Websites: *www.SavonHealth.com.* For more information about back pain: *www.SavonBackPain.com.*

Organizations: National Chronic Pain Outreach Association, P.O. Box 274, Millboro, VA 24460. 540-862-9437, M–F 10–3 EST.
■ Texas Back Institute, 6300 W. Parker Rd., Plano, TX 75093. 800-247-BACK, M–F 9–5 EST; *www.texasback.com.*

Website: Virtual Hospital, University of Iowa, *www.vh.org/patients/ihb/ortho/back patient/contents.html.*

Brochure: *Acute Low-Back Problems in Adults,* Agency for Health Care Policy and Research. Covers recent news in back pain research and care. For a free copy, call 800-358-9295, M–F 9–5 EST.

Books: *Back Pain: How to Relieve Low Back Pain and Sciatica,* by Loren Fishman, M.D. and Carol Ardman. Educates readers on sources of and cures for back pain. W. W. Norton, 1999, $13.95.
■ *The Back Pain Helpbook,* by James E. Moore, Ph.D., and Kate Lorig, R.N., Dr.P.H. Perseus Books, 1999, $15.

Muscle Cramps
www.SavonMuscleCramps.com

SIGNS AND SYMPTOMS

- A sudden tightening of a muscle, with sharp pain.
- A muscle that is hard to the touch.
- At times, twitching of the muscle.
- Heat cramps: sudden, severe spasms in the arms, legs, and sometimes the abdominal muscles.

A muscle cramp can happen anytime—in bed, during a walk, after working in the garden. The muscle contracts with great force and stays this way, most often for about a minute, before relaxing.

Muscle cramps occur mostly in the legs, often after exercise in the heat or when a limb is stuck in an awkward position for a long time. They may also result from an imbalance in minerals and fluids caused by dehydration. Abdominal cramps may be caused by lower back problems or menstruation. Medical conditions such as Parkinson's disease, untreated thyroid problems, or diabetes also can lead to cramps.

Muscle cramps are rarely serious, but heat cramps can be a sign of heat exhaustion. With dizziness or confusion, they can signal the onset of heatstroke, which can be fatal (see **heatstroke and heat exhaustion,** page 38).

WHAT YOU CAN DO NOW

➤ Stretch. For calf muscles, stand a little away from a wall and put your hands or forearms against it. Keep your feet flat on the floor and put your right foot forward, with leg bent, and extend your left leg behind you. Move your hips toward the wall until you feel the stretch in your calf. Hold for 10 to 20 seconds, and repeat on the other side.

➤ Massage. Begin at the edges of the cramp and move in toward the center, squeezing the muscle gently.

➤ For a stubborn cramp, immerse the area in warm water while stretching and massaging the muscle.

➤ If you have heat cramps, get out of the sun and sip cool water or a sports drink.

➤ For menstrual cramps, take warm baths or put a hot-water bottle or heating pad on your abdomen. Try ibuprofen to ease pain.

WHEN TO CALL THE DOCTOR

Call 911 or go to an emergency room **right away:**

➤ If you get a severe, cramping pain in your chest, shoulders, or arms; this can signal a heart attack.

➤ If you have heat cramps with dizziness or confusion; you may have heatstroke.

Call for advice and an appointment:

➤ If cramps are long-lasting or frequent.

HOW TO PREVENT IT

➤ Drink 6 to 8 glasses of water every day.

➤ Stretch often, and especially before bed.

➤ Warm up and stretch before exercising.

➤ To prevent heat cramps in hot weather, drink a small glass (about 4 ounces) of cool water before and after exercise and every 15 minutes during exercise. (Drinking lots of cold water at once may cause stomach upset.) If you use a sports beverage, drink one low in sugar.

➤ Take 400 IU of vitamin E daily and eat foods rich in potassium, such as bananas, to prevent muscle cramps.

FOR MORE HELP

Key Websites: *www.SavonHealth.com*. For more information on muscle cramps : *www.SavonMuscleCramps.com*.
Duke University Healthy Devil Online, *h-devilwww.mc.duke.edu/hdevil/women/women.htm*. Discusses causes of menstrual cramps and suggests treatment.
■ FYIowa, The Fitness Files, *fyiowa.webpoint.com/fitness/strindex.htm*. Shows how to keep your muscles stretched and limber to prevent cramps and injury.

Osteoporosis
www.SavonOsteoporosis.com

SIGNS AND SYMPTOMS

■ A broken bone (may be the first symptom), often in the spine, hip, ribs, or wrist.

■ Stooped and round-shouldered posture; loss of height (usually occurs after age 70).

■ Severe backache.

Osteoporosis means "porous bones." When you're young, your skeleton acts as a calcium bank for the rest of your body, taking in new deposits that help replace old bone. By the time you reach your mid-30s, though, it's easier to lose bone mass than to gain it. From then on, bones tend to become less dense and more brittle. (See color illustrations, page 167.)

Osteoporosis is most common in people over 70 and in women after menopause, when levels of bone-protecting estrogen drop. If you're thin, if you smoke or drink, or if others in your family have osteoporosis, you may have a high risk as well. It can get worse without symptoms until a bone breaks—often in the spine, causing severe backache and a stooped posture.

Major bone breaks may require surgery and bed rest, which can lead to further weakness and ailments such as blood clots or pneumonia.

That's the bad news. The good news? You can prevent osteoporosis, and if you have it, you can slow its progress. Self-care, including weight-bearing exercise and calcium supplements, is important. Hormone therapy for menopausal women can cut the risk of fractures in half, but it may also increase the risk of breast cancer (see **hormone replacement box,** page 235). Your doctor may prescribe physical therapy along with drugs that prevent bone loss or help build new bone.

WHAT YOU CAN DO NOW

➤ Ask your doctor about a bone density test; it can show whether you have lost bone (see **tests,** page 319).

➤ Get plenty of exercise. It lowers your risk of losing bone. And it can strengthen bones that have begun to thin. Weight-bearing exercise is best (see **get some exercise,** page 292), including racket sports, step aerobics, or climbing stairs. Strength training (lifting weights) also increases bone mass.

➤ Make sure you get lots of calcium and vitamin D in your diet. If you are past menopause, get at least 1,500 milligrams of calcium per day; men, younger women, or women on hormone replacement therapy should get 1,000 mg per day (see **the nutrition top ten,** page 298).

➤ If you're not sure your diet has enough calcium, take over-the-counter calcium supplements. Some common antacids are good sources. Check the label to see how much "elemental" (usable) calcium a supplement or antacid contains. (If you have a problem with kidney stones, talk with your doctor about calcium supplements; they may not be for you.)

➤ If you have osteoporosis that causes pain, take over-the-counter painkillers (see **pain relief** box, on page 315).

➤ To prevent falls: Install handrails on stairs and grab bars in the bathroom. Cover slippery floors with carpet, rubber mats, or nonskid wax. Use bright lamps and night-lights.

WHEN TO CALL THE DOCTOR

➤ If you fracture a bone.

➤ If you have stubborn pain in your back, ribs, spine, or feet.

➤ If you have a backache or are getting a curved back ("dowager's hump").

HOW TO PREVENT IT

➤ All the steps outlined in What You Can Do Now will help. Also:

➤ Try to gain a few pounds if you're underweight; being too thin puts you at risk.

➤ If you smoke, quit, and if you drink, don't drink much. Have no more than 1 drink a day (a "drink" is a 5-ounce glass of wine, a 12-ounce beer, or a 1.5-ounce shot of 80-proof liquor).

➤ If you are going through menopause, consider hormone replacement therapy (see **hormone replacement** box, page 235), which prevents bone loss and cuts the risk of fractures in half. It may increase breast-cancer risk in some women.

FOR MORE HELP

Key Websites: *www.SavonHealth.com*. For more information on osteoporosis: *www.SavonOsteoporosis.com*.

Organizations: Arthritis Foundation, 1330 W. Peachtree St., Atlanta, GA 30309. 800-283-7800, 24-hour recording, or 404-872-7100, M–F 9–5 EST; *www.arthritis.org*. Offers lists of local chapters.

■ National Institutes of Health, Osteoporosis and Related Bone Diseases National Resource Center, 1232 22nd St. NW, Washington, DC 20037-1292. 202-223-0344 or 800-624-BONE, M–F 9–5:30 EST, *www.osteo.org*. At Website, click on *Bone Health Information* and then on *Osteoporosis*. Click on *Bone Links* for resources.

■ National Osteoporosis Foundation, 1232 22nd St. NW, Washington, DC 20037-1292. 202-223-2226, M–F 9–5:30 EST, or 800-223-9994, M–F 7AM–midnight EST; *www.nof.org*.

Books: *The Osteoporosis Solution,* by Carl Germano, R.D., with William Cabot, M.D. Discusses the causes and prevention of osteoporosis. Kensington, 1999, $22.

■ *The Osteoporosis Book,* by Nancy E. Lane, M.D. Oxford University Press, 1998, $25.

■ *150 Most-Asked Questions About Osteoporosis: What Women Really Want to Know,* by Ruth S. Jacobowitz. William Morrow, 1996, $10.

MUSCLES, BONES & JOINTS

Overuse Injuries
www.SavonHealth.com

SIGNS AND SYMPTOMS

The tip-off to an overuse injury is pain that gets worse with activity. Often, it follows this pattern:

- At first, there is dull pain and general fatigue (the normal effects of exertion).
- Pain becomes sharper and more local (it's felt mostly in one place, such as the knee, hip, or arm).
- Pain lingers from one day to the next, often with swelling.
- Pain or swelling makes it hard to do the activity that caused it.
- Pain or swelling makes it hard to do normal activities of daily living, such as walking or standing.

Overuse injuries result from using bones, muscles, tendons, or joints in the same way, over and over again, without enough rest—often in the repeated motions of a sport. Runners are more likely than others to get overuse injuries of the knees and feet. For weekend warriors, throwing a ball or swinging a tennis racket can be hard on the shoulders and elbows. But these injuries can be caused by any repeated motion, such as typing, or by activities you do only now and then, such as trimming the hedge for the first time in the spring.

Overuse injuries can take longer to heal than other kinds. Without rest and therapy, they may come back or cause more serious problems, such as **arthritis** (see page 182).

WHAT YOU CAN DO NOW

- Stop or change what causes pain.
- Use the **RICE** treatment (see box below) on the sore spot.
- Take an over-the-counter painkiller (see **pain relief** box, page 315) for pain and swelling. But even if this helps, don't assume that it's okay to return to the activity that caused the pain in the first place. Allow plenty of time for the injury to heal.
- When pain and swelling have eased, slowly resume your normal activities. If doing this causes more pain, however, stop and rest some more. Find other things to do that don't hurt. For instance, if walking hurts your knee, try swimming until the pain in the knee is gone.

First Aid for Injuries: R•I•C•E

RICE stands for **Rest, Ice, Compression,** and **Elevation.** This is the best treatment for an overuse injury or a sprain. Start it as soon as you notice symptoms. If begun right away, it can save you days or even weeks of pain.

Rest: Try not to use the injured part until the pain and swelling go away (often 1 to 3 days).

Ice: Apply ice as soon as you can to reduce swelling and pain. Place a damp towel over the injured spot and a plastic bag full of ice on top of it. A bag of frozen peas also works well. Hold the cold pack in place for 10 to 30 minutes, then leave it off for 30 to 45 minutes. Repeat as often as you can. You should use ice for at least 3 days; for severe bruises, up to 7 days. For chronic pain, use ice whenever you have symptoms.

Compression: Use an elastic bandage to apply gentle but firm pressure until the swelling goes down. Wrap the bandage in an upward spiral, starting a few inches below the injured area. Apply even pressure to start, then wrap more loosely after you've passed the injured area. (To use ice and pressure at the same time, wrap a bandage over an ice pack.)

Elevation: For the first 1 to 3 days, keep the injured area raised above the heart to help drain any excess fluid from the area.

Note: Also for the first 1 to 3 days after an injury, to reduce swelling:
- Do not apply heat (hot showers, compresses, or baths).
- Do not work the injured part.
- Do not massage the injury.
- Do not drink alcohol.

Foot & Ankle Pain

The feet take a beating, especially when we stuff them into shoes that don't fit. That's why it's important to catch foot problems early, when they can be treated most easily.

SYMPTOMS	WHAT IT MIGHT BE	WHAT YOU CAN DO
Pain in ankle or foot after injury; maybe swelling, bruising, or bleeding; can't support weight.	Broken bone (see fractures and dislocations, page 35) or sprain.	Call doctor for prompt advice. If you can't get one, call 911 or go to emergency room.
Pain and fatigue in feet, legs, or hips when active; pain stops with rest; most common in older adults.	Peripheral vascular disease (see artery disease, page 104).	Call doctor for prompt appointment.
Pain, swelling, and stiffness, maybe with redness, in joints of ankles, feet, or toes.	Arthritis (see page 182).	Call doctor for advice and appointment.
Sharp pain or tender feeling under foot or heel; worse when walking or running, often worse in morning.	Plantar fasciitis—inflamed tissue that runs along heel and supports arch. Most often caused by stress on arch. Common among runners (see overuse injuries, facing page).	Stay off foot, take over-the-counter pain relievers to ease pain and swelling, and use RICE treatment (see box, facing page). Ask doctor or physical therapist about ways to stretch ligament.
Pain in Achilles tendon in back of ankle, or in other tendons in ankle or foot; may restrict foot movement.	Tendinitis (see page 202).	Call doctor for advice and appointment.
Hard, painful lump on side of foot, at base of big toe (bunion). Toe clenched and painful (hammertoe).	Bunion or hammertoe.	See bunions and hammertoes, page 185.
Patch of thickened skin on foot; may be painful.	Corn or callus.	See corns and calluses, page 148.
Wart on sole of foot, making walking painful. Tight shoes may make it worse.	Plantar wart.	See warts, page 180.

MUSCLES, BONES & JOINTS

Knee Pain

The knee is a hinge meant to swing one way—forward and back—within limits. Twisting to the side or bending too far back can cause injury. Most knee trouble can be prevented. When things do go wrong, treatment often gets good results.

SYMPTOMS	WHAT IT MIGHT BE	WHAT YOU CAN DO
Pain and perhaps a "pop" at moment of injury; swelling, stiffness, a "wobbly" knee, trouble walking.	Ligament sprain or rupture, and/or cartilage damage (see sprains and strains, page 44, and illustration, facing page).	Call doctor for prompt appointment. Use RICE treatment for pain and swelling (see box, page 198).
In teens: pain and swelling about 2 inches below kneecap; may cause limping or prevent running.	Osgood-Schlatter disease—inflamed tendon and bone.	Call doctor for advice and appointment. Use RICE treatment (see box, page 198).
Pain, swelling, and stiffness in knee joint.	Arthritis (see page 182).	Call doctor for advice and appointment.
Tender, stiff, and swollen knee; pain when bending knee; possibly fever or redness.	Bursitis (see page 187).	Call doctor for advice and appointment.
Pain just below kneecap, may be worse when sitting or straightening leg; may be felt after running or jumping; knee pain and tightness that worsen with movement.	Patellar tendinitis, "runner's" or "jumper's" knee" (see tendinitis, page 202, and overuse injuries, page 198).	Call doctor for advice and appointment. Use RICE treatment for pain and swelling (see box, page 198).

WHEN TO CALL THE DOCTOR

➤ If a week of home care doesn't help.

HOW TO PREVENT IT

➤ Allow at least 48 hours between hard workouts such as running, tennis, or swimming.

➤ Don't increase the time or intensity of a sport more than about 10 percent at one time. For example, if you walk or run 10 miles a week, increase your distance no more than about 1 mile each week.

➤ Know your body. Change your activities if you know you have a problem. For instance, people with flat feet may get knee or foot trouble from running; they can try swimming or tennis instead.

➤ Use the right gear. If you walk or run, your shoes should be sturdy enough to help absorb the shock. (If you have foot problems, ask your doctor about orthotics, shoe inserts that can help prevent knee and foot injuries.)

➤ If a certain motion makes trouble, change your technique. You may want to learn a new swimming stroke if you're prone to shoulder problems, for instance.

➤ Vary your routine so you don't keep working the same muscles and joints over and over. Jog one day, say, and swim the next.

➤ Warm up before exercise. Stretch gently and walk briskly for a few minutes. Warmed muscles, ligaments, and tendons are less likely to get hurt.

➤ Make sure your work site is comfortable and properly set up (see **carpal tunnel syndrome,** page 188).

FOR MORE HELP

Key Websites: *www.SavonHealth.com*. For more information on overuse injuries: *www.SavonHealth.com*.

Books: *Complete Guide to Sports Injuries,* by H. Winter Griffith, M.D. Describes how to avoid, treat, and recover from nearly 200 of the most common sports injuries. Perigee Books, 1997, $16.95.

■ *Dr. Scott's Knee Book,* by W. Norman Scott, M.D. A guide to symptoms, treatment, and prevention. Fireside, 1996, $11.

The Knee

Tendons (the ends of muscles attached to bone) and ligaments keep your knee bones in place; cartilage cushions the bones.

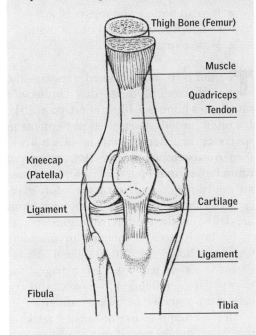

Thigh Bone (Femur)

Muscle

Quadriceps Tendon

Kneecap (Patella)

Ligament

Cartilage

Ligament

Fibula

Tibia

Temporomandibular Disorder
www.SavonPainManagement.com

SIGNS AND SYMPTOMS

■ Pain in the chewing muscles or jaw joint on either side of the head.
■ Headaches or earaches.
■ Clicking, popping, or grating sounds in the jaw joints when opening or closing the mouth.
■ Pain that spreads to the face, neck, or shoulders.
■ Jaw is locked shut or hurts to open.

Because we talk, chew, and yawn every day, the jaw is always busy. The hinges called temporomandibular joints, which connect the lower jaw to a bone on each side of the head, help the jawbone move smoothly (see illustration, page 202). Pain in or around these joints is known as temporomandibular disorder (TMD). About two-thirds of Americans have bouts of such pain.

Many things can cause TMD, including strain on the jaw muscles from clenching the teeth (see **tooth grinding,** page 83), **arthritis** (see page 182), injury to the jaw, and even **stress** (see page 218). Poor posture (from thrusting the chin forward) may also cause the problem.

TMD often clears up in a few days with rest and painkillers such as ibuprofen. When it is severe or chronic, treatments include physical therapy, anti-inflammatory drugs, tranquilizers to relieve muscle tension, and a bite guard to ease the strain on the joint. Surgery and injections are last resorts; there is little agreement on whether they really help.

WHAT YOU CAN DO NOW

➤ Take an anti-inflammatory painkiller such as ibuprofen (see **pain relief** box, page 315).

➤ Massage the muscles above and in front of your temples, as well as the large muscles along your jawline. Use small, circular motions.

➤ Limit talking and chewing for a few days. Rest your jaw by eating soft or liquid foods.

➤ Apply a hot or cold pack, available in drugstores, or a damp warm or cool towel for pain relief. Hold in place for a few minutes at a time.

➤ Don't clench your teeth.

WHEN TO CALL THE DOCTOR

➤ If the pain of TMD interferes with eating or talking.

➤ If you grind or clench your teeth and think you may need a bite guard to protect them. Your dentist can make one to fit your bite.

HOW TO PREVENT IT

➤ Whenever you find yourself clenching or grinding your teeth, stop.

➤ Reduce stress (see **relax,** page 303). This may be the best treatment.

➤ If you are prone to jaw pain, avoid hard foods such as carrots and apples, and chewy foods such as steak and bagels. Don't chew gum, pencils, or other objects.

➤ To lessen the strain on the jaw, don't sleep on your stomach.

➤ Never cradle a telephone receiver between your shoulder and jaw.

FOR MORE HELP

Key Websites: *www.SavonHealth.com*. For more information on temporomandibular disorder: *www.SavonPainManagement.com*.

Organizations: American Academy of Otolaryngology–Head and Neck Surgery, 1 Prince St., Alexandria, VA 22314. 703-836-4444, M–F 8:30–5 EST; *www.entnet.org*. Send a business-size self-addressed stamped envelope and ask for "Pain and TMJ" (temporomandibular joint).

■ National Oral Health Information Clearinghouse, 1 NOHIC Way, Bethesda, MD 20892-3500. 301-402-7364, M–F 9–5:30 EST; *www.aerie.com/nohicweb*. Offers free brochures on TMD.

Website: Healthtouch, *www.healthtouch.com*. Click on *Health Information,* then scroll to *TMJ & Jaw Joint Disorders.* Covers the symptoms and treatment of TMD.

Tendinitis
www.SavonTendinitis.com

SIGNS AND SYMPTOMS

■ Pain around a joint, often worse with movement and in bed at night.
■ Muscle spasms.

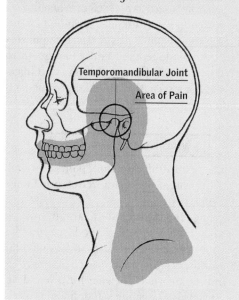

Temporomandibular Joint

Pain can spread far beyond the hinge that connects the jawbone and skull.

Temporomandibular Joint

Area of Pain

Tendinitis is an inflamed tendon—the tough band of tissue that connects a muscle to a bone (see illustration, page 201). It's often caused by repeated movements in sports or in assembly-line or office work. (See **overuse injuries,** page 198, and **carpal tunnel syndrome,** page 188.) Other causes are injury, not enough warm-up before exercise, calcium deposits in the tendon, and breakdown of the tendon from aging.

Tendinitis is most common in shoulders ("golfer's shoulder"), the outside of elbows ("tennis elbow," see box, facing page), the fingers ("trigger finger"), the wrist, and the back of the lower leg (Achilles tendinitis).

Most tendinitis heals with about 2 weeks of rest. More stubborn tendinitis can be treated with drugs to ease the pain and swelling, plus physical therapy, ice packs, ultrasound treatments, and gentle exercise.

WHAT YOU CAN DO NOW

➤ Rest the area until pain and swelling ease.
➤ Use a splint if the cause is overuse, and if you can't rest the painful joint.
➤ Take anti-inflammatories such as aspirin or ibuprofen to relieve the pain and swelling (see **pain relief** box, page 315).
➤ If tendinitis comes on quickly after an injury or heavy use, put an ice pack on the area for 10 to 30 minutes to reduce swelling. Wait 30 to 45 minutes, and repeat. Do so as often as you can. After 2 days, apply a towel soaked in hot water and wrung out, or a heat pack (available in drugstores), to relieve the pain. (See **RICE** treatment box, page 198.)
➤ After a few days, start to exercise gently.

WHEN TO CALL THE DOCTOR

➤ If the area around the joint appears discolored or deformed.
➤ If pain and swelling continue for more than 2 weeks despite rest and over-the-counter pain relievers. These could be early signs of arthritis.

HOW TO PREVENT IT

➤ When you have symptoms, rest the joint to prevent the problem from getting worse.
➤ If you perform the same tasks over and over during work—for instance, a lot of typing—ask your doctor or employer about an ergonomic specialist who can suggest ways to change your workplace to ease the stress on tender tendons.
➤ Stretch before and after work. When you have to repeat any movement over and over, take a 5-to-10-minute hourly break.
➤ Exercise often to maintain muscle and tendon strength to help prevent injuries.
➤ Always warm up before exercise and cool down after with gentle stretching.
➤ Wear shoes with flexible soles and good heel control when you exercise. If you have weak ankles, wear high-top shoes.
➤ Don't grip tools, pens, or sports gear too

Tennis Elbow

Anyone who uses elbows in sports or work can get tennis elbow. It results when the forearm is snapped, rolled, or twisted, or when people lift heavy objects with the elbow locked and the arm extended. In tennis, it can occur when the grip is wrong.

The symptoms of tennis elbow may last from 6 to 12 weeks. The best home care is rest and over-the-counter painkillers, then gentle exercise. You can also try wearing a Velcro tennis-elbow strap, sold in sporting goods stores, to support muscles and tendons. But don't wear the strap for long periods, because it can reduce blood flow.

Prevent tennis elbow the same way you prevent tendinitis. If tennis is the cause of your pain, try a more flexible racket or one with a slightly larger grip; ask a coach to help you change your grip to ease the stress on your elbow.

tightly. Wrap utensils in felt or rubber to create larger grips.
➤ Switch to low-impact exercise, such as swimming or low-impact aerobics, if you think higher-impact sports are to blame.

FOR MORE HELP

Key Websites: *www.SavonHealth.com*. For more information on tendinitis: *www.SavonTendinitis.com*.

Organization: Arthritis Foundation, 1330 W. Peachtree St., Atlanta, GA 30309. 800-283-7800, 24-hour recording, or 404-872-7100, M–F 9–5 EST; *www.arthritis.org*. Sends a brochure about tendinitis.

Website: American College of Rheumatology, *www.rheumatology.org/patients/factsheet.html*. Covers tendinitis and lists doctors near you.

MUSCLES, BONES & JOINTS

Behavior & Emotions

Alcohol Abuse & Alcoholism
www.SavonAlcoholAbuse.com

SIGNS AND SYMPTOMS

Alcohol abuse:
Problem drinking over the course of a year that is not an addiction but can include:

- Drinking in physically dangerous situations, such as driving a car or using heavy machinery.
- Repeated alcohol-related legal problems, such as arrests for driving under the influence or physically hurting others.
- Failure to fulfill work, home, or school obligations.

Alcoholism (alcohol addiction):
Same symptoms as those above, plus:

- Craving alcohol.
- Loss of control over drinking.
- A need for increasing amounts of alcohol to get "high."
- Drinking alone or early in the day.
- Broken capillaries, flushed face.
- Yellowish skin.
- Blackouts or memory loss.
- Personality changes, including depression, bad temper, irritability, and aggression.
- Shaky hands.
- Withdrawal—headaches, anxiety, insomnia, sweating, shakiness—when you stop drinking.

Alcohol causes more health problems in the United States than do all illegal drugs combined. Excessive drinking can disrupt a person's work, family, and social life, and can damage organs in every system of the body—the kidneys, liver, brain, heart, and digestive organs. It may increase the risk of many forms of cancer as well. Drinking during pregnancy can cause severe damage to the growing fetus. Alcohol also plays a role in about half the nation's homicides, suicides, and traffic fatalities.

The line between abuse and alcoholism can be hard to see. Alcoholism is a physical addiction, marked by loss of control: The alcoholic keeps drinking even when it causes physical, psychological, or social harm. Most experts define alcoholism as a chronic, progressive disease. Alcohol abuse, although it shares some of the symptoms of alcoholism, is not considered an addiction.

The causes of alcoholism are not known, but a person's risk is 3 to 4 times greater than normal if a parent is an alcoholic. The disease can be treated once an alcoholic agrees to seek help. A person with good basic health, a support system, and a desire to stop drinking has a good chance of staying sober. As one expert puts it, "Alcoholism is the most treatable untreated disease in America."

WHAT YOU CAN DO NOW

Alcohol abuse:
➤ If you think you might have an alcohol problem, keep careful track of how much you drink over a given time (a week or more), and don't fudge. Experts say that women should have no more than 1 drink a day, and men should have no more than 2.

Confusion

Everyone gets confused once in a while, but severe, frequent, or long-term confusion may be a sign of a problem. Confusion is the inability to think clearly or make decisions; in severe cases, people may not know where or who they are. Confusion can come on quickly or slowly. Depending on the cause—physical or mental illness, injury, poisoning, or drug side effects—it may require prompt medical care.

SYMPTOMS	WHAT IT MIGHT BE	WHAT YOU CAN DO
Confusion; headache; agitation; drowsiness, sluggishness, or loss of consciousness.	Poisoning from carbon monoxide fumes. Causes include car running in garage, or old-fashioned gas or kerosene appliances in poorly vented room.	Get person into open air **right away.** Call 911 or go to emergency room **right away.** Check for pulse and breathing; if none, begin CPR (see page 14).
Head wound or bruise, confusion, dizziness or loss of consciousness, slurred speech, nausea.	Head injury causing concussion or bleeding in the brain (see head, neck, and back injuries, page 36).	Call 911 or go to emergency room **right away.**
After being in cold air or water: shivering and numbness, confusion, slurred speech, stumbling, drowsiness, loss of consciousness.	Hypothermia (see page 39).	Call 911 or go to emergency room **right away.** Remove any wet clothing. Make person as warm as possible.
After being in a hot place for an extended period: dizziness, fever over 104, dry skin, confusion, loss of consciousness.	Heatstroke (see page 38)	Call 911 or go to emergency room **right away.** Move person to cooler place. Apply cool, wet cloths to person's body.
Confusion, anxiety, or loss of consciousness; weak or rapid pulse; cold, clammy, pale, or bluish skin; rapid, shallow breathing.	Shock—vital organs are deprived of blood due to sudden illness or injury, or severe allergic reaction (see page 22).	Call 911 or go to emergency room **right away.** Check for breathing and pulse; if none, begin CPR (see page 14). Loosen clothing.
Sudden, temporary confusion; dizziness; loss of coordination; tingling; lightheadedness; weakness or numbness, usually on one side of body; double vision or temporary blindness; speech problems; hearing loss; headache.	Transient ischemic attack (TIA) or stroke—blood flow to brain interrupted by temporary artery blockage (see stroke, pages 44 and 113).	Call 911 or go to emergency room **right away.**

(continued)

Confusion (continued)

SYMPTOMS	WHAT IT MIGHT BE	WHAT YOU CAN DO
Confusion, fever over 100, chills, fatigue, weakness; maybe nausea and vomiting, loss of appetite, headache, stiff neck.	Bacterial or viral infection, such as pneumonia (see page 97), meningitis (see page 55), toxic shock syndrome (see page 243), or kidney infection.	Call doctor for advice. If you can't get one, call 911 or go to emergency room.
Confusion, anxiety, dizziness, sweating, shakiness, hunger, headache, impaired vision, rapid heartbeat, numbness, lack of coordination.	Hypoglycemia—low blood sugar, especially in people who take insulin (see diabetes, page 277).	People with diabetes should eat or drink something with sugar; for others, sugarless foods. If symptoms persist, call doctor for advice. If seizures or loss of consciousness, call 911 or go to emergency room **right away.**
Confusion, sleepiness, loss of consciousness, muscle spasms, shortness of breath.	Chronic kidney disease.	Call doctor for prompt appointment.
Confusion, bruising or bleeding for no clear reason, jaundice.	Chronic liver disease.	Call doctor for prompt appointment.
Coming on over time: confusion; faulty judgment and thinking; inability to complete simple tasks; memory problems that get worse; tendency to lose things and to wander and become lost.	Alzheimer's disease (see page 48) or other dementia.	Call doctor for advice and appointment.
Confusion, drowsiness, chronic breathing or sleep problems.	High levels of carbon dioxide in blood from chronic lung disease, blocked airway, or obesity.	Call doctor for advice.
Forgetfulness, poor concentration, bad temper, anxiety, depression, falling asleep at wrong times.	Sleep deprivation or sleep apnea (see **sleep disorders**, page 286).	Call doctor for advice.

(A "drink" is a 5-ounce glass of wine, a 12-ounce beer, or a 1.5-ounce shot of 80-proof liquor.)

➤ Never have more than 1 drink in an hour.

The liver can't process more than an ounce of alcohol per hour.

➤ Don't drink on an empty stomach.

➤ If you notice yourself getting drunk often,

hoarding alcohol, saying you drink less than you do, or getting angry if someone confronts you, get professional help.

➤ Don't drink any alcohol if you are pregnant or trying to get pregnant.

Alcoholism:

➤ Admit the problem and resolve to stop drinking. If you can't, call your doctor or a treatment center. In most cases, early treatment improves chances of recovery.

➤ Join a self-help group or attend a meeting. Alcoholics Anonymous (AA) is the best known; it has groups throughout the country. If you are not at ease with AA's spiritual approach, you might want to explore programs such as Rational Recovery or Women for Sobriety. Family members may want to look into Al-Anon, a support program for family and friends.

➤ Exercise regularly. Exercise can provide a sense of well-being.

➤ Eat well. Alcohol robs your body of nutrients (see **eat well,** page 296).

➤ If you suspect that a partner or loved one depends on alcohol, talk to your doctor or contact an alcohol treatment program for advice.

WHEN TO CALL THE DOCTOR

➤ If you have symptoms of alcoholism or alcohol abuse.

➤ If you get drunk often and feel depressed.

➤ If you tried to stop drinking and had symptoms of withdrawal such as headache, anxiety, insomnia, nausea, or, in rare cases, shaking limbs and strange visions.

➤ If you are pregnant and you can't stop drinking.

HOW TO PREVENT IT

Alcohol abuse:

➤ Don't drink to try to escape anxiety and **depression** (see page 211).

➤ Try other, more healthful activities in place of social drinking if you find yourself eagerly waiting for a drink.

Alcoholism:

Most experts believe that staying away from alcohol completely is the key for alcoholics. That might not be easy. These steps may help prevent a relapse:

➤ Avoid places and events that you associate

with alcohol, and don't spend time with friends when they are drinking.

➤ Ask your family and friends to help. Tell them that you are trying not to drink, and let them know how they can support you.

➤ Replace your need for alcohol with other activities. Take a class, or volunteer.

➤ Get a checkup, and ask your doctor for advice about foods and vitamins that can aid your recovery.

➤ If you have a relapse, don't use it as an excuse to give up all your gains. Think about what led to the relapse and how to do things differently next time.

➤ Ask your doctor about prescription drugs that may reduce your desire for alcohol.

COMPLEMENTARY CHOICES

➤ A recent study suggests that the herbal remedy Saint-John's-wort may curb alcohol cravings by easing **depression** (see page 211). It may take a week or two for you to feel an effect. Also, be aware that some herbal extracts contain alcohol; choose a capsule, a tea, or an extract with glycerine instead. Check with your doctor first to find out about possible drug interactions (also see **drug combinations to avoid,** page 323).

➤ Acupuncture may help relieve the symptoms of withdrawal and prevent relapse once the alcoholic has stopped drinking (see **how to choose a natural healer,** page 310).

FOR MORE HELP

Key Websites: *www.SavonHealth.com*. For more information on alcohol abuse: *www.SavonAlcoholAbuse.com*.

Organizations: Al-Anon/Alateen Family Groups, 1600 Corporate Landing Pkwy., Virginia Beach, VA 23454. 800-356-9996, M–F 8–6 EST; *www.al-anon-alateen.org*. Al-Anon is a mutual support program for families and friends of alcoholics. Alateen is a support program for teenagers whose lives are affected by alcoholism.

■ Alcoholics Anonymous, P.O. Box 459, Grand Central Station, New York, NY 10163. 212-870-3400, M–F 8:30–4:45 EST; *www.aa.org*. Call for the number of a local

AA group, or look in your phone book under "Alcoholics Anonymous."

■ The National Alcohol and Drug Referral Line, 800-252-6465, 24-hour line. Staff answers questions and suggests inpatient treatment facilities.

■ National Clearinghouse for Alcohol and Drug Information, Box 2345, Rockville, MD 20847-2345. 800-729-6686, M–F 8–7 EST; *www.health.org.*

■ Rational Recovery, Box 800, Lotus, CA 95651-0800. 530-621-2667, M–F 8–4 PST; *www.rational.org/recovery.* A self-help program for people with alcohol or drug problems, with groups in 700 U.S. cities.

■ Women for Sobriety, Box 618, Quakertown, PA 18951. 215-536-8026, M–F 8:30– 3 EST; *www.womenforsobriety.org.* Mutual-help groups that address the special needs of women with alcohol problems.

Books: *Educating Yourself About Alcohol and Drugs: A People's Primer,* by Marc Alan Schuckit, M.D. A recovery guide for substance abusers and their loved ones. Plenum Publishing, 1998, $20.

■ *Alcohol: How to Give It Up and Be Glad You Did,* by Philip Tate, Ph.D. Detailed ideas to help people end alcohol or substance abuse problems. See Sharp Press, 1996, $12.95

Anxiety & Phobias
www.SavonAnxiety.com

SIGNS AND SYMPTOMS

Generalized anxiety disorder:
Severe long-term worry, tension, bad temper, or depression, for no clear reason, plus some of the following:
■ Inability to relax, sleep, or concentrate.
■ Fatigue.
■ Headaches.
■ Sweating or hot flashes.
■ Trembling or twitching.
■ Being easily startled.

Phobias:
■ Constant, irrational fear of certain things, such as heights, blood, insects, flying, or snakes.

■ Fear of social settings in which you think you will be shamed.
■ Upset stomach, general pains.

Panic disorder:
Feelings of terror—"panic attacks"— that strike suddenly, sometimes in times of stress but often for no clear reason, and typically last a couple of minutes. They are marked by:
■ Racing or pounding heart, sometimes with chest pain.
■ Shortness of breath.
■ Dizziness, weakness, or nausea.
■ Flushes, chills, sweating, and trembling.
■ Feelings of unreality or a sense of losing control.
■ Sense of doom or fear of dying.
Panic disorder often comes with fear of situations that might bring on a panic attack and would be hard to escape.

Obsessive-compulsive disorder:
■ Constant unwelcome thoughts of such things as germs, dirt, violence, sex, or loss.
■ Repeated actions and rituals performed in an effort to prevent or cast out unwelcome thoughts. Examples include washing the hands over and over, counting things, and rearranging objects.

Post-traumatic stress disorder:
■ Inability to escape thoughts about past ordeals such as war, disasters, rape, abuse, or illness.
■ Flashbacks and nightmares.
■ Trouble sleeping and focusing.
■ Frequent bad temper.
■ Aggressive or violent feelings and actions.
■ Withdrawal, numbness, or loss of interest in things that used to be enjoyable (see **depression,** page 211).

Feeling anxious sometimes is normal and healthy: It rouses you to action when you face a real threat. But too much worry disrupts daily life.

Anxiety can be mild or immobilizing. There is most likely more than one cause. Experts believe that heredity, along with life events, may cause it. Some believe it is a learned response stemming from past trauma and conflict. Recent research suggests it also has a physical basis: Studies show that chemical changes in the body can set off panic attacks and anxiety in some people.

Treatment can involve drugs, psychotherapy, stress reduction, biofeedback, or hypnosis, or a mix of these. Most people improve with treatment. If you are troubled by anxiety, call your doctor. You may want to be treated by a specialist in anxiety disorders.

WHAT YOU CAN DO NOW

➤ Be honest about how your anxiety affects you: Is it keeping you from doing things you want to do? If so, seek help.

➤ Learn about the problem from up-to-date books, tapes, and studies and by getting news from mental health groups.

➤ Talk to a friend about your fears and feelings. Telling others can release stress.

➤ Find a good therapist. Ask your friends or doctor to refer you to someone experienced in treating anxiety. Go to a session to see if you like the therapist's approach.

➤ Get some daily exercise, such as taking a brisk walk or a playing sport you enjoy. Research shows that people who get frequent exercise feel less anxious than those who don't.

➤ Cut down on alcohol and caffeine. Too much caffeine often causes anxiety and may trigger panic attacks. Don't use street drugs such as cocaine.

➤ Simplify your life by making your schedule less hectic (see **stress,** page 218).

➤ Spend less time on stressful projects. Do something you enjoy.

➤ Get enough rest. If you have trouble sleeping, see **sleep disorders,** page 286.

➤ Join a support group.

WHEN TO CALL YOUR DOCTOR

Call your doctor or a mental health professional for advice:

➤ If you feel troubled, anxious, or out of control, and can't function.

➤ If, along with being anxious, you have lost weight and your eyes seem to bulge; you may have a **thyroid problem** (see page 288) or other ailment.

COMPLEMENTARY CHOICES

➤ Deep breathing and relaxation exercises may help, especially when your anxiety level starts to rise. Learn yoga or meditation (see **relax,** page 303).

➤ Kava, an herbal remedy made from the root of a Polynesian pepper plant, seems to help ease anxiety in some people. Kava can be found in health food stores as a tea, capsule, or tincture. Do not mix it with prescription antianxiety drugs or alcohol.

➤ Studies show that acupuncture triggers the release of brain chemicals that may reduce anxiety and depression (see **how to choose a natural healer,** page 310).

FOR MORE HELP

Key Websites: *www.SavonHealth.com*. For more information on anxiety and phobias: *www.SavonAnxiety.com*.

Organizations: Anxiety Disorders Association of America, 11900 Parklawn Dr., Suite 100, Rockville, MD 20852-2624. 301-231-9350, M–F 9–5 EST; *www.adaa.org*. Offers newsletter and listings of therapists who treat anxiety disorders.

■ National Institute of Mental Health, Public Inquiries, 6001 Executive Blvd., Room 8184, MSC 9663, Bethesda, MD 20892. 301-443-4513, M–F 8:30–5 EST; *www.nimh.nih.gov*. Sends fact sheets on panic disorder and lists of resources. At Website, click on *For the Public,* then on *Anxiety Disorders.*

■ National Mental Health Association, 800-969-6642, 24-hour recording, or 703-684-7722, M–F 9–5 EST; *www.nmha.org*. Sends free pamphlets on anxiety and other mental health problems, provides counseling, and refers you to services and support groups.

■ "Vet Centers" of the Department of Veterans Affairs. Counseling centers for Vietnam veterans and other vets with post-traumatic stress disorder operate in many cities.

BEHAVIOR & EMOTIONS

Check your phone book or call local information for the number of the one nearest you.

Book: *The Sky Is Falling: Understanding and Coping With Phobias, Panic Attacks, and Obsessive-Compulsive Disorders,* by Raeann Dumont. Stories and advice about anxiety disorders. W. W. Norton, 1997, $13.

Attention Deficit Disorder
www.SavonADD.com

SIGNS AND SYMPTOMS

- Frequent inability to pay attention.
- Trouble focusing; daydreaming.
- Strong pattern of making careless mistakes or trouble following instructions.
- Impulsive actions.
- Talking too much and interrupting others frequently.
- Sometimes, hyperactivity— squirming and running around in quiet situations.
- Inability to get organized.

Attention deficit disorder (ADD) is one of the most frequently diagnosed behavioral problems. Because some experts believe it is widely overdiagnosed, it is also one of the most controversial. ADD is most common in children (more boys than girls), though adults also can have it. When people with symptoms of ADD are also hyperactive, they are said to have attention deficit hyperactivity disorder (ADHD).

Genuine ADD may run in families, although other factors can play a role in causing it. If a woman smokes, uses alcohol or drugs, or is exposed to lead during pregnancy, her fetus may be harmed, causing symptoms of ADD to appear in childhood. Children exposed directly to lead also can get ADD.

The symptoms should be seen as a problem only if they affect a person's ability to function in more than one setting—at school *and* at home, or at work *and* at play. Many children

are labeled with ADD when their behavior is quite normal for their age and their situation.

Also, symptoms of ADD can be triggered by problems other than ADD: Learning disabilities, physical or sexual abuse, tension, **depression** (see facing page), **stress** (see page 218), and family violence can all cause children to act in ways that look like ADD.

Children with ADD do not lack intelligence; rather, they have trouble focusing. As a result, they don't perform at their best. Life can be baffling for them: They have problems at school, they become known as slow learners or troublemakers, they often get angry and see themselves as bad or stupid.

Since there is no known cure for ADD, the normal treatment is to try to manage it with drugs, chiefly the stimulant methylphenidate (brand name Ritalin). This drug and other stimulants may help, but many experts think doctors prescribe them too often. Doctors may also prescribe antidepressants for some children.

Many doctors now believe that most children with ADD will continue to have some symptoms as adults. Adults may be highly disorganized, have wild temper outbursts, and feel unable to cope with the stresses of life, for example. They may have trouble getting along with other people, and problems with drug or alcohol abuse.

WHAT YOU CAN DO NOW

➤ If you suspect that you or your child has ADD, go to an expert you trust. Psychiatrists, pediatricians, neurologists, and psychologists are among those who work with ADD. Your family doctor may be able to refer you to one.

After diagnosis:

➤ Think about getting a second opinion if a doctor says you have ADD or your child does—especially if the doctor prescribes Ritalin or another drug, or does not specialize in psychological problems.

➤ Know your own or your child's patterns and habits, strengths and weaknesses. Some people with ADD do best with lots of planned time and few distractions, while others need lots of variety and do poorly if they are too controlled.

➤ Don't punish your child or belittle yourself for acting in ways that are hard to control.

➤ Join an ADD support group.

WHEN TO CALL THE DOCTOR

➤ If you or your child show symptoms of ADD that disrupt daily life, work, or school.

FOR MORE HELP

Key Websites: *www.SavonHealth.com*. For more information on attention deficit disorder: *www.SavonADD.com*.

Organizations: Children and Adults with Attention-Deficit/Hyperactivity Disorder (CHADD), 8181 Professional Pl., Suite 201, Landover, MD 20785. 800-233-4050, M–F 8–5 EST; *www.chadd.org*. Offers reports on ADD and a list of support groups.

■ National ADD Association, 1788 Second St., Suite 200, Highland Park, IL 60035. 847-432-ADDA, 24-hour recording; *www.add.org*. Leave a message to receive information on ADD.

■ National Institute of Mental Health, Public Inquiries, 6001 Executive Blvd., Room 8184, MSC 9663, Bethesda, MD 20892. 301-443-4513, M–F 8:30–5 EST; *www.nimh.nih.gov*. Ask for the booklet on ADHD. At Website, click on *For the Public*, then *Attention Deficit Hyperactivity Disorder.*

Books: *The ADDed Dimension: Celebrating the Opportunities, Rewards, and Challenges of the ADD Experience*, by Kate Kelly and Peggy Ramundo. Fireside, 1998, $12.

■ *The Misunderstood Child: Understanding and Coping With Your Child's Learning Disabilities*, 3rd edition, by Larry B. Silver, M.D. An updated guide for parents of children with learning disabilities and ADD. Times Books, 1998, $15.

■ *Driven to Distraction: Recognizing and Coping With Attention Deficit Disorder From Childhood Through Adulthood*, by Edward M. Hallowell, M.D., and John Ratey, M.D. An in-depth look at ADD's symptoms and treatment. Simon & Schuster, 1995, $13.

Depression
www.SavonDepression.com

SIGNS AND SYMPTOMS

■ Constant feelings of pessimism or sadness.

■ Feelings of worthlessness, hopelessness, guilt, or despair.

■ Lack of interest or pleasure in life—work, relationships, food, and sex.

■ Lack of energy; fatigue.

■ Sleep problems: insomnia, oversleeping, or frequent waking too early.

■ Trouble focusing, remembering, making decisions, and doing simple tasks; a feeling of moving in slow motion.

■ Unusual weight loss or gain.

■ Frequent thoughts of death.

■ Nagging ailments—such as headaches or stomach pain—that don't get better with treatment.

Feeling blue is normal—up to a point. When people are so unhappy they can't work, enjoy life, or even function normally, they have an ailment called depression.

The causes—and treatments—of depression are hotly debated, but clearly your genes, surroundings, brain chemistry, and life experiences each play a part. Depression can strike at any age, even in childhood, though its severe forms most often affect adults. Women are twice as likely as men to be diagnosed as depressed.

Depression can take many forms. Feelings such as sadness, pessimism, or self-pity in response to painful events are sometimes called **depressive reactions.** These feelings, which are normal, can be quite severe but most often go away in a short time without treatment.

There's also a form of chronic, low-level depression called **dysthymia.** People who have it aren't severely depressed or suicidal, but they have little joy in life and feel downcast about the future. Some suffer from fatigue, sleep problems, and low self-esteem, and tend to heap blame on themselves. They have a hard time making choices or shaking

BEHAVIOR & EMOTIONS

their gloomy mood, and they sometimes fall into major depression.

A woman may feel a letdown after childbirth. **Postpartum "blues"** may begin 3 to 10 days after delivery, last around 2 weeks, and require only emotional support from family and friends. **Postpartum depression** begins about 3 weeks after delivery and can last at least a month. If it is severe or lasts longer than that, it may need treatment.

People who suffer from **major depression** feel so miserable that they have trouble living day to day. They are often in despair and are troubled by guilt, sleep problems, fatigue, crushing sadness, and feelings of emptiness and worthlessness. They may be suicidal or obsessed with death.

In rare cases, they may lose touch with the real world and have delusions and hallucinations. Their depression—which may have started with a major loss and can last for months—may lift, only to return later. Research suggests that this kind of depression is linked to the brain chemicals that affect mood and behavior, and that it may run in families.

When depression comes in fall or winter and then fades in the spring or summer, it is called **seasonal affective disorder** (SAD). People with SAD are affected by the lack of sunlight and often go through major mood shifts between the seasons.

Mood swings are even more extreme for people with **manic depression,** also known as **bipolar affective disorder.** They go back and forth from being very active or "high" (though they may also be moody, unfocused, and paranoid) to feeling sluggish and beaten down by despair, with feelings of normalcy in between. Episodes usually occur once or twice a year.

WHAT YOU CAN DO NOW

➤ Get help. See your family doctor to rule out illness. Sometimes depression is a symptom of disease.
➤ Ask your doctor or pharmacist if any medicine you are taking could be causing your depression.
➤ Ask your doctor about counselors who work with depressed people, and about medication for depression.

➤ Get some physical exercise every day—join a class or group. Research shows that people who exercise regularly are less likely to be depressed or stressed.
➤ Try a support group. Many are peer-led groups for people who had traumas in childhood (for instance, alcoholic parents or abuse) or who have had major losses (see **grief,** page 217). It's important to get support from people who will treat you with respect and understanding.
➤ Find out as much as you can about depression from self-help and professional organizations. You can find many online.
➤ Don't use alcohol or street drugs to feel better: Alcohol is a depressant.
➤ If you have SAD, ask an expert about indoor lighting that mimics sunlight. Get out in the sun when you can, or take a trip to a sunny place.

WHEN TO CALL THE DOCTOR

Call your doctor or a mental health professional for advice:
➤ If you, your child, or someone close to you has suicidal thoughts or depression that doesn't seem to lift. (Check your phone book: Many cities have suicide hotlines.)
➤ If depression seriously disrupts work, school, or relationships. Psychologists, psychiatrists, social workers, and peer counselors all work with people who are depressed. They take varied approaches to treatment, from psychotherapy ("talk therapy") to medication.

HOW TO PREVENT IT

➤ Don't isolate yourself.
➤ When you're feeling blue, find a friend or someone to talk with about your troubles.
➤ Stay active. Research shows that regular exercise can improve your mood.
➤ Be sure to get enough sleep (see **sleep disorders,** page 286).
➤ Eat balanced meals.
➤ Take a break from watching, listening to, or reading the news.

COMPLEMENTARY CHOICES

➤ Some people find that taking an extract of the herb Saint-John's-wort each day helps ease depression. It may take a week or two to feel an effect. Don't combine the herb with prescribed antidepressants, and be aware that your skin may become more sensitive to sun exposure.

➤ Acupuncture may help. Studies show that it triggers the release of certain brain chemicals that relieve depression and anxiety (see **how to choose a natural healer,** page 310).

➤ Kava, an herbal remedy made from a Polynesian root, which is effective in treating anxiety, may also relieve depression in some people. You can find it as tea, capsules, or tincture at your local health food store.

FOR MORE HELP

Key Websites: *www.SavonHealth.com*. For more information on depression: *www.SavonDepression.com*.

Organizations: National Empowerment Center, 599 Canal St., 5th Floor E., Lawrence, MA 01840. 800-769-3728, M–F 8–4 EST; *www.power2u.org*. Mental health consumers' group lists support groups and drop-in centers and offers print and audio items.

■ National Institute of Mental Health, Public Inquiries, 6001 Executive Blvd., Room 8184, MSC 9663, Bethesda, MD 20892. 301-443-4513, M–F 8:30–5 EST; *www.nimh.nih.gov*. Offers brochures on depression. At Website, click on *For the Public,* then on *Depression.*

■ National Mental Health Association, 1021 Prince St., Alexandria, VA 22314-2971. 800-969-6642, 24-hour recording, or 703-684-7722, M–F 9–5 EST; *www. nmha.org*. Sends free pamphlets on depression, provides counseling, and suggests services and support groups.

Book: *Overcoming Depression,* 3rd edition, by Dimitri F. Papolos, M.D. A thorough guide to depression. Revised and updated. HarperCollins, 1997, $15.

Drug Abuse
www.SavonSubstanceAbuse.com

SIGNS AND SYMPTOMS

■ Changes in looks, dress, and/or attitude.
■ Behavior changes that affect work and relationships.
■ Bad temper or abrupt changes in mood.
■ Restlessness, or sometimes extreme lethargy.
■ Puzzling absences.
■ Odd money problems.
■ Blackouts and memory lapses.
■ Drug cravings, inability to stop using, lying about drug use, constant thoughts about getting a drug and using it.

The use of drugs to obtain pleasure, relieve pain, or alter reality has been common in most cultures throughout history. But drug use can lead to abuse and sometimes to addiction.

Drug abuse is the use of a substance—legal or illegal—often enough or in large enough doses to result in physical, mental, emotional, or social harm. Addiction is loss of control over drug use.

Experts still don't know why some people can use drugs now and then while others get hooked almost right away. Many experts agree that drug addiction is a disease, not simply a sign of weak character, and should be treated as such.

Abuse of illegal drugs can be risky and even fatal (see **street drugs** chart, page 214). But abuse of *legal* drugs is also a major problem. In the United States, some 21 million people have abused prescription drugs, such as painkillers, sleeping pills, and tranquilizers, at least once. Even mild over-the-counter drugs can be harmful when they are overused. And alcohol and tobacco claim more lives than all illegal drugs combined.

Like alcoholics, drug abusers can be hard to treat because they often deny their problem—even when it threatens to destroy their lives. Successful treatment aims to create social support, enhance self-esteem, and teach ways to avoid situations that can trigger relapse.

Street Drugs: Signs & Risks

Abuse of any drug can cause major personal and social problems. But street drugs, because they are illegal, carry special risks, the least of which is jail. The drugs themselves are dangerous and are often mixed with deadly fillers. Users have no way of knowing what they are really getting, how strong it is, or how it will affect them. New street drugs keep appearing. Here are some that are widely used.

TYPE OF DRUG	SIGNS OF USE	RISKS
Amphetamines (speed, uppers); methamphetamine (ice).	Restlessness; talkativeness; decreased appetite with weight loss; dilated pupils; insomnia; trembling; dry mouth; angry, paranoid, or violent behavior.	Stroke or heart failure; violence.
Opiates, including heroin (smack) and opium.	Fatigue, euphoria, weight loss, sweating, poor appetite, needle marks on arms (sometimes), slurred speech, mood swings.	Overdose can lead to coma and death. If injected, risk of HIV infection and hepatitis from contaminated needles.
Cocaine (coke), called crack or rock when smoked.	Decreased appetite; mood swings; talkativeness; dilated pupils; apparent intoxication; sniffling, runny nose and nosebleeds (if snorted); weight loss; paranoia; disconnected speech.	Holes in cartilage separating nostrils (if snorted); seizures and coma; death by cardiac arrest or respiratory failure; suicidal behavior after prolonged use.
Inhalants, including nitrous oxide (laughing gas), amyl nitrite (poppers), butyl nitrite (rush), chlorohydrocarbons (aerosol sprays), and hydrocarbons (glue, paint thinner).	Agitation, nausea, coughing, nosebleeds, fatigue, lack of coordination, violent behavior.	Suffocation; with glue or paint thinner, permanent damage to brain, kidneys, and nervous system. Sudden death from cardiac arrest.
Designer drugs, including synthetic heroin (China white), MPTP, MDMA (ecstasy), and ephedrine, pseudoephedrine, or the herb ephedra, mixed with caffeine (herbal ecstasy).	Euphoria, tremors, impaired speech, nausea, sweating, fainting, chills, hallucinations, fever.	Synthetic heroin can lead to Parkinson's-like symptoms, including tremors, paralysis, and impaired speech or permanent brain damage. Ecstasy may cause paranoia and depression.

Street Drugs: Signs & Risks

TYPE OF DRUG	SIGNS OF USE	RISKS
Sedatives (downers), including tranquilizers and barbiturates; Rohypnol (roofies); ketamine.	Lethargy, confused speech, lack of balance, impaired judgment and motor ability, memory loss.	Overdose. Combined with alcohol, can lead to coma and death.
Hallucinogens, including LSD (acid), mescaline, and PCP (angel dust).	Seeing things that aren't there, nausea, sweating and trembling, mood disorders, increased heart rate, paranoia, violent behavior (PCP).	PCP in large doses can lead to seizures, coma, and violence. LSD can cause panic or loss of control.
Cannabis, including marijuana (pot, grass) and hashish (hash).	Mood swings, increased appetite, red eyes, slowed time sense and reflexes, anxiety, lethargy, alienation (sometimes).	Not physically addictive, but may cause psychological dependence and damage to lungs from smoking.

WHAT YOU CAN DO NOW

➤ If you believe you have a drug problem and have tried to stop using but could not, call a drug treatment program or professional right away. It's hard to stop drug abuse on your own.

➤ If you see 2 or more of the listed signs in a family member or friend (especially a child or teenager) and suspect drug abuse, call your doctor or contact one of the organizations listed here for names of drug treatment centers.

WHEN TO CALL THE DOCTOR

Call for a prompt appointment:

➤ If you are pregnant (or think you might be) and have been abusing drugs.

➤ If someone (especially a child or teenager) shows signs of drug abuse.

HOW TO PREVENT IT

Staying drug-free frequently requires major changes in habits and lifestyle. Depending on the depth of the drug problem, recovery (the stage that follows withdrawal) can be difficult. Still, you can take steps to help yourself stay clean:

➤ Seek the support of family members, friends, and colleagues.

➤ Join a support group such as Narcotics Anonymous or Cocaine Anonymous.

➤ Avoid places and situations that you associate with drug use. Make new friends who don't use drugs, and try to stay away from friends when they are using drugs.

➤ Be careful not to substitute some other kind of addictive activity—such as gambling, smoking, or overeating—for the one you're quitting.

➤ Make sure your diet is healthy and that you exercise. Workouts help your body release chemicals that make you feel good.

➤ Remember, recovery doesn't happen in a day. If you have a relapse, don't use it as an excuse to go back to your old habits. Think about what led to the relapse, and plan how to avoid it next time.

FOR MORE HELP

Key Website: *www.SavonHealth.com*. For more information on substance abuse: *www.SavonSubstanceAbuse.com*.

BEHAVIOR & EMOTIONS

Organizations: Cocaine Anonymous National Referral Line, 800-347-8998, 24-hour line. A support program based on Alcoholics Anonymous. Call for meetings near you.

■ DrugHelp, 800-DRUGHELP, 24-hour immediate crisis intervention line; *www. drughelp.org.* Information and referral network that provides facts about drug treatment options, programs, and support groups.

■ Narcotics Anonymous, Box 9999, Van Nuys, CA 91409. 818-773-9999, M–F 8–5 PST; *www.na.org.* A self-help/mutual support program patterned on the Alcoholics Anonymous 12-step approach. Call about local meetings.

■ National Drug Information Treatment and Referral Hotline of the Center for Substance Abuse Treatment, 800-662-4357, M–F, 24-hour line. Refers callers to treatment programs.

■ Phoenix House, 800-262-2463, 24-hour line. Gives names and numbers of local treatment programs.

Book: *Educating Yourself About Alcohol and Drugs: A People's Primer,* by Marc Alan Schuckit, M.D. A recovery guide for substance abusers and their loved ones. Plenum Publishing, 1998, $20.

Eating Disorders
www.SavonEatingDisorders.com

SIGNS AND SYMPTOMS

Anorexia:
■ Eating very little food and dieting even while losing a lot of weight.
■ Feeling fat even when far below normal weight.
■ Compulsive exercising.
■ Irregular or no menstrual periods.
■ In women, increase in facial and body hair.
■ Dry, yellow, or sallow skin.
■ Depression, moodiness, impatience, social withdrawal.
■ Constant use of over-the-counter diet pills or laxatives.

Bulimia:
■ Frequent periods of overeating, followed by vomiting in secret.
■ Spending long times in the bathroom, especially after meals, and signs of frequent vomiting (such as bloodshot eyes) or laxative or diuretic use (dizziness).
■ Cavities, damage to tooth enamel, and gum disease caused by stomach acids from frequent vomiting.
■ Compulsive exercising.

As many as 8 million people in the United States are thought to have eating disorders: mental illnesses in which the person becomes obsessed with food and body image. Anorexia nervosa (self-starvation) and bulimia nervosa (binge eating and/or purging) are the most common. Both can be fatal, and they require prompt professional care.

Anorexia is most common in young women, but it can affect anyone. It often looks at first like a normal concern about weight. But it grows out of control as the person becomes locked into a vicious cycle of frantic dieting and overexercise. The person with anorexia views herself or himself as fat even when emaciated. A person with bulimia, in contrast, goes on eating binges—sometimes eating up to 20,000 calories at one sitting.

About one-fourth of people with bulimia have also had anorexia. The causes may involve low self-esteem, troubled family life, worries about body changes during adolescence, and social pressure to look thin. Both conditions seem to run in families.

Treatment may include nutrition counseling, individual or family therapy, and support groups. Antidepressant drugs can help with bulimia, even in people who aren't depressed. A serious eating disorder may need to be treated in a hospital.

WHAT YOU CAN DO NOW

➤ Get help from a doctor specializing in eating disorders as soon as you can. The longer an eating disorder goes untreated, the harder it is to reverse. Your family doctor may be able to refer you.

➤ Treat yourself or anyone who has the problem with love and understanding—be aware that this is a mental illness.

➤ Avoid diet pills, laxatives, and diuretics. Overuse of diet pills can result in stroke; taking too many laxatives and diuretics can cause heart failure.

WHEN TO CALL THE DOCTOR

➤ If you see symptoms of anorexia or bulimia, especially with depression or talk of suicide.

➤ If you find that you or a member of your family is constantly worrying about weight and appearance.

HOW TO PREVENT IT

➤ Give your children healthy attitudes toward food and body image. Handle issues of eating and weight with sensitivity. Don't criticize or joke about your child's looks.

➤ As a parent, be willing to admit your mistakes and to accept those of your children. Anorexia and bulimia are more common in families that value high achievement. Try to keep the pressure down.

FOR MORE HELP

Key Websites: *www.SavonHealth.com*. For more information on eating disorders: *www.SavonEatingDisorders.com*.

Organizations: Eating Disorders Awareness and Prevention, 603 Stewart St., Suite 803, Seattle, WA 98101. 800-931-2237, M–F 8–12 and 1–5 PST; *www.edap.org*. Promotes and creates prevention programs, distributes materials, and gives referrals to therapists.

■ National Association of Anorexia Nervosa and Associated Disorders, Box 7, Highland Park, IL 60035. 847-831-3438, M–F 9–5 CST; *www.anad.org*. Answers questions and refers callers to lists of experts and support groups.

■ Overeaters Anonymous, *www.overeaters anonymous.org*. A 12-step program with chapters around the world. Check the white pages for the chapter nearest you. If you don't find one, write OA's Worldwide Ser-

vice Office, 6075 Zenith Ct. NE, Rio Rancho, NM 87124, or call 505-891-2664, M–F 8–5 MST, for a list of chapters.

Book: *Fat Is a Feminist Issue: The Anti-Diet Guide for Women*, by Susie Orbach. Latest edition of a classic book. Budget Book Service, 1997, $8.99.

Grief

www.SavonGrief.com

SIGNS AND SYMPTOMS

Grief is normal after any deep loss. Symptoms vary, but may include:

■ Extreme depression and fatigue.

■ Sudden shifts in emotions—being numb and cool one minute and sobbing out of control the next.

■ Feeling helpless, confused, and lost.

■ Major changes in sleep patterns, such as trouble getting to sleep, waking up often at night, or wanting to sleep all the time.

■ Physical pain or discomfort.

■ Loss of appetite or overeating.

■ Lack of focus; trouble making choices or concentrating.

■ Self-destructive behavior, including reckless driving or abuse of drugs or alcohol.

■ Feelings of guilt.

Few things are as wrenching and as hard to get over as the death of a loved one. But other losses also leave people stunned with grief. These include divorce, miscarriage, the end of a friendship or serious relationship, a disabling illness or accident, losing a job, and even the loss of a pet.

Grieving often happens in stages. The first stage is usually marked by a mixture of numbness, shock, and denial. You may feel you're in a trance and unable to make decisions. Many people feel so drained, or they so badly neglect their own needs (such as eating or sleeping), that they get sick. Others try to pretend the shock is not so bad: "Don't worry about me. I'm fine."

After a while, you may go through phases of intense feeling. When someone close to you

BEHAVIOR & EMOTIONS

has died, feelings may include anger (at the unfairness of the death), fear (that you or other loved ones will also die), guilt (for having survived or for something you think you failed to do for the person who died), depression, and aimlessness.

Don't block your grief. Experts advise letting yourself (and others) feel numb, sad, angry, or depressed. Then, at your own pace, move on with your life. "Grief is not a sign of weakness," says the Theos Foundation, which sets up support groups for widowed people. "Allow grief to have its way for a while; then, gradually and gently, you can release yourself from its grip."

WHAT YOU CAN DO NOW

➤ Don't hide your grief from friends. Express your needs and ask for help.
➤ Find a support group. Being with others who are going through the same process can help. (Many groups work with people who have a loved one who is dying.)
➤ Find help for your children. If there is a death or other hurtful event in your family, your children need to grieve, too, and they need all the support you can give them. Grief groups for children exist but may be hard to find. For young children, counseling may be better.
➤ Put off making most major decisions—whether to move from your home, what to do with your loved one's possessions—while you're in the midst of grieving.
➤ Don't leave important things unsaid or undone before someone dies. Seek the person out and make sure that you resolve as much as you can; you'll spare yourself much grief and guilt later.
➤ If you know someone who is grieving, don't be afraid to talk with him or her.

WHEN TO CALL THE DOCTOR

➤ If you feel ill and think you need help. Ailments caused by grief are real.
➤ If symptoms of **depression** (see page 211) last longer than 2 months, or if you feel you might kill yourself.

FOR MORE HELP

Key Websites: *www.SavonHealth.com*. For more information on grief: *www.SavonGrief.com*.

Organizations: Compassionate Friends, P.O. Box 3696, Oak Brook, IL 60522-3696. 630-990-0010, M–F 9–4 CST; *www.compassionatefriends.org*. For families who are grieving the death of a child. Offers support, lists resources, and refers callers to community chapters.

■ Kara, 457 Kingsley Ave., Palo Alto, CA 94301. 650-321-5272, M–F 9–4 PST; *www.kara-grief.org*. Offers counseling, printed materials, and resources for children, adolescents, and adults suffering the death or serious illness of a loved one.

■ The International Theos Foundation, 322 Blvd. of the Allies, Suite 105, Pittsburgh, PA 15222-1919. 412-471-7779, M–Th 9–4 EST. For men and women newly widowed; connects callers with local support groups and sends printed information on grieving.

Website: The Hygeia Foundation for Prenatal Loss and Bereavement, *www.connix.com/~hygeia*. Offers support, resources, and an online journal for pregnancy and neonatal loss.

Book: *Parting Company: Understanding the Loss of a Loved One,* by Cynthia Pearson and Margaret L. Stubbs. Advice to caregivers on what to expect from and how to cope with caring for the dying. Seal Press, 1999, $18.95.

Stress
www.SavonStress.com

SIGNS AND SYMPTOMS

Physical:
■ Frequent headaches.
■ Trouble sleeping.
■ Fatigue.
■ Digestive illness.
■ Skin problems.
■ Back or neck pain.
■ Poor appetite or overeating, or heavy drinking.

Psychological:

- Anxiety, tension, or anger
- Withdrawal from social life.
- Pessimism or cynicism.
- Boredom.
- Bad temper or resentment.
- Loss of ability to concentrate or perform as usual.

Stress is our reaction to anything—good or bad—that upsets our balance. Stressful events trigger the body's release of the hormones—including adrenaline—that provide a quick supply of oxygen and energy.

But these hormone surges, if sparked again and again, can deplete the body's ability to bounce back and can cause problems such as ulcers, high blood pressure, and loss of appetite. Constant stress also puts you at risk of **headaches** (see page 52), **chronic fatigue syndrome** (see page 275), **depression** (see page 211), and digestive ailments. Stress can also upset your body's immune system and lower your resistance to disease.

Stress often comes from painful situations you feel you can't control: job burnout, money problems, grief, or divorce. Minor stresses range from arguments to traffic jams. But even a good event, such as marriage, a job promotion, or a new baby, can trigger stress. Other causes include illness, loneliness, pain, and the drive to be perfect.

WHAT YOU CAN DO NOW

➤ Do things that calm you. Take walks or long, hot baths. Talk with friends, or rent movies that make you laugh.

➤ Exercise 30 minutes a day at least 3 times a week. You'll reduce your level of stress hormones and gain a sense of well-being.

➤ Spend time outdoors. Some research shows that contact with nature can help reduce stress.

➤ Enroll in a stress reduction course. Ask your doctor to refer you, or check with the local hospital. Also, some employers offer courses or will send you to one.

➤ Learn relaxation techniques. These include deep breathing, stretching exercises, yoga, visualization, and meditation (see **relax,** page 303).

WHEN TO CALL THE DOCTOR

➤ If you are anxious, depressed, or troubled beyond routine stress (see **depression,** page 211, and **anxiety and phobias,** page 208).

➤ If you have symptoms of stress with any of these: new sleep patterns, mood swings, loss of sex drive, crying jags, exhaustion, great difficulty with minor tasks, agitated or slow movement, or a change in menstrual cycles. You may have a form of clinical depression.

➤ If your symptoms are long-lasting and trouble you.

HOW TO PREVENT IT

➤ Figure out what causes your stress and where you can make changes. Set reachable goals for yourself and be forthright with other people about what you can and can't do, and will and won't do.

➤ Don't try to be perfect. If you are juggling too many things, let a ball or two drop. Your house doesn't have to be spotless, and you don't always have to be the last one to leave the office. Practice giving yourself a break.

➤ Take a slow-paced, pressure-free vacation, leaving your work behind.

FOR MORE HELP

Key WebSites: *www.SavonHealth.com*. For more information on stress: *www.SavonStress.com*.

Organizations: American Institute of Stress, 124 Park Ave., Yonkers, NY 10703. 914-963-1200, M–F 9–5 EST; *www.stress.org*. Offers a monthly newsletter and a $35 informational packet.

- National Mental Health Association, 1021 Prince St., Alexandria, VA 22314-2971. 800-969-6642, 24-hour recording, or 703-684-7722, M–F 9–5 EST; *www. nmha.org*. Sends free pamphlets on stress and other mental health issues, provides counseling, and lists services and support groups.

Book: *Why Zebras Don't Get Ulcers: An Updated Guide to Stress, Stress-Related Diseases, and Coping,* by Robert M. Sapolsky. W. H. Freeman, 1998, $14.95.

BEHAVIOR & EMOTIONS

Sexual Health

Birth Control

Choosing a method of birth control takes careful thought about what will work best for you and your partner. Remember that no method is foolproof; to reduce your risk of getting pregnant, you may want to consider using more than one type.

Here are success rates, pros and cons, and costs of various birth control methods, listed in order of their numbers of users. (Success rates are for the first year of use.)

Sterilization

This is the most effective and most permanent form of birth control. For women, it involves surgery to close off the fallopian tubes (tubal ligation); for men it means a simpler, safer surgical procedure to block the flow of sperm into the penis (vasectomy).

Success rate: More than 99 percent; has failed in very rare cases.

Pros: Effective; no loss of sexual mood.

Cons: General anesthesia for tubal ligation has some risk; possible infection; hard to reverse; no defense against STDs.

Cost: Tubal ligation: $2,000–2,500; vasectomy: $240–520.

The Pill

With today's lower-estrogen pill, severe side effects are rare in nonsmokers. The Pill does pose risks, however. Among them are heart attack, blood clots in the veins, and stroke, as well as higher rates of breast cancer and cervical cancer. You are at higher risk if you or a close relative has any of those conditions. Before you start the Pill, discuss your complete health history with your doctor.

Success rate: 97 percent; higher if used "perfectly," without skipping days.

Pros: Effective; no loss of sexual mood.

Cons: Side effects (see above); must be taken daily; no defense against STDs.

Cost: $50–175 for exam; $16–25 monthly.

Condoms

Cheap and simple, the condom is the one contraceptive that also protects against most STDs—if the condom is latex.

Success rate: 90 percent for the male condom, 79 percent for the female condom (vaginal pouch). The success rate for condoms is much higher when they're used with foam spermicides. If you use a lubricant, opt for one that's water based; oil-based jellies and creams eat away at the latex. Handle carefully—watch the fingernails.

Pros: Best defense against STDs; low cost; easily available.

Cons: Can tear, slip, or come off during intercourse; may disrupt sexual mood.

Cost: 50 cents each for male condoms; up to $3 for the vaginal pouch.

Cervical Cap and Diaphragm

These devices pose few health risks, but they can be less effective than some other forms of birth control. Both must be used with a spermicide.

Success rate: 82–94 percent.

Pros: Low cost; few serious side effects; some defense against STDs.

Cons: Can interfere with mood; some spermicides may cause allergic reaction.

Cost: $70–175 for an exam; $15–40 for the device; $3–10 per tube for spermicide.

Sexually Transmitted Diseases

Each sexually transmitted disease (STD) listed here may produce no symptoms at first. When symptoms do show up, they may be confused with those of other diseases. If you are infected but don't have any symptoms, you can still pass an STD on to your partner. Note, too, that an open sore or irritated skin from an STD, either on the inside or outside of the genitals, puts you at greater risk of catching HIV. That's why if you have sex with more than one person, testing and checkups are vital, as is safe sex (see page 224).

SYMPTOMS	WHAT IT MIGHT BE	WHAT YOU CAN DO
Early to later: sore throat; fever; swollen glands in the neck, underarms, and groin. Fatigue, fever chills, and night sweats. Frequent colds, cold sores, oral fungal or yeast infections. Sudden weight loss, chronic diarrhea, dry cough, breathing problems, sores, vision loss. Confusion, memory loss.	AIDS—Caused by HIV (human immunodeficiency virus), found in blood, semen, and vaginal fluids, and sometimes in saliva and breast milk. HIV is spread mostly through sexual contact or by sharing needles. An infected woman can pass it to her child during childbirth or breast-feeding.	Call your doctor for a prompt appointment. Get an HIV test right away. In most cities, you can get the test without giving your name. If you are infected, the sooner you know it the better, so that you can start treatment to slow the onset of AIDS.
Watery mucus from penis or vagina, burning with urination, mild lower abdominal pain 1–3 weeks after infection. Some people (mostly women) may have no symptoms.	Chlamydia—bacterial disease. Can result in pelvic inflammatory disease in women (see page 236) or sterility. In newborns exposed during childbirth, can cause pneumonia, eye infections, and blindness.	Call doctor for prompt appointment. You and your partner(s) should be treated with antibiotics.
Itching or burning pain in genital area, then red bumps in or on genitals that may turn into blisters or open sores 2–10 days after infection. These go away within 3 weeks. Later attacks (with same symptoms) heal faster.	Genital herpes—viral infection spread through sex, from cold sores (see page 79), or, rarely, by hands that have herpes blisters or sores. Most contagious when symptoms are present. Can be transferred from mother to baby during childbirth.	Call doctor for prompt appointment. Medications shorten outbreaks and make them less severe. Don't have sex until sores heal. For more help: National Herpes Hotline: 919-361-8488, M–F 9–7 EST. American Social Health Association Resource Center, 800-230-6039, 24-hour recording.

(continued)

SEXUAL HEALTH

Sexually Transmitted Diseases (continued)

SYMPTOMS	WHAT IT MIGHT BE	WHAT YOU CAN DO
Small, round, red, flat, itchy bumps on genitals, around anus, or inside vagina; can also appear in mouth of someone who has had oral contact with genitals of infected person.	Genital warts—infection by human papillomavirus (HPV). Some strains of HPV raise risk of cervical cancer. After warts are removed, virus remains and can cause future outbreaks.	Call doctor for prompt appointment. Treatment can include drugs or laser surgery. Don't use over-the-counter wart treatments. Women who've had warts should get a Pap smear every 6 months.
Thick yellowish discharge from vagina or penis, burning and itching with urination, maybe discharge from rectum 2–10 days after infection. In later stages in women: abdominal pain, bleeding between periods.	Gonorrhea—bacterial infection. If left untreated, may spread to joints, tendons, or heart. May also cause pelvic inflammatory disease in women (see page 236). Infants exposed during birth can become blind.	Call doctor for prompt appointment. Treatment consists of antibiotics and painkillers. Don't have sex until doctor says it's safe. Your partner(s) should be tested and treated even if they have no symptoms.
Painless sores on or in genitals, rectal area, or mouth, and enlarged lymph nodes near sores 10 days to 3 months after infection. If untreated, in second stage (3 weeks to several months later): mild fever, rash, patchy hair loss, sore throat.	Syphilis—bacterial infection. Can damage brain, nervous system, and heart; can be fatal. Highly contagious in first 2 stages but not in third stage. Infected mothers may pass infection to infants during childbirth.	Call doctor for prompt appointment. Antibiotics can cure syphilis, although in later stages some damage cannot be reversed. Don't have sex during treatment. Your partner(s) should be tested and treated.
In women, heavy greenish-yellow or gray discharge from vagina, pain during intercourse, vaginal odor, painful urination 4–20 days after infection. Men may have no symptoms.	Trichomoniasis—infection caused by parasite. May increase risk that baby born to infected mother will be premature or underweight.	Call doctor for prompt appointment. You and your partner(s) will be treated with antibiotics. A man may have no symptoms but can infect others if not treated. Don't have sex until treatment is finished.

Sexually Transmitted Diseases

SEXUAL HEALTH

Implanted and Injected Hormones

The hormones found in the Pill can also be injected or implanted under the skin of a woman's arm. Because this option can have serious side effects, make sure your doctor knows your complete health history before you proceed.

Success rate: 99 percent.

Pros: Effective; no loss of sexual mood.

Cons: Expensive; no defense against STDs; possible side effects.

Cost: Implant: $500–750 for exam and insertion of 5-year implant; $120–150 for removal. Injection: $50–175 for exam and $35–55 injection (good for 90 days).

Spermicides

Available in foams, creams, jellies, and vaginal suppositories, spermicides are most effective when used with another form of birth control such as a condom, diaphragm, or cervical cap.

Success rate: 82 percent.

Pros: No side effects; easily available.

Cons: Some brands cause allergic reactions; no defense against STDs.

Cost: $3–10 for several applications.

Intrauterine Device (IUD)

A T-shaped device placed in the uterus that prevents implantation of an embryo, the IUD is hotly debated. Many doctors think the IUD is safe, but it has been linked to an increased risk of **pelvic inflammatory disease** (see page 236) and ectopic pregnancy (pregnancy outside the uterus) and may not be a good choice for women who want to have children later.

Success rate: 97–99 percent.

Pros: Effective; no loss of sexual mood.

Cons: Can cause PID; may impair future fer-

How to Have Safe Sex

➤ Have sex only with a person you know to be free of diseases.

➤ If you don't know your partner's sexual history, use a latex condom.

➤ If you have more than one sex partner, use latex condoms (even during oral sex). Never reuse a condom. A water-based lubricant will help prevent the condom from tearing.

➤ Don't have anal sex; it increases your risk of HIV and other STDs.

➤ It is safe to hug, kiss, massage, and touch others.

tility; no defense against STDs.

Cost: $300–400 for exam and insertion.

Natural Method

The withdrawal and rhythm methods are non-medicinal, but you could well end up dealing with an unwanted pregnancy.

Success rate: About 75 percent. (When you use no birth control, you and your partner have an 85 percent chance of a pregnancy over time.)

Pros: Low cost; natural.

Cons: Not effective; no STD protection.

Cost: None.

Emergency Contraception

Women sometimes need to take action after intercourse to avoid pregnancy. Your doctor can write a prescription for emergency contraceptive pills. If you don't have a doctor, call 888-NOT2LATE (888-668-2528). The hotline will give names and phone numbers of nearby doctors who can help; the sooner you take these pills, the better. For more advice, call the Emergency Contraception Hotline at 800-584-9911 (24-hour recording).

FOR MORE HELP

Key Websites: *www.SavonHealth.com*. For more information on birth control: *www.SavonBirthControl.com*.

Organizations: Office of Population Affairs Clearinghouse, P.O. Box 30686, Bethesda, MD 20824-0686. 301-654-

6190, M–F 9–5 EST. Ask for facts about birth control.

■ Planned Parenthood, 800-230-PLAN, 24-hour recording; *www.plannedparenthood.org*. Connects you to a local chapter, which offers information on birth control.

Website: Ann Rose's Ultimate Birth Control Links, *www.gynpages.com/ultimate*. Offers facts on birth control and a range of other links on the Web.

Books: *All About Birth Control: The Complete Guide,* by Jon Knowles and the Planned Parenthood Federation of America. Offers details on virtually all birth control methods available in the United States. Three Rivers, 1998, $12.

■ *The Birth Control Book,* by Samuel A. Pasquale, M.D., and Jennifer Cadoff. A woman's guide to choosing the safest and most effective method of birth control. Ballantine, 1996, $12.

Loss of Sexual Desire
www.SavonSexualHealth.com

SIGNS AND SYMPTOMS

■ Lack of interest in sex for more than 2 months.

■ In couples, sex less often than every other week, or anxiety about sex.

■ Sometimes, erection problems, premature ejaculation, painful intercourse, or trouble reaching orgasm.

A short-term loss of sexual desire is quite normal; people of all ages go through peaks and declines. A lack of desire is the most common complaint at sex therapy clinics. The problem is often caused by psychological factors: **depression** (see page 211), anger, boredom, conflict in a relationship, stress, fear of pregnancy, or memories of sexual abuse. It may also result from fatigue, **alcohol abuse** (see page 204), or the use of antidepressants, tranquilizers, or antihistamines. Less often, the cause is a hormonal imbalance or a disease such as **diabetes** (see page 277).

A marriage counselor or sex therapist

can often help if the problem is an emotional or psychological issue. Easing stress or treating any health problems may also help. Testosterone shots have helped some men, as well as some women who are past menopause. Sildenafil (Viagra) may help some men. It's the first oral prescription drug for erection problems. Sildenafil won't work in all cases, though, and it has side effects. Talk with your doctor to find out if it's right for you.

WHAT YOU CAN DO NOW

➤ See whether a drug you are taking might be the cause. Many drugs have side effects that can cause lack of desire. Ask your doctor.
➤ Cut back on alcohol or stop drinking (see **alcohol abuse and alcoholism,** page 204).
➤ Check your stress level (see **is stress putting your health at risk?** page 302). Worry and conflict chill interest in sex.
➤ Wait before you worry: If you have had a recent crisis—a loss, an illness, a major change—your sex drive may just be taking a rest (see **grief,** page 217, and **erection problems,** page 226).
➤ Try something new. Have sex at a different time or place, or try varied positions.
➤ Relax when making love. Take your time and try more foreplay. Tell your partner what arouses you.
➤ Share your feelings and worries about your sexual performance—but not while making love.
➤ Try reading or using erotic materials, watching videos, or playing out sexual fantasies, if this appeals to you.

WHEN TO CALL THE DOCTOR

➤ If loss of sexual desire is causing problems in your relationship.
➤ If you have erection problems or pain during intercourse.
➤ If your problem doesn't respond to self-help measures; you may have an illness.
➤ If you think a drug is the cause.
➤ If you are depressed.

HOW TO PREVENT IT

➤ Take steps to reduce **stress** (see page 218, and **relax,** page 303).
➤ Exercise regularly and eat good food (see **eat well,** page 296). Get plenty of sleep.
➤ Devote some time to your relationship. Set aside time to go out on "dates," or create romantic evenings at home.
➤ Try to solve problems in your relationship before they build up.

FOR MORE HELP

Key Websites: *www.SavonHealth.com.* for more information on loss of sexual desire: *www.SavonSexualHealth.com.*

Organizations: American Association of Marriage and Family Therapists, 1133 15th St. NW, Suite 300, Washington, DC 20005. 202-452-0109 M–F 9–5:30 EST; *www.aamft.org.* Send in a self-addressed stamped envelope for a list of counselors near you.

■ American Association of Sex Educators, Counselors, and Therapists, Box 238, Mount Vernon, IA 52314. *www.aasect.org.* A referral and credentialing service for sex therapists and counselors. Send a self-addressed stamped envelope if you want a list of nationally certified sex therapists and counselors in your area.

■ Sexuality Information and Education Council of the United States (SIECUS), 130 West 42nd St., Suite 350, New York, NY 10036-7802. 212-819-9770, M–F 9–5 EST; *www.siecus.org.* Refers people to organizations appropriate for their sexual questions and issues.

SEXUAL HEALTH

Men's Health

Erection Problems
www.SavonErectileDysfunction.com

www.SavonErectileDysfunction.com

SIGNS AND SYMPTOMS

- Frequent trouble getting and keeping an erection for intercourse.

Erection problems are more common than you might think—though people differ about what's a "problem." Many men have trouble getting an erection now and then, maybe more often as they age. If you are often unable to get erections and this bothers you, talk to your doctor.

An erection is a complex process, and many things can interfere with it. The most common are physical problems, including **diabetes** (see page 277); reduced blood flow to the penis (see **artery disease,** page 104); a sports injury; and too much alcohol (see **alcohol abuse and alcoholism,** page 204). Drugs prescribed for high blood pressure and depression, and psychological stresses such as **depression** (see page 211), worry, guilt, or "performance anxiety," can also cause trouble.

Although erection problems may upset you, they can almost always be treated. Sildenafil (Viagra) is the first oral prescription drug for erection problems, and it's the main remedy in most cases. However, this drug should *never* be taken if you're using nitroglycerin or any other nitrates to treat a heart problem. If you have heart disease, talk with your doctor before taking sildenafil.

Injections, implants, and other treatments may help if sildenafil doesn't, or if it's not an option.

WHAT YOU CAN DO NOW

- See if a drug you are taking might be the cause. Many blood pressure drugs, among others, can affect sexual function. Ask your doctor or pharmacist. There may be another drug that works as well, but without the side effects.
- Don't drink alcohol (see **alcohol abuse and alcoholism,** page 204) or smoke. Both make the problem worse.
- Check your stress level (see **is stress putting your health at risk?** page 302). Tension, worry, and conflict can chill interest in sex.
- Wait before you worry: If you have had a recent crisis—a loss, a breakup, a major change—your sex drive may just be taking a rest (see **loss of sexual desire,** page 224, and **grief,** page 217).
- Relax when making love. Take your time and try more foreplay. Tell your partner what arouses you.
- Share your feelings and worries about your performance—but not while making love. Set aside some time to talk with your partner about it.
- Try reading or using erotic materials, watching videos, or playing out sexual fantasies, if these appeal to you and your partner.
- See if you can get an erection while masturbating, when just waking up, or at other times when you aren't making love. If

Testicle Problems

Pain, swelling, and tenderness in the testicles can have any number of causes, ranging from sports injuries to illness (including mumps, when you get it as an adult). A lump can signal testicular cancer, the leading cancer for men between the ages of 20 and 35. Most doctors advise a monthly testicular self-exam (see **self-exams,** page 319).

SYMPTOMS	WHAT IT MIGHT BE	WHAT YOU CAN DO
Sudden extreme pain and tenderness in either testicle; may spread to lower abdomen. Scrotum may be swollen, firm, and red. Sometimes faintness and nausea.	Testicular torsion— twisting of testicle and tube that carries sperm to the prostate, cutting off blood supply to testicle.	Call doctor for prompt appointment. Can cause permanent damage if not treated promptly.
Firm, most often painless lump or swelling on one testicle. Testicle may feel heavy or hard, sometimes painful.	Testicular cancer. Most common in men between 15 and 34. Can almost always be cured when found early.	If you notice symptoms, call doctor for prompt appointment. Do a self-exam once a month after warm bath or shower. (See self-exams, page 319.)
Swelling and pain around testicle; comes on slowly, then becomes severe. Swollen area is hot and tender; swelling may spread to scrotum.	Epididymitis—inflamed sperm-storage tube (epididymis) behind each testicle. Causes include prostate infections and sexually transmitted diseases.	Call doctor for prompt appointment. Bed rest and ice packs may help. Antibiotics usually cure it; sex partners may also need treatment.
Soft, most often painless swelling in scrotum.	Hydrocele—excess fluid that builds up in membrane around each testicle. It's harmless.	Treatment of small hydroceles is most often not needed. If a hydrocele is very large or painful, call doctor for advice and appointment.
Swollen veins in scrotum, almost always on left side. Most often no pain. Swelling lessens when you lie down.	Varicocele—varicose or enlarged veins in scrotum. Very common and usually harmless. In 20% of cases, can cause infertility.	Call doctor for advice. Wear an athletic supporter to ease any discomfort.
Tenderness and pain in testicles or scrotum; not severe, may come and go.	Orchialgia—pain in testicles; no known cause, may be viral.	Take over-the-counter painkillers and warm baths. Call doctor for advice if pain lasts more than a week.

MEN'S HEALTH

you can, the problem is most likely not physical. Let your doctor know.

WHEN TO CALL THE DOCTOR

➤ If erection problems often keep you from having intercourse or cause tension with your partner.

➤ If you suspect one of your medicines is causing the problem.

➤ If physical causes have been ruled out; ask to be referred to a counselor or therapist.

HOW TO PREVENT IT

➤ Exercise regularly and eat well (see *Staying Healthy,* page 291).

➤ Reduce your stress: Try deep breathing, meditation, or yoga (see **relax,** page 303).

➤ Sometimes, daily pelvic-muscle exercises help men with artery disease or other circulation problems. Called Kegel exercises, they also tone the muscles that control urination. Begin by sensing which muscles you use to start and stop urination. Later, contract and release them in 15 to 20 squeezes, 3 times a day. Work up to holding the squeeze for at least 10 seconds each time.

FOR MORE HELP

Key Websites: *www.SavonHealth.com*. For more information on erectile dysfunction: *www.SavonErectileDysfunction.com*.

Organizations: American Foundation for Urologic Disease, 1128 North Charles St., Baltimore, MD 21201. 410-468-1800, M–F 8:30–5 EST; *www.afud.org*. Ask for brochure on erection problems.

■ Impotence Institute of America, P.O. Box 410, Bowie, MD 20718-0410. 800-669-1603, M–F 9–5 EST; *www.impotence-world.org*. Staff answers questions and sends brochures.

■ National Kidney and Urologic Diseases Information Clearinghouse, 3 Information Way, Bethesda, MD 20892. 301-654-4415, M–F 8:30–5 EST; *www.niddk.nih.gov/health/kidney/nkudic.htm*. Offers facts about erection problems. At

Website, click on *Urologic Diseases* and then on *Impotence.*

Books: *The Impotence Sourcebook,* by Christopher P. Steidle, M.D. Discusses the causes and treatments of impotence. Lowell House, 1999, $15.95.

■ *The Sexual Male: Problems and Solutions,* by Richard Milsten, M.D., and Julian Slowinski, Psy.D. Offers advice on a variety of male sexual problems. W. W. Norton, 1999, $25.95.

Prostate Problems
www.SavonProstate.com

SIGNS AND SYMPTOMS

General symptoms:
■ Frequent, urgent, sometimes painful need to urinate; urine may be bloody.
■ Weak or dribbling stream of urine.
■ Incontinence (sometimes).
■ Sometimes a feeling that the bladder is not emptied.

Prostate cancer:
Often no symptoms in early stages, sometimes followed by the symptoms above. In later stages:
■ Pain in the lower back or pelvis, or sometimes in other places.
■ Weight loss.

Prostatitis:
■ Pain between the anus and scrotum.
■ Discomfort when urinating.
■ Painful ejaculation; blood in the semen or urine.
■ Fever and chills (acute prostatitis).
■ Lower back pain.

The prostate is a chestnut-size gland that wraps around the urethra (the tube that runs between a man's bladder and the end of his penis; see color illustration, page 175). It makes most of the fluid in semen that carries sperm.

Enlarged prostate: In most men, the prostate gland grows larger with age—75 percent of men over 50 have somewhat larger

Do You Have a Prostate Problem?

Urinary problems are key signs of an enlarged prostate gland. The American Urological Association's Symptom Score Index, aimed at spotting such problems, can help a man check his prostate health. It does not detect prostate cancer.

Circle your response to each question. A total score of 7 or lower means no problem or no more than a mild problem; 8 to 19 is mild; 20 to 35 is severe. Note: The AUA advises that you ask your doctor to explain the results of this test.

In the last month, how often have you:	Never	Less than one time in five	Less than half the time	About half the time	More than half the time	Almost always
Had a feeling of not having emptied your bladder completely after you finished urinating?	0	1	2	3	4	5
Had to urinate again less than 2 hours after you last urinated?	0	1	2	3	4	5
Found your flow stopped and started again several times when you urinated?	0	1	2	3	4	5
Found it difficult to postpone urination?	0	1	2	3	4	5
Had a weak urinary stream?	0	1	2	3	4	5
Had to push or strain to begin urination?	0	1	2	3	4	5
In the last month, about how many times a night did you:	Never	One	Two	Three	Four	Five or more
Get up to urinate from the time you went to bed until you got up in the morning?	0	1	2	3	4	5

Adapted with the permission of the *Journal of Urology*

MEN'S HEALTH

Penis Problems

Most problems with the penis are rare.

An erection that won't go away (priapism): This painful problem occurs when blood cannot drain from the penis. It may result from treatments intended to produce erections (such as penile injections), diseases such as leukemia or sickle-cell anemia, side effects of some drugs, or injury. Priapism has nothing to do with arousal. If an erection does not subside after 4 hours, call your doctor for emergency advice. If you can't get him or her, call 911 or go to an emergency room.

A small, pimplelike sore: Most often on the head of the penis, a sore that lasts more than 1 or 2 weeks can be a sign of penis cancer or of a **sexually transmitted disease** (see chart on page 221). In later stages, cancer symptoms may include bleeding or discharge, pain with urination, and enlarged lymph nodes in the groin. Penis cancer is most common in uncircumcised men. Call your doctor for a prompt appointment if you detect any lasting sore or growth.

Blisters: One or more, on or around the penis, can mean a herpes infection. An outbreak can be itchy, painful, or both, and needs a doctor's care.

A bend in the penis (Peyronie's disease): This occurs during an erection and can be painful. It may be caused by scar tissue in the penis that does not stretch enough. The problem often goes away without treatment. In rare cases, it may require surgery.

Soreness and inflammation of the tip of the penis (balanitis): This can be caused by infection or by irritation from clothing, condoms, or spermicides. It's most common in men who are uncircumcised. Call your doctor for advice.

Tight foreskin (phimosis): Sometimes the foreskin in uncircumcised boys or men is too tight to retract easily; this may make erections painful. Phimosis can also be caused by an infection under the foreskin. Uncircumcised men and men with diabetes have a higher chance of getting such infections. Call your doctor for advice.

prostates, although fewer than half of them feel symptoms. As it grows, the prostate can squeeze the urethra and obstruct urine flow. Doctors call this benign prostatic hyperplasia. It isn't cancer. It doesn't lead to cancer. Nor does it need to be treated, unless difficult or frequent urination becomes a problem. Then surgery or drugs can help.

Prostate cancer: A tumor in the prostate is the most common cancer in American men. It can exist for many years without symptoms, until the tumor grows large enough to affect urination or cause pain by spreading to bones in the pelvis, lower back, or upper legs.

Prostate cancer grows slowly and can be treated best when caught early. If untreated, it may spread to other organs or bone. Treatment can include surgery, radiation, or hormone therapy. There is a risk of impotence or incontinence with these treatments, so some men who have prostate cancer that hasn't spread choose to watch and wait, after talking with their doctors. This is a reasonable option for men over 70.

Prostatitis: This is an inflamed prostate. One form is caused by bacteria, which can move to the prostate from the urinary system. In acute cases, an abscess may form that has to be drained. In chronic cases, the infection causes lasting discomfort and, rarely, a fever. Sometimes its only symptom is repeated bladder infections. Another, more common form of "prostatitis" is not caused by bacteria—it has no known cause—does not respond to antibiotics, and is better referred to as chronic pelvic pain syndrome; it is often related to the muscles of the pelvic floor and not the prostate.

WHAT YOU CAN DO NOW

➤ Drink water all day, as much as you can. If you're bothered by symptoms of an enlarged prostate, though, hold down the amount you drink between dinner and bedtime.
➤ If you are getting up often to urinate at night, avoid caffeine and alcohol.
➤ Be careful with cold and allergy medicines; they can worsen the symptoms of an enlarged prostate.
➤ Warm baths may help relieve pain.
➤ Take the prostate quiz (see page 229). Go over the results with your doctor.
➤ Try an over-the-counter painkiller for painful urination.

WHEN TO CALL THE DOCTOR

➤ If you have the symptoms listed.

HOW TO PREVENT IT

Enlarged prostate:
➤ There is no known way to prevent this.
Prostate cancer:
➤ Know your genes (see **a family tree,** page 316): If your father or brother had prostate cancer, your risk is much higher than if they didn't. This makes the next steps even more vital.
➤ Eat lots of fruits and vegetables. Also, cut down on animal fat in your diet; men who eat a lot of fat may increase their risk.
➤ Get a digital rectal exam each year beginning at age 50 to check for lumps on the gland. African Americans and men with a family history of prostate cancer should begin their yearly tests at age 40.
➤ Some doctors also advise a blood test for a substance called prostate-specific antigen (PSA) that can detect prostate cancer (see **tests,** page 319).
Prostatitis:
➤ Treat any urinary tract infection before it can spread.

COMPLEMENTARY CHOICES

➤ An extract of saw palmetto berries may work as well as some prescription drugs to relieve the symptoms of an enlarged prostate, with fewer side effects. Talk with your doctor before using saw palmetto if you're already taking medication for an enlarged prostate.

FOR MORE HELP

Key Websites: *www.SavonHealth.com*. For more information on prostate problems: *www.SavonProstate.com*.

Organizations: American Cancer Society, 800-ACS-2345, 24-hour line; *www.cancer.org*. At Website, click on *Prostate*.
■ American Foundation for Urologic Disease, 1128 North Charles St., Baltimore, MD 21201. 410-468-1800, M–F 8:30–5 EST; *www.afud.org*. Staff sends facts about prostate problems.
■ American Prostate Society, 7188 Ridge Rd., Hanover, MD 21076. 800-308-1106 or 410-859-3735, M–F 9–5 EST; *www.ameripros.org*. Volunteers answer questions and send out brochures.

Books: *The ABCs of Prostate Cancer: The Book That Could Save Your Life,* by Joseph Oesterling, M.D., and Mark. A. Moyad, M.P.H. Features positive messages from several well-known survivors. Madison Books, 1997, $19.95.
■ *The Prostate: A Guide for Men and the Women Who Love Them,* by Patrick C. Walsh, M.D., and Janet Farrar Worthington. Covers prostate problems and their treatment. Warner Books, 1997, $6.99.
■ *The Prostate Book: Sound Advice on Symptoms and Treatment,* by Stephen N. Rous, M.D. A guide to the male genital and urinary anatomy and prostate conditions. W. W. Norton, 1995, $13.

MEN'S HEALTH

Women's Health

Menopause

SIGNS AND SYMPTOMS

Many women have few or no signs that they are entering menopause. If you do feel some changes, they may include:

- Hot flashes or flushes—a sudden feeling of heat, mostly on the face, neck, and chest.
- Irregular periods. Menstrual flow may be very heavy or very light and then periods cease.
- Irritability and mood swings.
- Sleep disorders.
- Vaginal dryness.
- Urinary pain or incontinence.
- Pain during intercourse.

Sometime between a woman's late 30s and mid-40s, her body begins to prepare for menopause. The levels of hormones needed for pregnancy—estrogen and progesterone—decline. As a result, her periods become irregular. Her ovaries stop releasing eggs and, finally, she stops menstruating. Although a woman may experience the symptoms of menopause for many years before her periods stop, she has not officially reached menopause until she hasn't had a period for a year.

The average age for menopause is about 51, but it can come earlier or later. Surgery during which the ovaries are removed or illness can bring it on quickly, but it is most often a gradual process, taking between 2 and 10 years.

Some women notice no major changes in their bodies except the end of their periods.

Many have some or all of the other symptoms but don't find the process very uncomfortable. Others have a stronger response to the shift in hormone levels and may feel emotional or physical distress.

The declining level of estrogen can lead to health problems for some women. A shortage of this hormone can cause a decrease in bone mass (see **osteoporosis,** page 196). The drop in estrogen can also raise cholesterol levels, in turn raising the risk of heart disease. For these reasons, many doctors prescribe **hormone replacement therapy** (see box, page 235), but the treatment has some risks.

For many women, menopause is a positive life change that means freedom from menstrual periods and from concerns about birth control and pregnancy. It can also be a time of sadness and loss as a woman's parents enter old age or die and she faces signs of her own aging. If a woman has children, they may be leaving home at about the same time her fertility ends.

And all change—even good change—can lead to **stress** (see page 218). Exercise, diet, support systems, and lifestyle adjustments can help lower stress levels.

WHAT YOU CAN DO NOW

➤ Ask whether your local hospital has a menopause support group. Talk to your family and friends about the changes you are going through and how they affect your feelings.
➤ Don't stop using birth control when your periods get irregular—keep using it for at least a year after they stop, since you may still be releasing eggs and could get pregnant.

Menstrual Irregularities

All women should have pelvic exams as often as once a year if they are sexually active, so that any problems can be found and treated early. Be sure to tell your doctor about any changes in your menstrual cycle.

SYMPTOMS	WHAT IT MIGHT BE	WHAT YOU CAN DO
Missed or very heavy, painful menstrual periods; cramps, pain, or pressure in lower abdomen; vaginal spotting or bleeding. Sometimes no symptoms.	Ectopic pregnancy—pregnancy outside uterus, usually in fallopian tube (see color illustration, page 175).	Call doctor for prompt appointment. If bleeding or abdominal pain is severe, call 911 or go to emergency room **right away.**
Bleeding or spotting during pregnancy.	Common, but may signal a problem.	Call a doctor for prompt advice. If you can't get one, call 911 or go to emergency room **right away.**
Very heavy or painful periods, chiefly toward the end; pain in lower abdomen, vagina, or lower back that may begin just before period and worsen just after; pain during intercourse; blood in urine or stool while menstruating; nausea and vomiting just before period begins.	Endometriosis—disorder in which tissue that lines uterus grows outside uterus and becomes attached to other organs.	If you have symptoms for the first time or if pain is severe, call doctor for prompt appointment.
Very heavy, irregular, or missed menstrual periods; pain in lower abdomen or back; foul-smelling vaginal discharge; pain during intercourse; fever and sometimes chills.	Pelvic inflammatory disease (see page 236)—infection of reproductive organs, often caused by sexually transmitted diseases (see chart on page 221).	Call doctor for prompt appointment.
Changes in heaviness of flow, length of periods, or time between periods; aches or pain in abdomen; feeling of fullness, swelling, or pressure in abdomen; frequent urination.	Noncancerous ovarian cyst. ■ Noncancerous ovarian tumor. ■ Ovarian cancer.	Call doctor for prompt appointment. It's vital to diagnose cancer right away.

(continued)

WOMEN'S HEALTH

Menstrual Irregularities (continued)

SYMPTOMS	WHAT IT MIGHT BE	WHAT YOU CAN DO
Very heavy or painful menstrual period that begins a week or more late.	Early pregnancy and miscarriage.	If you think you may be pregnant and you are bleeding, call doctor for advice and appointment.
No menstrual period for several months.	Amenorrhea (absence of menstruation), which can be caused by emotional distress, hormone imbalance, dieting or eating disorders (see eating disorders, page 216), or strenuous athletic training. ■ Pregnancy (see page 238). ■ Breast-feeding. ■ Menopause (see page 232). ■ Abnormality of reproductive organs. ■ Use of certain drugs. ■ Stopping use of birth control pills.	Call doctor for advice. **Note:** If a young woman is over 16 and has never had a menstrual period, schedule appointment with doctor.
Very heavy periods; bleeding between periods; pain or discomfort in lower back or abdomen; frequent urination; constipation; possibly sudden, sharp pain in lower abdomen. Sometimes no symptoms.	Uterine fibroid tumors—common, noncancerous masses in uterus. Sometimes tumor becomes twisted, cutting off its blood supply and causing severe pain.	Call doctor for advice and appointment. Write down dates you are bleeding and how many pads or tampons you use each day.
Very heavy or painful menstrual periods while using IUD or after you stop taking birth control pills.	Common side effect of IUDs. ■ Hormonal changes caused by going off the Pill (see birth control health risks, page 220).	Call doctor for advice about your birth control method.
Very heavy menstrual period soon after childbirth.	Normal.	If you have more than 2 heavy periods after giving birth, call doctor for advice.
Menstrual flow that is always heavy; periods that last more than 7 days; large clots of blood.	Probably no problem, but heavy bleeding can result in anemia (see page 272).	If bleeding is very heavy (you use more than 1 pad or tampon in an hour), call doctor for advice.

➤ If you are on birth control pills, you may have periods even after menopause. If you are near 50 and taking the Pill, ask your doctor about a blood check, called an FSH test, that can tell if it's safe to stop.

➤ Wear cotton clothes if you are having night sweats or hot flashes. Nap during the day if night sweats cost you sleep.

➤ Dress in layers so you can cool down. Use a fan.

➤ Drink at least 8 glasses of water a day.

➤ For vaginal dryness, use a lubricant. If you and your partner use condoms, use a water-soluble lubricant rather than petroleum jelly, which breaks down latex.

➤ Reduce stress (see **relax,** page 303).

➤ Reduce your risk of heart disease by losing extra pounds if you are overweight, by quitting smoking, and by switching to a low-fat diet.

➤ Try to get 1,500 milligrams of calcium a day in your diet or from supplements. If you're on hormone replacement therapy, you still need at least 1,000 mg.

➤ Get regular weight-bearing exercise (such as jumping rope or lifting weights) to guard against osteoporosis.

➤ Cut back on caffeine and alcohol.

➤ Eat soy products, such as tofu and soy powders. Soy can reduce menopausal symptoms such as hot flashes and may help keep bones strong.

WHEN TO CALL THE DOCTOR

➤ If you have heavy bleeding for a long time, or any bleeding a year after your period stops. This could be a sign of uterine cancer.

➤ If you have any symptoms that bother you.

COMPLEMENTARY CHOICES

➤ Black cohosh may help relieve hot flashes. The usual dose is a 20 mg tablet twice daily for up to 6 months.

➤ Red clover tablets also may ease the discomfort of hot flashes. It may be up to 3 weeks before the herb takes effect.

➤ For symptoms such as fluid retention, insomnia, and nervousness, dong quai may help. This herb comes in tablets, tincture, or extract.

WOMEN'S HEALTH

Is Hormone Replacement Right for You?

As a woman enters menopause, she'll face a decision about whether to start hormone replacement therapy. Studies have shown that estrogen—the major ingredient in hormone therapy—can prevent bone loss and fractures, and can reduce the risk of heart disease. Hormone replacement therapy also helps ease the short-term effects of menopause.

Doctors often prescribe a mixture of estrogen and another female hormone, progestin, for women who have not had a hysterectomy. This protects women against endometrial cancer, which taking estrogen alone does not. Combined hormone therapy has also been shown to raise levels of HDL (good) cholesterol and to lower levels of LDL (bad) cholesterol, and to help prevent bone fractures in women who already have osteoporosis.

After menopause, women may take these hormones for the rest of their lives to protect against osteoporosis and heart disease. Questions remain about this therapy. Some studies have shown that it may slightly increase the risk of breast cancer if taken for more than 5 years. If you are thinking about hormone replacement therapy, be sure to discuss all the risks with your doctor.

Another option is to try medications such as raloxifene. While this drug won't cool hot flashes (it may actually worsen them), it offers the bone-protecting benefits of estrogen without increasing the risk of breast cancer.

Consult your doctor before trying any of these herbs.

FOR MORE HELP

Key Websites: *www.SavonHealth.com*. For more information on menopause: *www.SavonWomensHealth.com*.

Organizations: National Institute on Aging, Information Center, P.O. Box 8057, Gaithersburg, MD 20898. 800-222-2225, M–F 8:30–5 EST; *www.nih.gov/health/chip/nia/menop/men1.htm*. Call for fact sheets on menopause and estrogen therapy.

■ National Women's Health Resource Center, 120 Albany St., Suite 820, New Brunswick, NJ 08901. 877-986-9472, M–F 9–5 EST; *www.healthywomen.org*. Ask for the fact sheet on hormone replacement therapy ($5).

Website: Doctor's Guide to Menopause Information and Resources, *www.pslgroup.com/Menopause.htm*. Offers medical news, discussion groups, drug therapies, and links to other sites.

Books: *Dr. Susan Love's Hormone Book*, by Susan M. Love, M.D. Helps women weigh pros and cons of hormone therapy to treat menopause. Random House, 1998, $15.

■ *American Medical Association Essential Guide to Menopause*, edited by Angela Perry. Reliable information on menopause and its treatments. Pocket Books, 1998, $14.

Pelvic Inflammatory Disease

www.SavonPelvicInflammatoryDisease

SIGNS AND SYMPTOMS

Often PID has no symptoms. Sometimes it can cause:
■ Mild to severe aching in the lower abdomen, sometimes with backache.
■ Pain during intercourse.
■ Fever, sometimes with chills.
■ Absent or irregular periods, or very heavy bleeding.
■ Heavy or foul-smelling discharge from the vagina.
■ Frequent urination with burning pain.
■ Nausea and vomiting.
■ Trouble getting pregnant (chronic or prior PID).

Pelvic inflammatory disease (PID) is an infection of the female reproductive organs, including the ovaries, the fallopian tubes, the cervix, and the uterus. Untreated, it can result in fatal illnesses, such as blood poisoning or infection of the abdominal cavity. It can also cause infertility or ectopic pregnancy (in which a fertilized egg settles outside the uterus).

PID is often caused by the bacteria that produce gonorrhea and chlamydia (see **sexually transmitted diseases** chart, page 221). It may also be brought on by other bacteria that get into the upper genital region through sexual intercourse, abortion, miscarriage, childbirth, or hysterectomy.

Sexually active teens, women with more than one sex partner, and those with a partner who has sex with others are most likely to get PID. Some experts believe that frequent douching may also increase the risk by pushing bacteria farther up into the reproductive system. Intrauterine devices (IUDs) increase the risk. Birth control pills, however, hinder the passage of bacteria and may slightly lower the chance of getting PID or may keep it from getting more severe.

PID can be treated with antibiotics, but it often comes back and may become chronic (you may have it for a long time, with symptoms that come and go). When antibiotics don't help, a doctor may have to remove or repair infected tissue.

WHAT YOU CAN DO NOW

After diagnosis:
➤ Take all of the drugs your doctor prescribes, even if symptoms are gone.
➤ If gonorrhea or chlamydia caused your PID, make sure your partner is treated. Otherwise, he may reinfect you.
➤ Don't have sex until all symptoms are completely gone.

Breast Pain or Lumps

Breasts change with puberty, the menstrual cycle, and pregnancy, and they change with age. Starting at puberty, women should examine their breasts every month so that they know the breasts' structure and can detect any masses or lumps (see **breast self-exam** box, page 239). Most changes in breasts are normal and no cause for concern. But some require medical care.

SYMPTOMS	WHAT IT MIGHT BE	WHAT YOU CAN DO
Lump (usually painless) in breast or underarm area; flat area or indentation on breast; change in contour, texture, size, or symmetry of breast; change in nipple (such as indrawn or dimpled look, itching or burning feeling, or discharge that may be dark or bloody).	Noncancerous cyst. ■ Noncancerous tumor. ■ Breast cancer (if breast is painful, could signal advanced stage).	Call doctor for prompt appointment. Most lumps are not cancerous, but it is very important to have an exam. Biopsy may be needed to diagnose or rule out breast cancer.
After having just given birth: pain and tenderness in breast, hard or swollen breast, fever, area with redness and pain.	Infection of breast (mastitis), caused by bacteria. Redness and pain can mean an abscess.	Call doctor for advice and appointment. Keep on breast-feeding. If you get an abscess, use a breast pump on infected side and feed on uninfected side. If you have a fever, rest in bed and drink plenty of fluids.
Pain, tenderness, or swelling in breasts; missed period; fatigue; nausea.	Pregnancy (see page 238).	Call doctor for advice and appointment for pregnancy test. Wear support bra.
Less than 5 days after giving birth: tenderness, hardness, or swelling in breast. Also, when breast-feeding mother cannot keep to feeding schedule.	Swelling with milk.	Nurse more often, or try using warm compresses to reduce discomfort. Call doctor for advice if symptoms persist.
In women who are breast-feeding: sore nipple or sharp pain in nipple while nursing.	Sore or cracked nipples, common during first few weeks of breast-feeding.	Gently wash nipples after nursing and apply pure vitamin E oil. With fever, call doctor for advice.
Breast pain while taking estrogen.	Drug side effect.	Call doctor for advice.

(continued)

WOMEN'S HEALTH

Breast Pain or Lumps (continued)

SYMPTOMS	WHAT IT MIGHT BE	WHAT YOU CAN DO
Lumpy or swollen breasts; pain or discomfort, chiefly in the week before menstrual period.	Fibrocystic breasts. More than half of all women develop this harmless condition, most often between ages of 25 and 50.	Call doctor for advice if you notice lumps for first time; if you notice a new lump; or if a lump becomes larger, harder, or more painful. Limit intake of caffeine. Wear support bra.
Pain or tenderness in breasts before menstrual period.	Premenstrual syndrome. ■ Irregular periods.	See premenstrual syndrome, page 241, and menstrual irregularities chart, page 233.

➤ Get plenty of bed rest.
➤ If needed, take an over-the-counter painkiller such as ibuprofen.

WHEN TO CALL THE DOCTOR

➤ If you have symptoms of PID.

HOW TO PREVENT IT

➤ Practice safe sex to protect yourself from STDs by using a barrier method, such as a condom.
➤ Have regular medical checkups if you are sexually active.
➤ To prevent infection after you have had pelvic surgery or a minor gynecologic procedure, don't douche or have intercourse for a week.

FOR MORE HELP

Key Websites: *www.SavonHealth.com*. For more information on pelvic inflammatory disease: *www.SavonPelvicInflammatoryDisease.com*.
Organizations: American College of Obstetricians and Gynecologists, Resource Center, 409 12th St. SW, P.O. Box 96920, Washington, DC 20090-6920. 202-638-5577, M–F 9–5 EST; *www.acog.org*. Send a business-size self-addressed stamped envelope; ask for the brochure on PID.

■ National STD Hotline, Centers for Disease Control and Prevention, P.O. Box 13827, RTP, NC 27709. 800-227-8922, M–F 8AM–11PM EST; *www.ashastd.org* for general information or *www.iwannaknow.org* for teen questions about STDs. Staff answers questions, sends out written information about STDs, and refers callers for testing.
Website: Duke University Healthy Devil Online, *h-devil-www.mc.duke.edu/h-devil/women/women.htm*. Covers PID, the STDs that cause it, symptoms, treatment, contraception, and pelvic exams.

Pregnancy
www.SavonPregnancy.com

The best time to start taking better care of your health is before you become pregnant. The first few weeks of your pregnancy can be crucial for the rapidly growing fetus. If you eat poorly, drink, smoke, or take drugs, you can harm your baby.

Good health habits and good prenatal care help assure a healthy baby. They also help you cope with the stress that comes with pregnancy, childbirth, and parenthood. If you are planning a pregnancy, you may want to visit your health care provider to discuss your diet, lifestyle, past pregnan-

How to Do a Breast Self-Exam

A regular breast self-exam is one of the best ways to find a cancerous tumor when it is small, before the cancer has a chance to spread. Check yourself at the same time every month, 2 to 3 days after your period. (Remember, self-examination is not a substitute for regular exams by a doctor; see **tests,** page 319.)

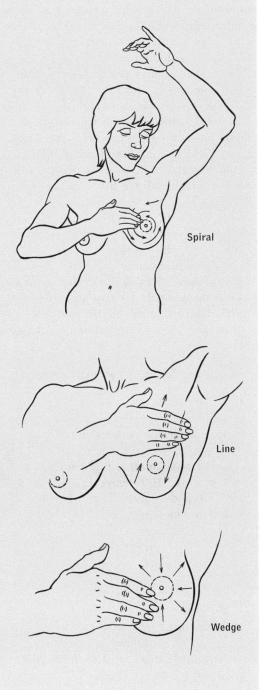

Spiral

Line

Wedge

1 Stand facing a mirror with your arms at your sides. Look for anything unusual on your breasts: dimples, scaly patches, puckers, or discharge coming from a nipple.

2 Check for changes in the contours of your breasts. Watch in the mirror as you lift your hands behind your head, clasp your hands, and press them against the back of your head.

3 Check again with your hands on your hips and your elbows pulled forward.

4 Squeeze your nipples gently to check for discharge.

5 With one arm raised, use the fingertips of your other hand to feel your breast for any lumps under the skin. Start in your armpit and move toward your breast, pressing in small areas about the size of a quarter. (Try this in the shower; your fingers will slide more easily over soapy skin.)

Use a definite pattern—a spiral, line, or wedge. Cover the entire breast, as well as the upper chest and underarm. Repeat on other side.

Spiral: Start at the outer edges of the breast and slowly work your way around it in smaller and smaller circles.

Line: Start under your arm and slowly make up and down strokes, progressing across the breast.

Wedge: Start at the outer edge of the breast and move slowly toward the middle, then back to the edge.

6 Repeat step 5 lying on your back, with one arm over your head and a pillow under your shoulder. Use one of the patterns above to check each breast.

If you find a lump, unusual firmness, a change in shape, or any discharge from a nipple, call your doctor.

WOMEN'S HEALTH

cies, medical history, and any medicines you are taking.

Diet, Rest, and Exercise

During your pregnancy, get plenty of rest and exercise, eat well-balanced foods, and avoid anything that could harm the fetus. Follow your health care provider's advice, as well as these guidelines:

➤ Get enough calories, protein, iron, calcium, and folic acid in your diet. (Ask about any changes you should make and which foods are good sources of the nutrients you need.)

➤ Take any vitamin and mineral supplements prescribed for you, but no more than the amount prescribed. Too much of some vitamins and minerals can harm the baby. (Research shows that women who take more than 10,000 IU of vitamin A per day are more likely to have babies with major heart defects and other problems.)

➤ Avoid things known to cause birth defects, miscarriages, or other harm to the fetus: Don't drink, smoke, or take any drugs not prescribed or approved by your doctor. That includes any over-the-counter drugs,

such as aspirin and cold medicines. (You should also avoid those that include alcohol when you are trying to get pregnant or when you are breast-feeding. Consult your health care provider.)

➤ Cut down on caffeine (in coffee and sodas).

➤ Be aware of hazards in your workplace, such as radiation or heavy metals like lead and mercury. If you can't avoid them, think about changing jobs.

➤ Avoid paint fumes, gas, and other chemical vapors.

➤ Don't touch cat feces or litter boxes, and cook meat until it is well-done. Cat feces and raw meat can spread toxoplasmosis, a disease that may cause miscarriage or birth defects.

➤ Exercise at least 3 times a week. Brisk walking, jogging, swimming, yoga, and low-impact aerobics are all good during pregnancy. Avoid heavy exercise, though, especially in hot weather. Wear a support bra to protect your breasts.

➤ Get enough rest. Go to bed early, and take breaks throughout the day to relax and put your feet up. Share more of the housework or child care with your partner, family, or friends.

Danger Signs in Pregnancy

Call your doctor for a prompt appointment if you have:

➤ Vaginal bleeding or spotting. This is common, but it sometimes signals a miscarriage or other problem.

➤ Fever over 100 degrees; backache; chills; and frequent, burning urination or blood in the urine. This may mean a kidney infection.

➤ Sudden weight gain, swelling of the hands and face, severe headache with blurred vision. These are signs of preeclampsia, a form of high blood pressure that can be very dangerous.

➤ Less fetal movement or none at all for more than a day (if the fetus has begun to move). The fetus may be in trouble.

Staying Comfortable

Try the following for some of the common discomforts of pregnancy:

Abdominal pain:

➤ Use a hot-water bottle or heating pad to relieve pain or cramps from stretched abdominal muscles.

➤ Don't change positions quickly, especially when turning at the waist.

➤ Call your doctor for advice if your pain persists or gets worse.

Backache:

➤ Don't take any over-the-counter drugs. Instead, use a hot-water bottle or a heating pad to relieve pain.

➤ Don't stand for a long time.

➤ Sit in chairs that have good support for your back, or use a small pillow behind the lower back. Keep your back straight and put your feet up.

➤ Sleep on a firm bed, on your side, with a pillow between your knees for support.

➤ Wear low-heeled shoes with good support, or shoe inserts made for pregnant women. Don't wear high heels.

➤ Try pregnancy underwear, or an elastic sling for abdominal support.

Breast discomfort:

➤ Wear a support bra.

Constipation: See page 116.

Headache: See page 52.

➤ Get enough rest.

➤ Eat small meals often, and drink at least 8 glasses of water a day.

➤ Learn yoga or meditation.

➤ Call your doctor if your headache is severe or lasts, or if it comes with nausea or blurred vision.

Heartburn: See page 124.

Hemorrhoids: See page 126.

➤ Don't use over-the-counter hemorrhoid treatments without asking your health care provider.

Nausea and vomiting (morning sickness): See page 133.

➤ Eat crackers or plain toast as soon as you wake up. Sit on your bed for a few minutes before getting up.

➤ Try to eat often so you never have an empty stomach. Snack all day rather than eating 3 full meals. (The best snacks are high-protein foods such as nuts, yogurt, and granola, and peanut butter on apple slices or celery.) Have a snack at bedtime and when you get up during the night.

➤ Drink plenty of water and other liquids, but avoid milk, citrus juices, coffee, tea, and sodas with caffeine.

➤ Try papaya juice or almonds to ease nausea. Also try fresh ginger—put a small piece on your tongue or make a tea by grating and steeping ginger in hot water.

➤ Call your doctor if you have severe nausea and vomiting; rapid heartbeat; pale, dry skin; or signs of dehydration (dry mouth, sticky saliva, dizziness, decreased urination, sometimes thirst).

Urinary tract infections:

➤ Call your doctor if you have pain when you urinate, or if you think you have a bladder or other urinary tract infection (see **painful urination,** page 138).

➤ Use a hot-water bottle or heating pad on your lower abdomen for pain.

➤ Drink at least 8 to 10 glasses of water a day.

➤ Drink cranberry juice daily to help prevent urinary tract infections.

Varicose veins and swelling in the legs: See page 115.

➤ Exercise daily.

➤ Don't stand or sit for long periods.

➤ Put your legs up when you can.

FOR MORE HELP

Key Websites: *www.SavonHealth.com.* For more information on pregnancy: *www.SavonPregnancy.com.*

Organization: National Healthy Mothers, Healthy Babies Coalition, 121 N. Washington St., Suite 300, Alexandria, VA 22314. 703-836-6110 or 877-289-9039, M–F 9–5 EST; *www.hmhb.org.* Offers information about prenatal and baby health education programs.

Website: *www.childbirth.org.* Offers pregnancy and childbirth information, personal stories, resources, and links to other sites.

Book: *What to Expect When You're Expecting,* by Arlene Eisenberg, Heidi E. Murkoff, and Sandee E. Hathaway, B.S.N. Workman, 1996, $12.95.

Premenstrual Syndrome
www.SavonPMS.com

SIGNS AND SYMPTOMS

■ Bloating and weight gain.

■ Breast swelling or tenderness.

■ Headaches.

■ Dizziness.

■ Fatigue.

■ Decrease or increase in sex drive.

■ Outbreaks of acne.

■ Mood swings, bad temper, nervousness, or depression.

■ Food cravings.

■ Diarrhea or constipation.

Premenstrual syndrome, or PMS, affects many women some of the time, and some women nearly every month. It is marked by a range of physical and emotional changes that

WOMEN'S HEALTH

begin 1 to 2 weeks before a woman's period and stop when her period starts. The symptoms can be mild or severe. Some women feel just a little low on energy, while a small number get so depressed or tense that they can barely function.

No one knows for sure what causes PMS. It may result from changes in hormone levels, monthly changes in brain chemicals, or poor diet.

WHAT YOU CAN DO NOW

➤ Change your diet. The week before your period, skip salt, sugar, and caffeine (found in coffee, tea, sodas, and chocolate). Limit fats, and add grains, fruits, and vegetables.

➤ Cut out alcohol in the week before your period—it can worsen headaches, fatigue, and depression.

➤ Eat small meals often—6 times a day—and snack to maintain a steady level of blood sugar.

➤ Exercise daily. Raising your body temperature helps your body balance hormones.

➤ Reduce stress (see **stress,** page 218). Practice yoga or meditation. Take a stress reduction course.

➤ Take good care of yourself. Get enough sleep. Take warm baths. Get a massage.

➤ Try PMS medication or an over-the-counter painkiller to help with bloating, cramps, and aches.

➤ Take 50 to 100 milligrams of vitamin B6 and 250 mg of magnesium daily; increase gradually if necessary. This may help relieve PMS symptoms.

➤ Get enough calcium, zinc, copper, and vitamins A and E. Some amino acids and enzymes may also help.

➤ Join a PMS support or self-help group.

WHEN TO CALL THE DOCTOR

➤ If you've followed the advice above, but your symptoms still bother you.

HOW TO PREVENT IT

There is no way to prevent PMS, but taking steps to control your diet and to get enough rest and exercise can help soften the impact.

COMPLEMENTARY CHOICES

➤ The herb chaste tree may help balance your hormones and reduce anxiety and depression. You can buy it as berries, powder, capsules, and tinctures. To make a tea, pour 1 cup boiling water onto 1 teaspoon ripe berries and let steep for 15 minutes. Drink 3 times a day.

➤ Dandelion seems to ease bloating and breast swelling. Steep 1 tablespoon dried or 2 teaspoons fresh leaves per cup boiling water. Drink up to 4 cups a day. You can also sprinkle fresh leaves in salads or blend in juices.

➤ Another herb, skullcap, may help calm tension and irritability. Mix one-half to 1 teaspoon of the liquid form into 8 ounces of water. Or steep 2 teaspoons dried leaves in 1 cup boiling water for 10 to 15 minutes. Consult your doctor before taking any of these herbs.

FOR MORE HELP

Key Websites: *www.SavonHealth.com.* For more information on premenstrual syndrome: *www.SavonPMS.com.*

Organizations: National Women's Health Network, 514 10th St. NW, Suite 400, Washington, DC 20004. 202-628-7814, M–F 9–5:30 EST; *www.womenshealthnetwork.org.* Staff answers questions on PMS and sends fact packet for a small fee. At Website, click on *Health Info* and then on *Premenstrual Syndrome (PMS).*

■ PMS Research Foundation, Box 14574, Las Vegas, NV 89114. Offers resource information. Write and describe your specific concerns or symptoms, and enclose $5, to receive related resource materials.

Website: Duke University Healthy Devil Online, *h-devil-www.mc.duke.edu/h-devil/women/women.htm.* Covers PMS and cramps.

Books: *Once a Month: Understanding and Treating PMS,* by Katharina Dalton, M.D. Discusses common symptoms and offers self-help tips. Hunter House, 1999, $15.95.

■ *Self-Help for Premenstrual Syndrome,* 3rd edition, by Michelle Harrison, M.D. Explains how to manage PMS, with current information and advice. Random House, 1999, $15.

Toxic Shock Syndrome

www.SavonToxicShock.com

SIGNS AND SYMPTOMS

Call 911 or go to an emergency room **right away** if you have:

- Sudden fever (over 102 degrees).
- Diarrhea.
- Vomiting.
- A deep red, sunburnlike rash, most often on the palms of the hands or soles of the feet.
- Headache, confusion, or dizziness.
- Weakness or fainting.

Toxic shock syndrome comes on suddenly and can cause severe illness. It is caused by common bacteria *(Staphylococcus aureus)* that release toxins into the bloodstream.

Toxic shock occurs chiefly among menstruating women who use tampons—most of all superabsorbent tampons. When a tampon is left in place for a long time, it can trap the bacteria and give them an ideal place to grow. Toxic shock has also been linked to the use of birth control sponges and—very rarely—to diaphragms and cervical caps.

The disease can also affect children, men, and women of all ages who are exposed to the bacteria through surgery, a burn, or an open wound.

Toxic shock syndrome requires emergency care. In most cases, people are hospitalized and given intravenous antibiotics to kill the bacteria. If untreated, it can cause liver or kidney failure, severe shock, and—in rare cases—death. Most patients recover, though, if they are treated quickly.

WHAT YOU CAN DO NOW

➤ If you have symptoms of toxic shock, call 911 or go to an emergency room **right away.** If you have a tampon, a menstrual sponge, a birth control sponge, a diaphragm, or a cervical cap inside you, remove it right away.

WHEN TO CALL THE DOCTOR

Call 911 or go to an emergency room **right away:**

➤ If you have symptoms of toxic shock syndrome—especially if you are menstruating and have been using tampons.

Call for a prompt appointment:

➤ If you are being treated for toxic shock syndrome and you get new symptoms. Drugs used to treat the illness may produce side effects.

HOW TO PREVENT IT

➤ Use tampons less often. If you don't want to stop using them, be sure your tampons are made of cotton; they pose the least risk. Switch between tampons and sanitary pads. If you've ever had toxic shock syndrome, don't use tampons at all.

➤ Don't use superabsorbent tampons.

➤ Change tampons at least every 4 to 6 hours.

➤ Don't use tampons or menstrual sponges overnight.

➤ If you use a diaphragm or cervical cap, never leave the diaphragm in for more than 24 hours (8 hours during your period) or the cervical cap in for more than 48 hours.

➤ Wash your diaphragm or cervical cap after each use in warm, soapy water. Rinse and dry it well with a clean towel.

➤ Wash your hands well before you insert a tampon or any other device.

➤ Always clean and disinfect cuts or scrapes anywhere on your body. If a wound appears to be infected, get medical help.

FOR MORE HELP

Key Websites: *www.SavonHealth.com*. For more information on toxic shock syndrome: *www.SavonToxicShock.com*.

Organization: National Women's Health Network, 514 Tenth St. NW, Suite 400, Washington, DC 20004. 202-628-7814, M–F 9–5:30 EST; *www.womenshealthnetwork.org*. Staff answers questions on toxic shock syndrome and, for a small fee, sends a fact packet.

Vaginal Problems
www.SavonWomensHealth.com

SIGNS AND SYMPTOMS

Yeast infection:
- Redness, itching, and sometimes burning during urination.
- Pain during intercourse.
- White, cheesy, odorless discharge (sometimes).

Bacterial vaginosis:
- Watery, grayish white or yellow discharge with a fishy odor.
- Mild burning or irritation.

Contact dermatitis:
- Redness and itching of the vulva (the outer genital area).

The term *vaginitis* refers to many irritations of a woman's genital area.

A **yeast infection** is the most common. It's caused by overgrowth of a fungus normally found in the vagina. It can be brought on by pregnancy, diabetes, use of antibiotics, and sometimes use of the Pill. Some experts believe that feminine hygiene products also cause it. If you get frequent yeast infections, your doctor can prescribe antifungal pills.

Bacterial vaginosis occurs when bacteria normally found in the vagina grow out of control or when bacteria normally found in the rectum get into the vagina. Poor health, poor hygiene, or clothing made of material that does not allow air to reach the skin can make it more likely.

Contact dermatitis may be caused by chemicals in latex condoms, spermicides, or diaphragms; feminine hygiene sprays; colored or scented toilet tissue; soaps, detergents, or fabric softeners; and deodorant tampons or sanitary pads (see **dermatitis,** page 149). Your doctor can prescribe an ointment that will help.

WHAT YOU CAN DO NOW

For all vaginitis:
- Don't have intercourse for 2 weeks, or until all soreness is gone.
- Don't scratch. Use cool compresses or sitz baths to ease itching.

- Use plain yogurt with live acidophilus cultures (check the label) to make a compress or to put in the vagina. You can apply it as a douche, or with a spoon or applicator made for vaginal treatments.
- Keep your vulva clean, and dry it well after urinating or showering. You can use a hair dryer set on low to blow warm, dry air on the sore area—just be careful of the heat.
- Wash all underwear in mild, fragrance-free soap or detergent (soap made for baby laundry is good) and rinse twice. Don't use fabric softener or bleach.

Yeast infection:
- If you are sure that you have a yeast infection, use an over-the-counter antifungal cream made for yeast infections. Be sure to use all of the cream as directed, even after your symptoms are gone.
- The infection can spread, so stop having sex until you finish treatment. Your sexual partner also may need treatment to keep from reinfecting you.

WHEN TO CALL THE DOCTOR

Call for a prompt appointment:
- If you have bleeding between menstrual periods or after menopause; a firm, raised lesion or bump on the vulva or inside the vagina; or vaginal pain and itching that doesn't go away. These may be signs of cancer of the vagina or vulva.
- If you notice a vaginal discharge that is yellow or green and foul-smelling. This may be a symptom of a **sexually transmitted disease** (see chart on page 221).

Call for advice and an appointment:
- If you have symptoms of bacterial vaginosis. Your doctor can treat the infection with an oral antibiotic. It can spread, so be sure your partner is also treated.
- If you have any vaginal symptoms for the first time, or if they recur more than twice a year.
- If symptoms don't go away after treatment, or are severe.

HOW TO PREVENT IT

- Wipe from front to back after a bowel movement to avoid spreading bacteria

Women's Health Resources

Organizations: American College of Obstetricians and Gynecologists, Resource Center, 409 12th St. SW, P.O. Box 16920, Washington, DC 20024-6920. 202-638-5777, M–F 9–5 EST, *www.acog.org*. Offers pamphlets on topics such as birth control, pregnancy, menopause, PMS, and cancer. Send a business-size self-addressed stamped envelope and request the topic you want.

■ National Women's Health Resource Center, 120 Albany St., Suite 820, New Brunswick, NJ 08901. 877-986-9472, M–F 8–5 EST; *www.healthywomen.org*. Offers reports on women's health issues and publishes the *National Women's Health Report* newsletter (6 issues for $30). Staff members will give referrals to women's centers near you.

Websites: The Breast Cancer Network, *www.breastcancer.net*. Has information on breast-cancer detection and treatment.

■ HealthWeb: Women's Health, *www.medsch.wisc.edu/chslib/hw/womens*. University of Wisconsin at Madison's resource site devoted to women's health.

Books: *Our Bodies, Ourselves for the New Century: A Book by and for Women,* by the Boston Women's Health Book Collective. The revised and updated bible of women's self-help medical books. Touchstone,1998, $24.

■ *American Medical Association Complete Guide to Women's Health,* with medical editor Ramona Slupik, M.D. Covers health issues, from safe sex and weight control to depression and hormone replacement therapy. Random House, 1996, $39.95.

■ *Dr. Susan Love's Breast Book,* 2nd edition, by Susan M. Love, M.D. Classic breast-care guide. Perseus, 1995, $18.

from the rectum to the vagina.

➤ Don't use scented toilet paper, perfumed soaps, or feminine hygiene products.

➤ Change tampons and sanitary pads at least 4 times a day.

➤ Clean diaphragms, cervical caps, and spermicide applicators well after each use.

➤ Don't wear tight pants, clothing that can trap moisture, or underwear or panty hose with a crotch that's not cotton.

➤ If you are taking antibiotics, ask your doctor whether you should use an antifungal cream in your vagina to prevent a yeast infection.

➤ Try eating a cup of yogurt that has live cultures every day (check the label). Studies show that yogurt may prevent yeast infections.

➤ Check your vulva monthly for changes.

| **FOR MORE HELP** |

Key Websites: *www.SavonHealth.com*. For more information on vaginal problems: *www.SavonWomensHealth.com*.

Organization: National Women's Health Network, *www.womenshealthnetwork.org*. Staff answers questions and sends facts about vaginitis and yeast infections.

Website: Duke University Healthy Devil Online, *h-devil-www.mc.duke.edu/hdevil/women/women.htm*. Covers vaginal and urinary tract infections.

Book: *Our Bodies, Ourselves for the New Century: A Book by and for Women,* by the Boston Women's Health Book Collective. An updated version of the classic guide to women's health. Touchstone, 1998, $24.

Children's Health

Bed-Wetting

SIGNS AND SYMPTOMS

Bed-wetting now and then is normal. It may be a problem:

- If your child is 6 or older and seldom stays dry overnight.
- If you are concerned about it, or if your child is.

Bed-wetting is common, even well after a child has learned to use the toilet. About 1 child in 10 will wet the bed after the age of 5. Boys are more likely to have the problem than are girls, and it tends to run in families. Some children who wet the bed simply have small bladders, or their nerves and muscles are not mature enough to control their bladders all night. Less often, a child doesn't have enough of a hormone that helps the kidneys hold urine. Most children outgrow these problems by their teens.

If your child has been dry during the night for a while and then begins wetting the bed, it may be a sign of something such as diabetes or a bladder infection. Or it may be a reaction to a recent stressful event, such as the birth of a brother or sister.

WHAT YOU CAN DO NOW

- Remind your child to use the bathroom just before going to bed each night.
- Limit the amount your child drinks before bedtime.
- Don't give your child drinks with caffeine, such as colas and teas. Caffeine increases the flow of urine.
- If your child has been sleeping for more than an hour, wake him or her to use the toilet again before you go to bed.
- Praise your child for staying dry. Never scold or embarrass a child for wetting the bed; you may make the problem worse.

WHEN TO CALL THE DOCTOR

Call for a prompt appointment:
- If it is painful for your child to urinate, or if your child has bloody or very cloudy urine, a very narrow urine stream, or abdominal pain. Any of these could signal a bladder infection.

Call for advice:
- If your child feels frustrated, or if you do.

HOW TO PREVENT IT

- Try bladder training: Once a day, tell your child to hold his or her urine for a few minutes past the first feeling of a full bladder. Be patient: It may take a few months for your child to master it.

FOR MORE HELP

Key Websites: *www.SavonHealth.com*. For more information on bed wetting problems: *www.SavonBedWetting.com*.
Organization: National Kidney Foundation Information Center, 800-622-9010, M–F 8:30–5 EST; *www.kidney.org*. Sends reports on bed-wetting and a list of physicians in your area.
Further resources: See box on page 271.

Children's Rashes

It can be hard to tell if a childhood rash is a sign of a serious disease or a minor ailment. Also, babies and young children have delicate skin that may become inflamed and then clear up on its own. Look for other symptoms, and any changes in the rash—these are clues to its cause.

SYMPTOMS	WHAT IT MIGHT BE	WHAT YOU CAN DO
Itchy red welts with pale centers, anywhere on body.	Hives (see page 155).	If child begins wheezing or has trouble swallowing, call 911 or go to emergency room **right away.** Otherwise, call doctor for advice.
Purple rash, pale skin, overall fatigue, headache, aching limbs, swollen glands, many infections, mouth sores.	Childhood leukemia.	Call doctor for prompt appointment.
First symptoms: sore throat, slight fever; 2 weeks later: painless, purple, spotted rash on ankles, elbows, shins, or buttocks.	Allergic purpura—a reaction that causes bleeding under the skin, forming a rash.	Call doctor for prompt appointment.
First symptoms: low fever, swollen glands; 2–3 days later: slightly raised red rash on face that spreads to rest of body.	German measles (rubella) (see page 257).	Call doctor for advice. Keep child away from pregnant women (this virus can damage a fetus).
First symptoms: fever as high as 105, cough, runny nose, overall sick feeling; 2–3 days later: rash of small red spots that starts on face and neck, then spreads to rest of body.	Measles (see page 262).	Call doctor for advice. If bumps are dark red and appear to be filled with blood or if seizures occur (very rare), call 911 or go to emergency room **right away.**
First symptoms: sore throat, fever of 101–104, headache; 1–2 days later: bright red rash begins on face and groin, spreads to torso, arms, and legs.	Scarlet fever (see page 266).	Call doctor for appointment.

(continued)

CHILDREN'S HEALTH

Children's Rashes (continued)

SYMPTOMS	WHAT IT MIGHT BE	WHAT YOU CAN DO
Whitish patches in mouth and throat, or red patches in genital area.	Thrush (in mouth) or yeast infection (see fungal infections, page 153).	Call doctor for advice.
Blisters in mouth; blistering rash on hands, feet, and sometimes buttocks; fever up to 102; sore throat; fatigue.	Hand, foot, and mouth disease (see page 258).	Call doctor for prompt appointment if child has trouble swallowing.
Small red itchy spots that turn into fluid-filled blisters; slight fever. Rash starts on face and torso.	Chicken pox (see facing page).	Call doctor for advice. Ease itching with oatmeal baths or calamine lotion.
Fever as high as 102; sometimes sore throat, headache, or fatigue. Bright red rash that starts on face ("slapped-cheeks"), then spreads, may itch.	Fifth disease (see page 257).	Call doctor for advice.
First symptoms: Fever as high as 105 (in children 3 and younger), mild cough, runny nose; 3–6 days later: red, spreading rash that disappears in a few hours to a few days.	Roseola (see page 265).	Call doctor for advice. If child's fever is 102 or higher, call doctor right away.
Round, itchy rash that appears mainly on scalp, feet, or around nails; creates bald patches on scalp.	Ringworm—a contagious fungal infection.	Call doctor for advice.
Dry, scaly skin; itchy red bumps; rash may cover small area or most of body; common on knees and elbows.	Eczema (see page 152).	If spreading, call doctor for advice. Soothe mild cases with cream; avoid lotions with preservatives, oils, or perfume.
Rash of small blisters, mostly on face, legs, or arms; blisters break and weep, forming golden crust.	Impetigo (see page 259).	Very contagious; keep rash and places around it clean with soap and water. If rash persists or gets worse, call doctor for advice.

Children's Rashes

SYMPTOMS	WHAT IT MIGHT BE	WHAT YOU CAN DO
Light red rash in spots or large blotches; occurs in hot weather.	Heat rash.	Remove clothing. Call doctor for prompt appointment if rash lasts 24 hours or other symptoms appear.
Dry scales that turn into yellow, greasy patches; may be itchy. On scalp (in cradle cap); or in creases of neck, behind ears, in armpits, on face, or in diaper area (in seborrheic dermatitis).	Cradle cap. ■ Seborrheic dermatitis (see dermatitis, page 149).	For cradle cap, loosen scales by rubbing with baby oil and combing hair with a fine-tooth comb. If it persists, call doctor for advice.
Bright red, tight, and/or sore skin in diaper area; rash that may consist of small bumps.	Diaper rash (see page 253).	Change wet diapers often, and right away after bowel movement. If rash doesn't improve in 3 days, call doctor for advice.

Chicken Pox
www.SavonVaricella-Zoster.com

SIGNS AND SYMPTOMS

- An itchy rash that usually begins on the face and torso. It starts out as small red spots; these turn into fluid-filled blisters. In the final stage of the rash, the blisters burst and scab over. The rash most often lasts 7 to 10 days.

Sometimes:
- Painful blisters in the mouth or vagina, or around the eyes.
- A low fever.

Chicken pox is a highly contagious childhood disease that affects about three-fourths of children before the age of 15. The rash and other symptoms appear 1 to 3 weeks after a person gets the virus. Infected people can give the disease to others for a day or two before the spots appear and 5 to 6 days after.

Most of the time, chicken pox is not serious. But it can lead to eye and lung prob-lems in newborns and other people with weak immune systems, and it tends to be more severe in adults. A vaccine can now help prevent it.

You can do many simple things to help your child feel better. Above all, try to relieve the itching, since scratching can cause infections and scars.

WHAT YOU CAN DO NOW

➤ Give acetaminophen for pain. (Never give aspirin to a child or teenager who has chicken pox, a cold, the flu, or any other illness you suspect of being caused by a virus; see box on **Reye's syndrome,** page 95.) Don't give ibuprofen to a child with chicken pox. Some studies suggest it can increase the risk of strep infections.
➤ If your child wears diapers, leave them off when you can to let the blisters dry.
➤ Make sure your child gets plenty of rest and lots to drink.

To relieve itching:
➤ Apply calamine lotion to the rash, and try adding a handful of oatmeal, baking soda, or an over-the-counter anti-itch

CHILDREN'S HEALTH

Childhood Immunization Schedule

Throughout childhood, routine pediatric checkups include immunizations. These vaccines protect against a range of major diseases—from polio to diphtheria—that once were widespread and deadly. Most states require that children get their shots before starting school. If a child is sick, has had a serious reaction to a previous vaccine, or is allergic to neomycin or eggs, tell your doctor before the child is given any shot. Serious reactions to immunizations are rare, but ask about what to watch for.

CHILD'S AGE	VACCINE(S)	RECORD
Birth–2 months	Hep B (hepatitis B)—dose 1	
1–4 months	Hep B—dose 2	
2 months	DTaP (diphtheria/tetanus/pertussis [whooping cough])—dose 1	
	IPV (polio)—dose 1	
	Hib (protects against *Haemophilus influenzae* type B, which can cause meningitis)—dose 1	
4 months	DTaP—dose 2	
	Hib—dose 2	
	IPV—dose 2	
6 months	Hep B—dose 3 (given from 6–18 months)	
	DTaP—dose 3	
	Hib—dose 3	
	IPV—dose 3	
12–18 months	DTaP—dose 4	
	Hib—dose 4	
	MMR (measles, mumps, rubella [German measles])—dose 1	
	Var (varicella zoster virus; protects against chicken pox)	
4–6 years	DTaP—dose 5	
	MMR—dose 2	
	IPV—dose 4	
11–12 years	Hep B (3 doses if not given during infancy)	
	Td (tetanus/diphtheria, if at least 5 years since last dose). In all cases, every 10 years thereafter.	
	MMR—dose 2 (if not given at 4–6 years)	
	Var (if not previously given and child hasn't had chicken pox)	

This chart is based on recommendations by the American Academy of Pediatrics. These recommendations are subject to change, so be sure to ask your pediatrician for the current schedule.

bath powder to your child's bathwater.

➤ Try a child's dose of an over-the-counter antihistamine.

➤ For sores inside the mouth, see **canker sores,** page 78. Make a mouthwash of one-half teaspoon salt in an 8-ounce glass of warm water. Let your child suck on ice chips and juice bars; they ease pain and add fluids.

To help prevent skin infections:

➤ Keep your child's skin, clothes, and bed linens clean.

➤ To keep your child from breaking the blisters, trim the fingernails or cover his or her hands with socks or mittens.

WHEN TO CALL THE DOCTOR

Call 911 or go to an emergency room **right away:**

➤ If your child is drowsy and also has eye pain, speech problems, loss of hearing, a stiff neck or back, a severe cough, or extreme sensitivity to light. These may be symptoms of acute encephalitis, an inflammation of the brain sometimes brought on by chicken pox (see **meningitis and encephalitis,** page 55).

➤ If it's hard for your child to breathe; this may be a symptom of **pneumonia** (see page 97), a rare complication of chicken pox (more common in adults).

Call for advice and an appointment:

➤ If areas of your child's rash get redder or more swollen or tender, or produce a yellow discharge.

➤ If your child still has a fever over 102 after 3 to 4 days; it may be a symptom of strep.

HOW TO PREVENT IT

➤ Children 1 year and older can get a chicken pox vaccine. Children under 13 need only a single shot. Anyone 13 and older needs 2 shots, 4 to 8 weeks apart.

FOR MORE HELP

For a list of resources on children's health, see box on page 271.

Colic
www.SavonColic.com

SIGNS AND SYMPTOMS

In a healthy infant under 3 months:

■ Crying that goes on for 3 hours or more at a time, despite efforts to comfort the baby. Crying is often worse in the evening and at night.

When gas pain is the cause:

■ Baby extends legs or pulls them up to the abdomen.

■ Baby passes gas.

If your baby is acting colicky, don't despair. About 1 infant in 5 has colic. Often it seems to have no cause. But sometimes it can be the result of gas pains from certain foods in the nursing mother's diet or the type of milk in the baby's formula.

Although colic is harmless, it can be very tiring for parents. This phase of your baby's life may seem endless, but most colicky babies grow out of it by about the time they are 3 months old. Sometimes, though, colicky crying may signal an illness, such as an **ear infection** (see page 71) or a **hernia** (see page 127).

WHAT YOU CAN DO NOW

➤ Stay calm. Never shake a baby—you can cause brain damage.

➤ Make sure a wet diaper or hunger is not the problem. See if the baby is too hot or cold—or bored.

➤ If gas pain seems to be the problem, place your baby stomach-down on your lap and gently massage the baby's back.

➤ Rhythmic motion often soothes babies. Walk with your baby in your arms or in a body carrier. Rock him or her in a rocking chair or swing. Take him or her for a ride in a car.

➤ Try putting the baby near the sound of a clothes dryer or a vacuum cleaner. Some babies are calmed by "white noise" or rhythmic sounds.

➤ Wrap your baby snugly in a blanket for security and warmth.

CHILDREN'S HEALTH

➤ Spend 10 minutes alone, relaxing, while someone else holds the baby. When you feel yourself getting near the breaking point, ask a friend or neighbor for help.

➤ Don't give up. What doesn't work one time may work the next. And it's a short-term problem.

WHEN TO CALL THE DOCTOR

Call for advice:

➤ If this is the first time your baby has had colic. Your doctor will want to rule out any illness.

➤ If the colic keeps getting worse.

➤ If your baby is more than 3 months old and is still colicky.

➤ If your colicky baby is not hungry and is not gaining weight.

HOW TO PREVENT IT

➤ If you're nursing, notice whether your baby is colicky after you eat certain foods, so that you can avoid them. Frequent problem foods include cabbage, onions, garlic, broccoli, and turnips, and the caffeine in coffee, tea, chocolate, cocoa, and some sodas.

➤ For a colicky bottle-fed baby, switch to a formula without cow's milk. Use nipples with a larger hole so your baby doesn't swallow air.

➤ Always burp your baby after a feeding.

➤ Try feeding your infant smaller amounts more often.

FOR MORE HELP

For a list of resources on children's health, see box on page 271.

Croup
www.SavonCroup.com

SIGNS AND SYMPTOMS

■ Loud, barking, seal-like cough.
■ Trouble breathing.
■ Shrill wheezing or grunting noise while breathing.
■ Hoarseness.
■ Sometimes fever.

Children who have croup find it hard to breathe because their airways have become swollen and narrow. Croup usually starts as a viral respiratory infection. Some children may get croup every time they have a cold or other illness, most often between October and March.

Children between the ages of 6 months and 3 years are the most likely to get croup. Those over 5 tend not to get it because their airways have grown larger, so swelling is less likely to affect breathing. Boys are more prone to croup than girls.

Croup most often clears up in about 6 days. Meanwhile, you can help your child feel better with simple at-home measures. But in rare cases, your child's airways may swell so much that he or she can barely breathe. If so, you may need to take him or her to the hospital.

WHAT YOU CAN DO NOW

➤ Have your child breathe moist air, either from a bowl filled with steaming water, a humidifier, or a hot shower (see **hints on humidifiers and vaporizers,** page 92). Your child's breathing should ease after 15 to 20 minutes.

➤ Take your child outside briefly—dressed warmly if it's cold out. Cold, moist air may ease breathing. A drive with the car windows open also may help.

➤ Sit your child up straight to ease breathing. For a baby, use an infant seat.

➤ Stay calm, and try to keep your child calm.

WHEN TO CALL THE DOCTOR

Call for advice **right away** (if you can't get it, call 911 or go to an emergency room):

➤ If your child starts to make loud, high-pitched wheezing noises while inhaling.

➤ If your child struggles to get a breath or can't speak for lack of breath.

➤ If your child has trouble swallowing.

Call for a prompt appointment:

➤ If your child breathes quickly and noisily.

➤ If your child has a fever of 102 or higher.

HOW TO PREVENT IT

➤ Get prompt treatment for any child with a respiratory illness.

➤ Make sure your children wash their hands often to reduce the chance of spreading illness.

FOR MORE HELP

For a list of resources on children's health, see box on page 271.

Diaper Rash

www.SavonDiaperRash.com

SIGNS AND SYMPTOMS

■ Red skin or small bumps on a baby's buttocks, genitals, lower abdomen, thigh folds, or any place in contact with wet or soiled diapers.

■ In the same areas, shiny, bright red skin or tight, paperlike skin.

■ Strong ammonia odor (sometimes).

Most babies will get diaper rash at least once. Babies between 8 and 10 months old, or those just starting to eat solid foods, are most likely to get it. Formula-fed babies tend to get diaper rash more often than do breast-fed babies.

Most diaper rash is caused by too much contact with moisture, urine, or feces. Skin lotions and soaps, and detergents used to wash cloth diapers, also can cause rashes.

Back to Sleep

Sudden Infant Death Syndrome (SIDS), the unexplained death of a baby in the first year of life, is the major cause of death of infants between 1 month and 1 year old. No one knows exactly what causes SIDS, but parents and caregivers can make their babies safer by following just a few simple steps.

➤ Put your child on his or her back to sleep, whether it's for a nap or for the night. In the few years since back-sleeping has been advised, the SIDS rate has fallen sharply.

➤ Make sure your baby sleeps on a firm mattress or other firm surface; avoid waterbeds, beanbag furniture, or other soft materials.

➤ Don't use sheepskins, fluffy blankets, or comforters either under the baby or as coverings. Keep pillows and stuffed toys out of your baby's crib. Babies can be smothered by soft materials.

➤ Don't overbundle your baby or overheat a room. The temperature in a baby's room should feel comfortable to an adult.

➤ Keep your baby away from cigarette smoke.

If home care doesn't get rid of diaper rash in 2 or 3 days, your baby may have a fungal or bacterial infection. Babies on antibiotics are very prone to fungal rashes (see **fungal infections,** page 153).

WHAT YOU CAN DO NOW

➤ Keep your baby's bottom as clean and dry as you can. When possible, let your baby go diaperless.

➤ Use a hair-dryer set on low to blow warm, dry air on your baby's bottom.

➤ After washing and drying your baby, apply an over-the-counter zinc oxide ointment. Baby powder doesn't work well and can harm the lungs if inhaled.

Antibiotics: Use With Care

Ear infections are the most common childhood ailment for which doctors prescribe antibiotics. These drugs can work wonders, halting pain, speeding healing, and preventing complications. But there's another side to the miracle cures: Overuse of antibiotics is producing drug-resistant bacteria that are growing harder and harder to kill.

If your child has an infection, he or she should not be given an antibiotic unless your doctor believes it is necessary. Many bacterial ear infections clear up on their own. Up to 20 percent of ear infections are caused by viruses, and in those cases antibiotics are useless. According to a survey published in 1999 in the journal of the American Academy of Pediatrics, more than half the physicians questioned said that pressure from parents was a major reason for oral antibiotic overuse. Even when a doctor thought antibiotics were not necessary, parents often requested them.

You can help reduce antibiotic overuse. The key is to work with your doctor. Don't ask for an antibiotic if he or she thinks it's not needed. Likewise, if your doctor does prescribe one, ask what it is and why you or your child is getting it. Once you're given a prescription, use all the medicine, as directed, even if you or your child feels better before it's gone—stubborn germs can linger and cause more trouble later.

WHEN TO CALL THE DOCTOR

➤ If the rash doesn't improve after 3 days of home treatment.
➤ If your baby's rash covers more than the diaper area.
➤ If the diaper area has red or pus-filled blisters that crust over.
➤ If a baby boy's foreskin becomes very red and inflamed.

HOW TO PREVENT IT

➤ Change soiled or wet diapers as soon as you can.
➤ Expose your baby's bottom to the air whenever possible.
➤ Don't use plastic pants or paper diapers that are tight around the legs or tummy.
➤ If you wash cloth diapers yourself, use a mild laundry soap, and avoid fabric softeners. Put the diapers through at least 2 rinse cycles to remove all traces of soap. Add 2 tablespoons of vinegar to the rinse water. This helps fight bacteria.

FOR MORE HELP

For a list of resources on children's health, see box on page 271.

Diarrhea in Children
www.SavonDiarrhea.com

See **diarrhea,** page 119.

Ear Infections in Children
www.SavonEarInfections.com

SIGNS AND SYMPTOMS

In young children, especially those who aren't yet talking, watch for:
■ Tugging at the ear (sometimes).
■ Bad temper.
■ Restlessness.
■ Lack of appetite.
■ Rectal temperature of 100 degrees or higher (99 or higher oral).
■ Discharge from the nose or ear.

For treatment, prevention, and more help, see **ear infections,** page 71.

Fever in Children
www.SavonFever.com

- Oral temperature higher than 99 degrees; rectal temperature above 100.2.
- Hot forehead.
- Flushed face.
- Sweating.
- Crying, irritability, or lack of appetite.

Although an oral temperature of 98.6 degrees is considered normal, body temperature varies with age, activity, and the time of day (it's most often lower in the morning and higher in the late afternoon). A temperature of 97 to 99 is no reason to worry; an oral reading higher than 99 is often the first sign that your child is sick.

A fever can be a sign of a childhood ailment, including viral or bacterial illnesses. In a baby or young child, fever can lead to a **seizure** (see box, page 256).

How to Take a Temperature

Taking a sick child's temperature is no fun for anyone, but following the suggestions below may make it easier. You can measure your child's body heat by way of the mouth (over age 5 only), ear (over 3 months), rectum, or armpit.

Some tips:

➤ Never leave a child or baby alone with a thermometer in place.
➤ For oral readings: Don't take a temperature right after your child eats, drinks, or takes a hot bath. You'll get a false reading.
➤ For oral readings with a glass thermometer: Shake it down below 95 degrees. Put it under the tongue toward one side of the mouth. The child should hold it for 3 minutes with the lips and tongue—not the teeth—and breathe through his or her nose. This reading will be 1 degree lower than the rectal temperature.
➤ For rectal readings: Use only a rectal thermometer. Lubricate the end with petroleum jelly. Place the child face down (over your lap is good) and gently insert the thermometer three-fourths of an inch into the rectum at a 90-degree angle. Hold it in place for 2 minutes (if your baby will not lie still, remove the thermometer right away).
➤ For underarm reading: Put the thermometer in the deepest part of the armpit. Hold it in place by gently pressing the baby's elbow against his or her side for 4 to 5 minutes. The reading will be 1.8 degrees lower than the rectal temperature.

Choosing a thermometer. Here's what experts say about the accuracy, speed, and ease of various options:

➤ **Glass** (cost: $1 to $3) comes as an oral type, and a thicker rectal type for babies and small children. Very accurate, but hard to read, bothersome to small children, and breakable. It has to be shaken down, and it has to be held in the mouth 2 to 3 minutes, the rectum 2 minutes, or the underarm 4 to 5 minutes.
➤ **Digital** (cost: $4 to $10) works in the mouth, rectum, or underarm in about the same time as the glass type. It's very accurate and easy to read and use, but the battery could wear out when you need it most.
➤ **Digital ear** (cost: $55 to $70) is the fastest and least trouble to use (even on a sleeping baby): Put the tip in the ear, then hold the button for 2 seconds. It's costly, though, and it may not be accurate unless you make a tight seal with the ear.
➤ **Contact strips** (held on the child's forehead for 2 minutes) or pacifier styles ($2 to $3 each) are easy to use, but not always accurate. The pacifier shows only whether the temperature is higher than normal.

Fever Seizures

Watching a feverish child have a convulsion (febrile seizure) can be terrifying. These seizures are common in children from 6 months to 5 years old whose temperatures have risen quickly. Despite the violence of a seizure, it is rarely harmful.

The signs of seizure include shaking or jerking of the arms and legs, a fixed stare or the eyes rolling back, drooling, heavy breathing, and the skin turning blue, mainly on the face. A seizure can last for less than a minute, more than 5 minutes, or, rarely, up to 20 minutes.

Take prompt action to prevent injury. Lay your child on a flat surface on his or her side, away from any sharp or hard objects. Turn your child's head to the side so that vomit or saliva can drain. If your child does vomit, use your finger to clean out the mouth. Make sure the airway is clear, but don't force anything into your child's mouth. To reduce fever, take off his or her clothing and sponge the body with lukewarm water.

If the seizure lasts for more than a few minutes or is severe, call 911 or go to an emergency room **right away.**

Some of the childhood illnesses marked by fever are chicken pox, croup, measles, mumps, rheumatic fever, strep throat, and whooping cough. (See the entry for each illness, and **fever** chart, page 273.)

WHAT YOU CAN DO NOW

➤ Check your child's temperature with a thermometer (see **how to take a temperature,** page 255).
➤ Make sure your child is not overdressed or in a place that's too hot. Remove extra clothing, and cool the room if you can.
➤ If a child is eating and sleeping well and is playful, there most likely is no serious problem. But complaints of feeling sick or tired, lack of appetite, and crying for no clear reason are often signs of illness.

➤ Have your child drink plenty of cool fluids to help lower body temperature and prevent dehydration.
➤ Give your child acetaminophen to help lower the fever. (Never give aspirin to a child or teenager who has a fever, a cold, chicken pox, the flu, or any other illness you suspect of being caused by a virus; see box on **Reye's syndrome,** page 95.) Ask your doctor before giving medication to an infant under 3 months old.
➤ To lower body temperature, sponge your child with lukewarm water, especially if he or she has had seizures before or is vomiting. Don't use cold water or alcohol.

WHEN TO CALL THE DOCTOR

Take your child's temperature before you call the doctor (see **how to take a temperature,** page 255).

Call 911 or go to an emergency room **right away:**

➤ If your child has other symptoms, such as vomiting, diarrhea, trouble breathing, a rash, or a stiff neck; or if he or she cries a lot and is confused or delirious. These may be signs of **meningitis** (see page 263).
➤ If your child has a temperature of 105 degrees after spending time on a hot beach or in a closed car or other hot place. This is not really a fever; it is **heatstroke** (see page 38). It needs emergency treatment.

Call for a prompt appointment:

➤ If an infant younger than 3 months has a rectal temperature of 100.4 or higher; if a child 3 months to 5 years has a rectal temperature of 102 or higher; if a child 5 years and older has an oral temperature of 102 or higher.

Call for advice :

➤ If your child has a fever that lasts more than 3 days.

HOW TO PREVENT IT

There is no way to prevent most fevers. To avoid fevers caused by overheating:

➤ Don't overdress your child, and never leave your child alone in a closed car.

➤ Have your child drink lots of water and wear a hat when in hot sun.

➤ Keep your child's room at a safe temperature. Use a fan if the room is hot or stuffy, and never put a crib next to a radiator, heater, or heating vent.

FOR MORE HELP

For a list of resources on children's health, see box on page 271.

Fifth Disease
www.SavonInfections.com

SIGNS AND SYMPTOMS

■ Rectal temperature as high as 102 degrees (101 oral).

■ Later, a bright red rash on the cheeks; they may look as if they've been slapped. Over the next few days, rash spreads to the buttocks, torso, arms, and thighs. Activity or heat may make the rash worse.

■ Coldlike symptoms, including sore throat, headache, reddish eyes, and fatigue (sometimes).

■ Itchiness (sometimes).

Fifth disease, a viral childhood illness, is among the 6 common infections—along with measles, German measles (rubella), roseola, chicken pox, and scarlet fever—that cause a rash and fever, and that are contagious (see entry for each illness). It is also called "slapped cheek." Children between the ages of 5 and 14 are most likely to get fifth disease, and outbreaks occur most often in the spring and early summer.

Once the virus has taken hold, the rash may not appear for up to 14 days. Meanwhile, your child, who may have symptoms of a cold, can spread the disease to other children through the air. Your child is contagious before the rash shows up, but not while he or she has the rash or after it's gone.

Fifth disease is mild. Most children feel fine even while they have the rash, and the illness often clears up in about 10 days. But the virus (named parvovirus) can cause arthritis in older children and adults and miscarriages in pregnant women. It can also lead to other illnesses in children and teens who have sickle-cell anemia.

WHAT YOU CAN DO NOW

➤ If your child feels sick, have him or her rest in bed and drink plenty of fluids.

➤ If the rash is itchy, apply an over-the-counter cream such as calamine lotion.

➤ For minor aches or pains, or for fever, you can give your child acetaminophen. (Never give aspirin to a child or teenager who has fifth disease, a cold, chicken pox, flu, or any other illness you suspect of being caused by a virus; see box on **Reye's syndrome,** page 95.)

WHEN TO CALL THE DOCTOR

Call for advice:

➤ If your child has new symptoms or a fever of 102 degrees or higher.

HOW TO PREVENT IT

➤ Make sure your children wash their hands often to reduce the chance of spreading disease.

FOR MORE HELP

For a list of resources on children's health, see box on page 271.

German Measles (Rubella)
www.SavonMeasles.com

SIGNS AND SYMPTOMS

■ Rectal temperature as high as 102 degrees (101 oral).

■ Swollen glands, most often in the neck.

■ By the second or third day, a rash that starts on the face and spreads to the chest and back, then the legs and arms. Rash can appear as tiny

red or pink spots or as irregular blotches. It lasts only a few days.
- Painful, aching joints, especially in teens.

German measles, also known as rubella, is a mild viral illness that used to be one of the milestones of early childhood. Now that a vaccine exists, rubella is very rare.

The virus spreads through the air when a person who has it coughs or sneezes. A child who catches it may feel no worse than he or she would with a simple cold. But an adult who catches it may feel much more sick. Rubella most often clears up on its own 5 to 7 days after the first symptoms appear.

The infection presents a serious threat to a growing fetus in early pregnancy. If a woman gets rubella in her first 3 months of pregnancy, her child has a 50 percent chance of being born with birth defects. These can include blindness, deafness, mental retardation, and heart problems.

WHAT YOU CAN DO NOW

➤ Keep your child quiet and provide a lot of liquids.
➤ Give your child acetaminophen for discomfort. (Never give aspirin to a child or teenager who has rubella, a cold, chicken pox, the flu, or any other illness you suspect of being caused by a virus; see box on **Reye's syndrome,** page 95.)
➤ If you think your child has rubella, keep him or her away from others, especially pregnant women. Rubella is contagious 2 days before and up to a week after the rash appears.

WHEN TO CALL THE DOCTOR

Call for advice:
➤ If you suspect your child has rubella.
➤ If you are pregnant and believe you have been exposed to rubella, even if you have been immunized in the past. You need to find out if you are still immune.

HOW TO PREVENT IT

➤ Make sure your children get the MMR (measles, mumps, and rubella) vaccine, a routine part of early childhood immunizations (see **childhood immunization schedule,** page 250).
➤ If you're a woman of childbearing age and you weren't immunized in childhood, and never had German measles, get the rubella vaccine. If you aren't sure whether you had the disease or were immunized, ask your doctor for a test.

You should have the shot at least 3 months before you get pregnant; the vaccine should never be given to a pregnant woman. Use birth control for 3 months after the shot to make sure you don't get pregnant while the vaccine is still present and could affect your baby.

FOR MORE HELP

For a list of resources on children's health, see box on page 271.

Hand, Foot & Mouth Disease
www.SavonInfections.com

SIGNS AND SYMPTOMS

- Painful small, raw, cankerlike sores on the tongue and insides of the cheeks.
- An itchy rash with red spots, bumps, and/or small blisters on the hands and feet, between the fingers and toes, sometimes on the buttocks.
- Sometimes fever (under 102 degrees rectal, 101 oral).
- Tiredness.

Like many childhood illnesses, hand, foot, and mouth disease is caused by a virus. Most often spread by the feces-to-mouth route, the virus is also spread in the air. Once it takes hold, symptoms show up in 3 to 6 days.

Outbreaks of hand, foot, and mouth disease occur most often in the summer and fall, when the virus grows best. The disease usually clears up by itself within a week. There's no treatment, but you can help your child feel better at home.

WHAT YOU CAN DO NOW

➤ Don't give your child citrus fruits, spicy foods, or other foods that might make his or her mouth more sore. Serve liquids, such as chicken or vegetable broth, and soft foods, such as oatmeal or mashed banana, if solid foods are too painful for your child to chew.

➤ Saltwater rinses and gargles can soothe mouth sores. Mix one-half teaspoon salt in 1 cup (8 ounces) of warm water, and have your child rinse his or her mouth after eating. Be sure your child is old enough to rinse and then spit out rather than swallow the salt water.

➤ Boil utensils (or run dishwasher on hot cycle) or use disposable cups, forks, and spoons to avoid spreading the disease.

➤ Be sure your child drinks plenty of fluids. Water and juice (not citrus) are best. Popsicles and ice chips are also good choices. They can ease pain and add fluids.

➤ If the rash is itchy, apply an over-the-counter anti-itch cream.

➤ To help relieve pain or reduce your child's fever, give acetaminophen. (Never give aspirin to a child or teenager who has hand, foot, and mouth disease, a cold, chicken pox, the flu, or any other illness you suspect of being caused by a virus; see box on **Reye's syndrome,** page 95.)

WHEN TO CALL THE DOCTOR

Call for a prompt appointment:
➤ If your child has trouble swallowing.

HOW TO PREVENT IT

➤ Make sure children wash their hands after using the toilet.

➤ See that children don't share glasses, silverware, or toys that have been in other children's mouths.

➤ Choose a babysitter or day care center with high standards of cleanliness. Check that the staff members wash their hands often, especially after they change children's diapers.

FOR MORE HELP

For a list of resources on children's health, see box on page 271.

Impetigo
www.SavonImpetigo.com

SIGNS AND SYMPTOMS

■ Small patches of red or pus-filled blisters, most often on the face, legs, or arms; blisters range from the size of a matchstick head to the size of a quarter.

■ After blisters pop, a sticky golden crust.

■ Itching.

Impetigo is a skin infection most common in children because they're prone to scrapes, skinned knees, and other minor breaks in the skin that give bacteria a place to thrive. Children with colds or runny noses often get it because the skin around the mouth and nose becomes raw. Usually caused by streptococcus or staphylococcus bacteria, impetigo is very contagious and spreads quickly over the body and from one person to others through touching or sharing towels.

The bacteria that cause it are harmless until they enter the skin through a cut, insect bite, or other break. Impetigo occurs most often in the summer, chiefly in hot, humid climates. It's also common in hospitals, day care centers, and schools. Impetigo is unattractive and uncomfortable, but easy to treat.

WHAT YOU CAN DO NOW

➤ Gently wash away the crusty discharge with warm water and soap.

➤ If it's a minor case, apply an over-the-counter antibiotic ointment.

➤ Warn other people not to touch your

child's sores, towels and washcloths, and unwashed clothing. Change linens daily; wash them in hot water and detergent, with bleach.

➤ Do what you can to help your child avoid touching or scratching the blisters.

➤ To keep the bacteria from growing, expose blisters to air; don't bandage them.

➤ Bathe your child in lukewarm water. Use an antibacterial soap.

➤ Dress your child in long-sleeved shirts and long pants to go to school or day care until the crusts are gone and the skin clears, which takes 7 to 10 days.

WHEN TO CALL THE DOCTOR

Call for a prompt appointment:

➤ At the first sign of impetigo. This is a strep or staph infection, so your doctor will need to prescribe an antibiotic.

➤ If your child's urine turns red or dark brown. This signals a rare related kidney ailment.

Call for advice:

➤ If the impetigo covers a large area or keeps spreading after 3 days.

➤ If your child gets a fever higher than 100 degrees or has a blister wider than 1 inch. This may mean a deeper infection.

HOW TO PREVENT IT

➤ Wash all cuts, scrapes, and wounds with antibacterial soap and water. Keep them clean and dry while they heal.

➤ Make sure children wash their hands often and keep their nails trimmed. Remind them not to scratch insect bites, scabs, or other skin irritations.

➤ Don't have children share towels, washcloths, or bedding.

FOR MORE HELP

For a list of resources on children's health, see box on page 271.

Lead Poisoning
www.SavonFirstAid.com

SIGNS AND SYMPTOMS

Most children with low levels of lead poisoning show no distinct symptoms. Sometimes, though, they will have:

■ Constipation.
■ Vomiting.
■ Loss of appetite.
■ Fatigue.
■ Learning disabilities and/or behavior problems.

Severe lead poisoning:

■ Stomach pain.
■ Headaches.
■ Loss of coordination.
■ Loss of recently learned skills.

One in 11 American children has a high level of lead in his or her blood. Lead poisoning does not occur only in inner-city families trapped in poor housing; it also strikes middle- and upper-income families living in older houses (most often houses being repaired). Children between the ages of 6 months and 6 years are at highest risk. Lead can harm a fetus as well, so pregnant women also should avoid it.

Almost three-quarters of the houses built before 1980 have lead paint either inside or outside. Most children are exposed through lead-based paint and paint dust. Lead may also be present in the water from your faucet, in the dishes in your cabinets, and in your backyard soil.

Severe lead poisoning can cause mental retardation, intestinal problems, hearing loss, anemia, and even death. At low but chronic levels, it can result in learning disabilities, behavior problems, and reduced IQ.

The Centers for Disease Control and Prevention (CDC) advises parents to have their children's blood tested for lead by the time the children are 1 year old.

WHAT YOU CAN DO NOW

➤ Ask your doctor to test your child's blood for lead. This is the only way to know your child's lead level.

For Your Child's Safety

The biggest threat to your child's life is an accident. In the United States, nearly 300 children under age 4 die every month as the result of accidents, and more school-age children die of injuries than of all diseases combined. Most of these tragedies can be prevented. Here are a few safety tips recommended by the American Academy of Pediatrics.

Around the house:

➤ Protect your baby and toddler from falls by putting gates on stairways and doors and installing window guards on all windows above the first floor.

➤ Install a smoke alarm in the kitchen, outside each bedroom, at the head of each staircase, and in the basement and/or attic. Test the batteries every month and change them once a year.

➤ Keep medications and chemical household products out of sight and reach of children. If your child swallows something that could be poisonous, call your doctor or local poison control center right away.

➤ It is safest to keep all guns out of the home. If you must have a gun, keep it unloaded and in a locked place separate from the ammunition. If there are guns in the homes of your child's friends, ask if they are safely stored before you let your child play there.

➤ Keep a list of emergency numbers on or by your phone. Learn first aid and **CPR** (see page 14, 16, or 17).

In the car:

➤ Children under the age of 5 should be securely buckled in a car safety seat or a booster seat. Be sure that the seat is installed correctly and is the right size for your child's age, height, and weight.

➤ The air bag that saves your life can kill your child. The safest place for all children to ride is in the back seat. Never put a baby in the front seat of a car with a passenger-side air bag. Infants should ride in a rear-facing car seat in the back seat until they are at least 20 pounds and 1 year old.

➤ Children age 5 and over should be taught to use a lap belt and shoulder belt. Serious injuries can occur with lap belts alone—if your car doesn't have shoulder belts in the back seat, it's a good idea to have them installed.

Around the water:

➤ Never leave a young child alone in or near a bathtub, pail of water, wading or swimming pool, or any other water, even for a moment. Your child can drown in less than 2 inches of water.

➤ If you have a swimming pool, fence it on all sides—including between the house and the pool—and keep the gate locks in working order.

➤ Even if your child knows how to swim, never let her or him swim alone.

➤ When in any boat, make sure your child wears a life vest.

Out and about:

➤ Make sure your child wears a helmet every time he or she rides a bike. Buy the helmet when you buy the bike.

➤ Teach your child always to stop at the curb and never to cross the street without a grown-up.

➤ When your child plays sports, be sure he or she always wears the proper protective equipment for the activity, such as shin pads, mouth guards, or helmets.

➤ If lead levels in the blood are high—10 micrograms per deciliter or more—talk to your doctor about how to keep your child from being exposed further.

➤ For severe cases (more than 45 micrograms per deciliter), a treatment called chelation therapy can help the body get rid of lead.

➤ If you believe your child has been exposed to lead—if your house paint is old and peeling or if work has recently been done on your house.

HOW TO PREVENT IT

Have the paint, water, and soil in and around your home tested. You may find you need to rid it of lead hazards. Other steps to take:

➤ If your house was built before 1980, keep it as clean and dust-free as you can.

➤ If your house was built before 1980 and you plan to repaint or repair it, ask your local health department for advice on how to get the job done safely.

➤ Have your tap water tested for lead. If any shows up, use bottled water or a filter that removes lead (get the maker's certification that it does). Use only cold tap water (if it passes the lead test), bottled water, or filtered water for drinking, cooking, and making baby formula.

➤ Feed your child meals that include plenty of calcium- and iron-rich foods; these can reduce lead absorption.

➤ Avoid foods canned in other countries. They may contain lead.

➤ Have painted toys and glazed dishes that were made outside the United States tested for lead, or get rid of them. Never use imported dishware to store foods.

FOR MORE HELP

Key Websites: *www.SavonHealth.com*. For more information on lead poisoning: *www.SavonFirstAid.com*.

Organizations: The Alliance to End Childhood Lead Poisoning, 227 Massachusetts Ave. NE, Suite 200, Washington, DC 20002. 202-543-1147, M–F 8:30–5:30 EST; *www.aeclp.org*. Provides publications and referrals.

■ Lead Poisoning Prevention Branch, Centers for Disease Control and Prevention, 1600 Clifton Rd. NE, Mailstop E25, Atlanta, GA 30333. 404-639-2510, M–F 8–4:30 EST; *www.cdc.gov*. Provides facts about lead poisoning.

Websites: National Safety Council, *www.nsc.org*. In the Environment section under Resource Topics, click on *Lead Poisoning*. Gives information on how to prevent lead poisoning in your community.

■ Parentsplace.com, *www.parentsplace.com/readroom/lead*. Search for *lead poisoning*. Offers information about the hazards of lead and a guide to poison prevention.

Book: *Getting the Lead Out: The Complete Resource on How to Prevent and Cope With Lead Poisoning*, by Irene Kessel and John T. O'Connor. Describes the major sources of lead and offers prevention strategies. Plenum, 1997, $28.95.

Further resources: See box on page 271.

Measles
www.SavonMeasles.com

SIGNS AND SYMPTOMS

First 2 to 3 days:

■ Very high fever (up to 105 degrees rectal, 104 oral).

■ Coldlike symptoms, including a runny nose; a dry cough; swollen glands; red, watery eyes; loss of appetite; and aching muscles.

A day or two later:

■ Inside the mouth, painless small gray or white bumps, like grains of salt surrounded by red rings.

In another day or so:

■ Small red spots that first appear on the face and neck. As they spread down the body, they join to form large blotches.

Measles is a very contagious viral illness that can be quite severe. One to 2 weeks after your child has been exposed, coldlike symptoms show up. During this time, the disease is most contagious, although it can be spread until the fever and rash are gone, about 5 to 8 days later. Infected children most often pass measles to others through coughing or sneezing. Today, though, few children in the United States get measles, thanks to a vaccine.

There's no cure for measles, but you can help your child feel better. Rarely, measles can go on to become a more serious problem, such as **pneumonia** (see page 97). Even less often, measles can trigger **encephalitis** (see page 55), an inflammation of the brain.

WHAT YOU CAN DO NOW

➤ Give your child lots of fluids.
➤ Help your child rest in bed.
➤ Use a cool-mist humidifier in your child's bedroom (see **hints on humidifiers and vaporizers,** page 92).
➤ If your child's eyes are sensitive to light, darken the bedroom.
➤ If your child has minor aches or pains, give acetaminophen. (Never give aspirin to a child or teenager who has measles, a cold, chicken pox, the flu, or any other illness you suspect of being caused by a virus; see box on **Reye's syndrome,** page 95.)
➤ Keep your child away from others.

WHEN TO CALL THE DOCTOR

Call 911 or go to an emergency room **right away:**
➤ If your child has a headache, can't stand bright light, and feels so drowsy that he or she is hard to wake up. These can be warning signs of **encephalitis** (see page 55).
➤ If bumps are dark red and appear to be filled with blood or if seizures occur.
Call for a prompt appointment:
➤ If your child has a feeling of fullness in the ear, and maybe some pain. He or she may have an ear infection.
➤ If your child is short of breath while resting. He or she may also have chills, sweating, and chest pain. This can be a sign of pneumonia.

HOW TO PREVENT IT

➤ Make sure your child gets the MMR vaccine for measles, mumps, and rubella (see **childhood immunization schedule,** page 250). The shot is most often given at 12 to 18 months, with a booster at 4 to 6 years.

FOR MORE HELP

For a list of resources on children's health, see box on page 271.

Meningitis in Children
www.SavonMeningitis.com

SIGNS AND SYMPTOMS

The following symptoms need immediate treatment. If your doctor is not available, call 911 or take your child to an emergency room **right away.**
■ Rectal temperature of 100 degrees or higher (99 oral); with:
■ Headache or stiff neck. When child is lying down, the head can't be bent toward the chest (except in infants less than 12 months old) because of shooting pain in the neck and back.
■ Bad temper or listlessness.
■ Loss of appetite.
■ Turning away from bright lights.
■ Maybe nausea and vomiting.
■ In infants, bulging of the soft spot of the skull.

Meningitis is an inflammation of the brain and spinal cord. The bacterial form is especially dangerous for infants and young children. To prevent permanent damage—or death—meningitis must be treated promptly.

For more information on the disease, see **meningitis and encephalitis,** page 55.

CHILDREN'S HEALTH

Mumps

www.SavonMumps.com

SIGNS AND SYMPTOMS

- Low fever (101 degrees rectal).
- Headache.
- Loss of appetite.
- Fatigue.
- Swollen glands in the neck below the ear near the jawbone, on one or both sides.
- Earache (sometimes).
- Nausea and vomiting (sometimes).
- Swelling in one or both testes in men and boys or swelling of ovaries in women and girls (sometimes).

Mumps is a viral infection of the salivary glands that is most common in children between the ages of 2 and 12. (Unvaccinated adults who have never had mumps can also get it.) The virus is spread through the air when an infected person coughs or sneezes. Mumps is uncomfortable but not often serious, and symptoms should go away in 7 to 10 days.

Infected adults are prone to a very painful symptom: inflamed testes in men and inflamed ovaries in women. While the symptom is more common in adults, a young boy can also have pain in his testes, while a girl may feel pain in the lower abdomen. The discomfort should pass within 4 days. Occasionally, the swelling causes sterility, so check with your doctor if you have concerns.

Because of an effective vaccine, mumps is uncommon. Once a person has had mumps, she or he is immune and is not likely to get it again.

WHAT YOU CAN DO NOW

➤ Call your doctor for advice if you suspect your child has mumps.
➤ Be sure your child gets lots of rest while he or she has a fever. That doesn't have to mean staying in bed—quiet play is okay.
➤ Provide plenty of liquids and soft foods, such as soups, cooked vegetables, and fruits. Don't offer sour fruits, foods, or

juices—they can make swollen salivary glands more sore.
➤ To soothe swollen places, try cold or warm packs—whichever feels best. Apply ice packs (a bag of frozen peas wrapped in a washcloth works well), or warm cloths or heating pads.
➤ Give acetaminophen or ibuprofen to ease pain and reduce fever. (Never give aspirin to a child or teenager who has mumps, a cold, chicken pox, the flu, or any other illness you suspect of being caused by a virus; see the box on **Reye's syndrome, page 95.**)

WHEN TO CALL THE DOCTOR

Call for emergency advice (if you can't get any, call 911 or go to an emergency room):
➤ If your child has the symptoms of mumps and a severe headache or neck pain, is listless, or behaves oddly. This could mean **meningitis** (see page 55).
Call for a prompt appointment:
➤ If your child has mumps and feels severe abdominal pain or vomits. This could signal an inflamed pancreas.

HOW TO PREVENT IT

➤ Make sure your child gets the MMR vaccine for measles, mumps, and rubella (see **childhood immunization schedule,** page 250). The shot is most often given at 12 to 18 months, with a booster at 4 to 6 years.
➤ To prevent others from catching mumps, keep your child home from school or day care for 7 to 10 days after the swelling appears.

FOR MORE HELP

Websites: *www.SavonHealth.com.* For more information about mumps: *www.SavonMumps.com.*
ECBT (Every Child By Two), *www.ecbt.org/mumps.htm.* From the Centers for Disease Control and Prevention. Covers mumps and proper immunization.
Further resources: See box on page 271.

Rheumatic Fever

www.SavonRheumaticFever.com

Early symptoms (usually 1 to 6 weeks before other symptoms):
- Sore throat, with swollen glands in the neck (sometimes).

Later:
- Rectal temperature of 100 degrees or higher (99 or higher oral).
- Pain and swelling that moves from joint to joint.
- Fatigue and shortness of breath.
- Loss of appetite.
- Rash on chest, back, and abdomen (sometimes).

Rheumatic fever is a rare but sometimes dangerous offshoot of a strep infection, most often **strep throat** (see page 267). It's most common in children between the ages of 5 and 15, although adults can also get it.

Rheumatic fever occurs as part of the body's immune response to strep. Antibodies made to destroy the bacteria instead attack the joints or, in some cases, the valves of the heart. If rheumatic fever follows a strep infection, symptoms most often appear 1 to 6 weeks later.

If treated promptly with antibiotics, rheumatic fever poses little threat and passes within 2 to 12 weeks. If the heart has been affected, symptoms may last as long as 6 months. Any damage to the heart valves may not show up until years later.

WHAT YOU CAN DO NOW

- Have your child rest in bed and drink plenty of liquids.
- When your doctor confirms rheumatic fever, he or she may advise aspirin for joint pain. That's all right, because this illness comes from bacteria. But never give aspirin to a child or teenager who has a cold, chicken pox, the flu, or any other illness you suspect of being caused by a virus (see box on **Reye's syndrome,** page 95).

WHEN TO CALL THE DOCTOR

- If a child or an adult has just had strep and then shows symptoms of rheumatic fever.
- If a child or an adult has a fever, sore throat, and swollen glands that last for 48 hours or more; these symptoms could signal a strep infection.
- If new symptoms appear after treatment has begun. This could be a reaction to a prescribed drug.

HOW TO PREVENT IT

- Get prompt tests and treatment for **strep throat** (see page 267) or any other strep infection.

FOR MORE HELP

For a list of resources on children's health, see box on page 271.

Roseola

www.SavonRoseola.com

Early symptoms:
- Sudden high fever (only in children 3 years and younger; older children have no fever).
- Decreased appetite.
- Mild diarrhea.
- Slight cough.
- Runny nose.
- Mild irritability, drowsiness.
- Swollen glands (rarely).

Later symptoms:
- Normal temperature after 3 to 6 days. At the same time, a spotty, slightly raised red rash appears on the torso.
- Rash may spread to the arms, neck, legs, and face. It disappears in a few hours to a few days.

CHILDREN'S HEALTH

Roseola is also called "baby measles" because children get it most often between the ages of 6 months and 2 years. It often frightens parents because of its alarming symptoms, but in fact this common viral ailment poses little risk.

Beware Dr. Web

Millions of people turn to the Internet for medical advice, and they find plenty of health sites to choose from—at least 15,000, by some estimates. But just how reliable is the information on those Web pages?

The answer is not very soothing. Several recent studies—including a few that focused specifically on children's medical problems—indicate that much of the health information on the Internet is incomplete, out of date, or just plain wrong. In a study of Web advice on treating diarrhea in children, 80 percent of the 60 sites sampled gave inaccurate or obsolete information.

So when looking for online health care, be skeptical. Here are a few questions worth asking:

➤ **Who put the site together?** Be wary of sites sponsored by someone who might profit from your taking the site's advice. The most reliable information tends to come from government health agencies and medical specialty groups; even these, however, will have biases.
➤ **Where did the information come from?** Web pages are not required to meet any medical standards. Look for background information on authors and sources, references such as peer-reviewed journals, and links to other reputable sites.
➤ **How current is the information?** A site should state when it was last updated—and it should be within the last month.

Finally, don't start any treatments recommended on the Web until you've checked with your doctor.

This illness usually passes within a week of the first symptoms. When the rash is gone, the child is no longer contagious and can return to school and playing with others.

WHAT YOU CAN DO NOW

➤ Give your child plenty of fluids.
➤ Have your child rest as long as he or she has a fever.
➤ Sponge a feverish child with lukewarm water—not cold water or alcohol.
➤ Ask your doctor if you should give acetaminophen to reduce fever. (Never give aspirin to a child or teenager who has roseola, a cold, chicken pox, the flu, or any other illness you suspect of being caused by a virus; see box on **Reye's syndrome,** page 95.)

WHEN TO CALL THE DOCTOR

Call for a prompt appointment:
➤ If your child has a rectal temperature of 102 or higher (101 or higher oral).
➤ If your child has seizures.

HOW TO PREVENT IT

➤ Don't let a child with roseola play with other children until the rash clears up.
➤ Make sure all family members wash their hands often—always before touching food and after using the bathroom.

FOR MORE HELP

For a list of resources on children's health, see box on page 271.

Scarlet Fever
www.SavonScarletFever.com

SIGNS AND SYMPTOMS

Symptoms vary, but most go as follows:
■ First day: rectal temperature as high as 104 degrees (103 oral), red and sore throat, fuzzy tongue,

white coating on tonsils, headache, swollen neck glands, vomiting (sometimes).
- By the second day: bright red rash that breaks out on face (except right around mouth) and in groin area.
- By the third day: rash, which feels like sandpaper to the touch and may itch, spreads to rest of body. Temperature falls, and tongue turns bright red.
- By the sixth day: rash fades and skin and tongue may peel, leaving raw, tender skin.

Scarlet fever is caused by strep bacteria. Children between the ages of 2 and 10 get it most often. It's **strep throat** (see this page) with a rash, and it is contagious.

If not treated, scarlet fever can lead to abscesses on the tonsils or, rarely, **rheumatic fever** (see page 265), which may develop 2 to 3 weeks after the rash appears.

Prompt treatment with antibiotics usually results in full recovery.

WHAT YOU CAN DO NOW

➤ Make sure your child gets plenty of rest and drinks lots of liquids. Give soft foods that won't hurt a raw throat.
➤ Your doctor may advise acetaminophen to reduce fever and relieve pain (see **pain relief,** page 315). Never give aspirin to a child or teenager who has a cold, chicken pox, the flu, or any illness you suspect is caused by a virus (see box on **Reye's syndrome,** page 95).

WHEN TO CALL THE DOCTOR

Call for a prompt appointment:
➤ If your child has a sore throat with a rash, or if he or she has other symptoms of strep throat or scarlet fever. Your child needs antibiotics if he or she has a strep infection.
Call for advice:
➤ If your child does not improve with treatment.

HOW TO PREVENT IT

➤ Get prompt tests and treatment for strep throat or other strep illnesses.
➤ Keep your child away from anyone who has strep.
➤ Once your doctor confirms scarlet fever, make sure other family members are tested for strep if they develop a sore throat, with or without a rash.

FOR MORE HELP

For a list of resources on children's health, see box on page 271.

Strep Throat
www.SavonStrepThroat.com

SIGNS AND SYMPTOMS

Young children:
- Mild sore throat.
- Swollen glands in throat.
- Rectal temperature of 101 degrees.
- Irritability.
- Loss of appetite.

Older children and adults:
- Sudden severe sore throat.
- Swollen glands in throat.
- Oral temperature of 102 degrees or higher.

The streptococcus bacteria that cause strep throat are spread by contact or through the air. Strep throat is most common in 5-to-15-year-olds but it can affect adults. It's rare in children under 3.

If strep throat goes untreated, it can lead to **rheumatic fever** (see page 265), kidney problems, and other illnesses. It's easy to mistake strep symptoms for signs of a cold or flu. A throat culture or strep test can show whether it's strep.

Prompt treatment with antibiotics such as penicillin or erythromycin most often eases symptoms within a day or so.

CHILDREN'S HEALTH

WHAT YOU CAN DO NOW

➤ Your child should rest, drink liquids, and eat foods that won't hurt a raw throat.

➤ Give your child acetaminophen for pain relief. (Never give aspirin to a child or teenager who has a cold, chicken pox, the flu, or any other illness you suspect of being caused by a virus; see box on **Reye's syndrome,** page 95.)

➤ For children 3 and older, gargling with warm salt water can ease throat pain.

➤ Don't smoke or let others smoke in the room with a sick child.

➤ Over-the-counter throat lozenges may help. Some have a local painkiller—ask your doctor or pharmacist.

➤ Take all antibiotics as prescribed, even after symptoms are gone.

WHEN TO CALL THE DOCTOR

➤ If a child or an adult has the symptoms listed or a sore throat that lasts 48 hours or longer. If your child tests positive for strep, he or she will be given antibiotics.

HOW TO PREVENT IT

➤ Stay away from people who are coughing and sneezing.

➤ To prevent your sick child from infecting others, wait until he or she has been on antibiotics for 48 hours before you send him or her back to school or day care.

FOR MORE HELP

For a list of resources on children's health, see box on page 271.

Teething
www.SavonTeething.com

SIGNS AND SYMPTOMS

Sometime in the first year, baby teeth appear, often with:

■ Fussy, clingy behavior, and night-time crying.

■ Lots of drooling.

■ Chewing on fingers, teething rings, and other objects.

■ Red, swollen, and inflamed gums.

■ More demand for nursing or bottle-feeding, or child may refuse breast or bottle because sucking action hurts sore gums.

■ Poor appetite.

Few parents forget the arrival of their baby's first teeth, and in most cases, the memories can be as painful as they are sweet. Your normally sunny child, who appears otherwise healthy, may suddenly be crabby and restless all night long.

Children teethe at different ages. The front teeth tend to appear during the child's first year, and the first and second molars appear between the ages of 1 and 3.

For most children, the front teeth cause less trouble, though some children fuss with each tooth. The first and second molars, which seem to cause more pain, often disrupt eating and sleeping routines. The pain is likely to last a few days with each new tooth.

WHAT YOU CAN DO NOW

➤ When your child seems to be in pain, rub his or her gums with a clean finger. A chilled (but not frozen) washcloth or teething ring can ease soreness and provide something to chew on.

➤ Wrap an ice cube in a soft cloth and rub it gently on your child's gums to reduce inflammation. Keep the ice moving over the gums to avoid hurting tissue.

➤ Comfort and distract your child with holding, cuddling, and rocking.

➤ If the pain lasts, ask your doctor about using acetaminophen. (Never give aspirin to a child or teenager who has a cold, chicken pox, the flu, or any other illness you suspect of being caused by a virus; see box on **Reye's syndrome,** page 95.)

➤ The drooling that comes with teething can cause a rash on the face, neck, and up-

Caring for Those First Teeth

Here are some simple steps you can take to protect your baby's new teeth and ensure healthful habits later on:

➤ As soon as the first teeth appear, make toothbrushing part of your child's daily routine. Use either a gauze pad or a child's toothbrush with soft bristles. Gently rub the teeth bottom to top, front and back.

➤ Never put your baby to bed with a bottle. Juice and milk contain sugars that if left in the mouth for long can lead to tooth decay.

➤ Try to limit the amount of sweets your child eats.

➤ Begin visits to the dentist when all 20 baby teeth have appeared (around age 3).

For more help:

■ American Academy of Pediatric Dentistry, 211 E. Chicago Ave., Suite 700, Chicago, IL 60611. Send in a business-size self-addressed stamped envelope for "The Pediatric Dentist" pamphlet.

■ American Academy of Pediatrics, *www.aap.org*. First click on *You and Your Family*, then on *AAP Public Education Brochures*, and then on *Baby Bottle Tooth Decay*.

per chest. Using an infant cream can help. Change wet clothing often, or use bibs.

➤ Never rub brandy or any other alcoholic drink on your child's gums (no matter what you might have heard). Alcohol, even in small amounts, is bad for children.

WHEN TO CALL THE DOCTOR

➤ If your child runs a fever that lasts more than 48 hours or is higher than 100 degrees, has diarrhea, or is lethargic. These symptoms may signal something more serious than teething.

➤ If your child has no teeth by 12 months of age. This could mean a harmless, inherited tendency to late teething, but it might mean delayed bone growth.

FOR MORE HELP

For a list of resources on children's health, see box on page 271.

Vomiting in Children
www.SavonNauseaandVomiting.com

See **nausea and vomiting,** page 133.

Whooping Cough
www.SavonCough.com

SIGNS AND SYMPTOMS

First stage (lasts 1 to 2 weeks):
■ Runny nose and sneezing.
■ Dry cough.
■ Low fever (101 degrees rectal).

Second stage (lasts 2 to 10 weeks):
■ Frequent, severe coughing spasms, sometimes followed by a whooping sound when breathing in (as air is forced over the swollen voice box). Babies may have repeated coughing fits without making the whooping sound.
■ Red or blue face during coughing spells. If your child turns blue or stops breathing, call 911 and give CPR **right away.** (See page 14, 16, or 17 for how to do **CPR.**)
■ Vomiting may follow coughing fits.

Third stage (may last months):
■ Cough that slowly becomes less frequent and severe.

Whooping cough, also called pertussis, is one of the most serious of the classic childhood ailments. This illness is a

CHILDREN'S HEALTH

highly contagious bacterial infection that attacks the throat and lungs and is spread through the air by coughing or sneezing. If left untreated, it can cause pneumonia and lung damage.

Because of widespread immunization, whooping cough is less common among children in the United States than it once was. Those who do get it are most often infants and children under 4 who haven't had shots to prevent it. (The vaccine, however, is only 80 percent effective.)

Even if they've had their shots, teenagers and adults also can get whooping cough. In fact, experts have recently reported a surprisingly large number of cases in adults who were vaccinated as children. Because they don't make the whooping sound that children do, adults may think they have **bronchitis** (see page 90). The danger this poses is that adults may pass the illness to children. If you have a cough for more than 2 weeks, call your doctor for advice.

An antibiotic can prevent the spasms of coughing if it's given during the first stage of the illness. Once the whooping type of cough starts, antibiotics will not get rid of it, but they can make the illness less contagious.

Infants may need to be taken to a hospital to get rid of mucus blocking the nose and airways. They may also need oxygen.

WHAT YOU CAN DO NOW

After diagnosis:
➤ Keep your child calm.
➤ Give lots of liquids to prevent dehydration. Water and juice are good choices.
➤ Make sure your child gets enough to eat. Frequent small meals may reduce the chance of vomiting. Even though whooping cough can be tiring and a child may not feel like eating, it's important to keep him or her well nourished.
➤ To keep a baby from inhaling mucus while coughing, place the baby on his or her stomach with the head turned to the

side. Older children may breathe more easily if they sit up and lean forward.
➤ Don't give your child a cough suppressant, as it may prevent the clearing of mucus from blocked airways.
➤ Give acetaminophen for pain relief. (Never give aspirin to a child or teenager who has a cold, chicken pox, the flu, or any other illness you suspect of being caused by a virus; see box on **Reye's syndrome,** page 95.)

WHEN TO CALL THE DOCTOR

Call 911 **right away** and give CPR:
➤ If your child turns blue or stops breathing during or after coughing (see page 14, 16, or 17 for how to do **CPR**).
Call for a prompt appointment:
➤ If your child's cough becomes more severe and frequent.

HOW TO PREVENT IT

➤ Starting at the age of 2 months, a child should get shots against whooping cough (see **childhood immunization schedule,** page 250).
➤ Your doctor may advise preventive antibiotics for housemates or schoolmates of a child who has whooping cough, even if they have been immunized.
➤ Don't expose your child to anyone who has whooping cough. Call your doctor if your child is exposed, even if he or she has been immunized.

FOR MORE HELP

For a list of resources on children's health, see the next page.

Children's Health Resources

General Health

Key Websites: *www.SavonHealth.com*. For more information on any particular illness, see *www.SavonChildren.com*. See each illness heading for the exact Website address.

Websites: American Academy of Pediatrics, *www.aap.org*. Click on *You and Your Family*, then on *AAP Public Education Brochures*. Covers many issues, from diaper rash to single parenting.

■ ParentsPlace.com, *www.parentsplace. com*. Offers articles, support groups for parents, and links to other sites.

■ Pediatric Points of Interest, *www. med.jhu.edu/peds/neonatology/poi.html*. From the Department of Pediatrics and Residency at Johns Hopkins University. Click on *Organizations in Pediatrics Medicine* or *Parenting Resources* for a list of children's health resources and links to other sites.

Books: *The American Academy of Pediatrics, Caring for Your School-Age Child: Ages 5 to 12,* edited by Edward L. Schor, M.D. Broadway Books, 1999, $17.95.

■ *The American Academy of Pediatrics, Caring for Your Baby and Young Child: Birth to Age 5,* edited by Steven P. Shelov, M.D. Bantam, 1998, $17.95.

■ *Dr. Spock's Baby and Child Care,* by Benjamin M. Spock, M.D. Revised edition of the child-care bible. Pocket Books, 1997, $7.99.

■ *You and Your Adolescent: A Parents' Guide for Ages 10 to 20,* by Laurence Steinberg, Ph.D., and Ann Levine. HarperPerennial, 1997, $15.

■ *Your Baby and Child: From Birth to Age 5,* by Penelope Leach. Alfred A. Knopf, 1997, $20.

■ *What to Expect: The First Year,* by Arlene Eisenberg, Heidi Murkoff, and Sandee E. Hathaway. Workman, 1996, $14.95.

■ *What to Expect: The Toddler Years,* by Arlene Eisenberg, Heidi Murkoff, and Sandee E. Hathaway. Workman, 1996, $15.95.

Food and Health

Organization: Weight-control Information Network, 1 Win Way, Bethesda, MD 20892-3665. 800-946-8098, M–F 8:30–5 EST; *www.niddk.nih.gov/health/ nutrit/win.htm*. At Website, click on *Publications* and then on *Helping Your Overweight Child*. Call or write for reports on childhood obesity.

Website: Johns Hopkins University Cardiovascular Health Promotion for Children, *www.jhbmc.jhu.edu/cardiology/partner ship/kids/kids.html*. Offers heart-healthy tips, research data, and links.

Book: *Feeding Your Child for Lifelong Health: Birth Through Age 6,* by Susan B. Roberts, Ph.D., and Melvin B. Heyman, M.D. Bantam Doubleday Dell, 1999, $15.95.

Mental Health

Organizations: The American Academy of Child and Adolescent Psychiatry, 3615 Wisconsin Ave. NW, Washington, DC 20016-3007. 202-966-7300, 8:30–5 EST; *www.aacap.org*. At Web site, click on *Facts for Families and Other Resources*, then on *Facts for Families*, for fact sheets on child-hood psychiatric issues.

■ National Clearinghouse on Family Support and Children's Mental Health, Portland State University, P.O. Box 751, Portland, OR 97207-0751. 800-628-1696, 24-hour recording. Sends reports on many emotional issues children face.

■ Parents Anonymous, 675 West Foothill Blvd., Suite 220, Claremont, CA 91711. 909-621-6184, M–F 8–4:30 PST; *www.parentsanonymous-natl.org*. Lists resources and support groups for parents who want to break cycles of abuse.

■ Parents Leadership Institute, Box 50492, Palo Alto, CA 94303. 650-322-5323, 24-hour recording; *www.parent leaders.org*. Ask about workshops, publications, and videos. Brochure series Listening to Children includes "Crying," "Healing Children's Fears," and "Reaching for Your Angry Child."

Book: *Growing Up Sad: Childhood Depression and Its Treatment,* by Leon Cytryn, M.D., and Donald H. McKnew, M.D. W. W. Norton, 1998, $13.95.

CHILDREN'S HEALTH

General Problems

Anemia
www.SavonAnemia.com

SIGNS AND SYMPTOMS

Main symptoms:
- Feeling tired and weak.
- Pasty skin; pale gums, nail beds, and eyelid linings.
- Shortness of breath, dizziness, and fainting.
- Headaches and trouble focusing.

Iron deficiency anemia:
Main symptoms, plus:
- Brittle nails.
- Black or bloody stools from bleeding in the intestines.

Folic acid deficiency anemia:
Main symptoms, plus:
- Sore mouth and tongue.
- Loss of appetite.
- Swollen abdomen.
- Nausea and diarrhea.

Vitamin B12 deficiency anemia:
Main symptoms, plus:
- Sore mouth and tongue.
- Problems with walking and balance.
- Tingling in hands and feet.
- Memory loss and confusion.

If you are anemic, your blood has trouble carrying oxygen to your tissues and taking away carbon dioxide. You become anemic either because you don't have enough red blood cells or because your red blood cells lack a protein that lets them carry oxygen. There are many kinds of anemia.

Women who have heavy menstrual flow, or who are pregnant or nursing, may get **iron deficiency anemia.** It is most often handled with iron supplements. But if the anemia stems from ailments that cause blood loss, such as **ulcers** (see page 134) or stomach or colon cancer, the problem behind it needs to be treated.

Lack of folic acid, a vitamin needed to make red blood cells, can cause **folic acid deficiency anemia.** Teens, pregnant women, smokers, alcoholics, and people who don't eat well are at risk.

Vitamin B12 deficiency anemia (the most common type is called pernicious anemia) may affect the brain, spinal cord, and mental functions for life. In the United States, B12 anemia is rarely caused by a lack of B12 in the diet. Instead, it most often comes on if you're unable to absorb the vitamin from food—a problem that can be genetic. Conditions such as **inflammatory bowel disease** (see page 128) also can reduce absorption of B12.

A rare form, **aplastic anemia,** isn't related to diet; it can be caused by a virus or by radiation, powerful medicines, or toxins such as benzene.

Anemia can sometimes be a sign of leukemia, lymphoma (cancer in the lymph system), chronic kidney disease, or other chronic ailments.

WHAT YOU CAN DO NOW

If you think you have anemia, call your doctor. **Note:** Don't take over-the-counter iron pills. Too much iron can cause symptoms like those of anemia and make you feel worse, and may make it hard to tell what's really wrong.

Fever

The average body temperature is 98.6 degrees, but some people have higher or lower normal levels. Temperatures also tend to rise as the day goes on. In adults, a fever is a temperature of 100 or above. An oral reading will do for anyone over age 5; you'll need a rectal reading for children 5 and under. Call your doctor for advice if you see a temperature of 100.4 in infants under 3 months, 102 rectal in children 3 months through 5 years old or 102 oral in children over 5, or 104 in adults. Many of us try to detect a fever by feeling the forehead, but that isn't the best way. Use a thermometer (see **how to take a temperature** and **fever in children,** page 255).

SYMPTOMS	WHAT IT MIGHT BE	WHAT YOU CAN DO
Fever after some hours in a hot place, no sweating, rapid heartbeat, confusion, loss of consciousness.	Heatstroke (see page 38).	Call 911 or go to emergency room **right away.**
Fever with very painful headache, stiff neck, nausea, aversion to light, drowsiness, confusion, red or purple rash (sometimes).	Meningitis (see page 55).	Call 911 or go to emergency room **right away.**
Fever and stiff jaw, muscle spasms and pain, sweating, trouble swallowing.	Tetanus (sometimes called lockjaw)—bacterial infection from a wound.	Call 911 or go to emergency room **right away.**
Sudden, high fever; vomiting and diarrhea; red rash; fatigue; headache, confusion, and dizziness.	Toxic shock syndrome (see page 243).	Call 911 or go to emergency room **right away.**
In children: fever, sudden seizures; turning blue in face (maybe).	Fever seizure (see fever in children, page 255, and fever seizures box, page 256).	If seizure is severe or lasts more than a few minutes, call 911 or go to emergency room **right away.** Otherwise, lay child on side or stomach, away from sharp objects. Most often harmless.
Rapid onset of fever, chills, pounding heart, confusion, signs of infection.	Blood poisoning (see box on page 29).	Call doctor **right away;** if you can't get one, call 911 or go to emergency room.
Low fever, pain in lower right part of abdomen, nausea and vomiting.	Appendicitis (see page 24).	Call doctor for prompt appointment. Meanwhile, don't eat or take laxatives; surgery may be needed.

(continued)

GENERAL PROBLEMS

Fever (continued)

SYMPTOMS	WHAT IT MIGHT BE	WHAT YOU CAN DO
Low fever at first, higher 1–3 weeks later; pain in lower pelvis; foul discharge from vagina; painful urination.	Pelvic inflammatory disease (see page 236).	Call doctor for prompt appointment.
Fever and cough with or without sputum; chest pain; shortness of breath.	Pneumonia (see page 97).	Call doctor for prompt appointment.
Sudden onset of fever and sore throat with white coating on tonsils; bright red rash about 24 hours later.	Scarlet fever (see page 266).	Call doctor for prompt appointment.
Fevers, night sweats, swollen lymph nodes, repeat infections, weight loss, fatigue, diarrhea, sores.	HIV infection. ■ AIDS.	Call doctor for advice and testing appointment.
Low fever, nausea or loss of appetite, yellowish skin or eyes (jaundice), dark urine, light-colored stools, fatigue.	Hepatitis (see page 279).	Call doctor for advice and appointment.
Fatigue lasting weeks or months, bad sore throat, fever, swollen lymph glands.	Mononucleosis—viral illness spread by close contact such as kissing; attacks breathing system, liver, spleen, and lymph glands; most common in teens and young adults.	Call doctor for advice and appointment. Getting well takes 10 days to 6 months. Go back to normal activities over time.
Persistent low fever; coughing, sometimes with bloody sputum; chest pain; weight loss; heavy night sweats.	Tuberculosis.	Call doctor for advice and appointment.
High fever (over 103), weakness, headache, chills, raw throat, dry cough, runny nose, aching muscles.	Flu (see page 95).	Call doctor for advice. In children, fever of 102 or higher may be risky.
In children: fever with dry cough, loud breathing, runny nose, red eyes, blisters, swelling, or rash.	Any of many childhood diseases (see children's health chapter, page 246).	See fever in children, page 255.

WHEN TO CALL THE DOCTOR

Call 911 or go to an emergency room **right away:**

➤ If, after taking iron pills, you get bloody diarrhea, fever, fatigue, vomiting, or seizures. Too much iron in your system can be fatal.

Call for advice:

➤ If you have symptoms of anemia.

➤ If you are being treated for diet-related anemia and don't get better in 2 weeks.

HOW TO PREVENT IT

To get enough iron:

➤ Eat plenty of iron-rich foods, including potatoes, broccoli, raisins, beans, oatmeal, and blackstrap molasses.

➤ Include lean red meat, liver, and shellfish in your diet.

➤ Don't drink coffee or tea with meals. They contain a substance that makes it hard for your body to absorb iron.

To get enough folic acid:

➤ Eat plenty of citrus fruits (grapefruit, oranges), beans, and green vegetables.

➤ Include liver, eggs, and milk in your diet.

➤ If you drink alcohol, drink just a little—no more than 2 drinks a day for men, 1 for women. (A drink is a 12-ounce beer, a 5-ounce glass of wine, or a 1.5-ounce shot of hard liquor.) Alcohol can affect how well your body absorbs folic acid.

➤ If you're pregnant or nursing, or if you have very heavy periods, discuss your diet with your doctor.

To get enough vitamin B12:

➤ Include meat, chicken, fish, and dairy products in your diet. Buy cereals with added B12.

FOR MORE HELP

Key Websites: *www.SavonHealth.com*. For more information on anemia: *www.SavonAnemia.com*.

Organization: National Heart, Lung, and Blood Institute Information Center, 31 Center Dr., MSC 2480, Room 4A21, Bethesda, MD 20892-2480. 301-592-8573, M–F 8:30–5 EST; *www.nhlbi.nih.gov*. Staff answers questions and sends brochures about anemia.

Chronic Fatigue Syndrome
www.SavonCFS.com

SIGNS AND SYMPTOMS

■ Flulike symptoms; severe fatigue that lasts longer than 6 months and is not caused by work or exercise.

■ Weakness and fatigue that last for more than 24 hours after mild exercise (sometimes fatigue occurs 1 or 2 days later).

■ Sore throat.

■ Low fever (temperature as high as 101 degrees) or chills.

■ Painful lymph nodes.

■ Headaches of a new type, pattern, or severity.

■ Pains that spread to joints without causing redness or swelling.

■ Short-term blind spots and trouble looking at light.

■ Trouble thinking or staying focused; forgetting things; being moody and confused.

■ Trouble sleeping.

Little is known about chronic fatigue syndrome (CFS). Its causes are unclear, and it is diagnosed by ruling out other diseases. But researchers are beginning to untangle some aspects of it. CFS strikes people of all ages and races, and of both sexes, although most people diagnosed with it are women. There's no proof that you can catch it from other people.

The pain, fatigue, and problems with thinking that mark the ailment often keep people out of work or school. This can lead to depression. Symptoms often ease up or go away after a number of months or years, but they may come and go indefinitely.

Treatment stresses plenty of rest, gentle exercise, and a healthful diet. Drugs such as antidepressants and over-the-counter pain relievers can help ease some symptoms. Also, medicines that target some of the underlying problems are being tested.

Fibromyalgia

Fibromyalgia may come with chronic fatigue syndrome and is sometimes confused with it. Symptoms include pain in muscles, tendons, and ligaments (though not in joints), fatigue, and sleep problems. Unlike chronic fatigue syndrome, fibromyalgia can be spotted with the "18 Tender Points" test, which applies pressure to 18 body parts. Tenderness in at least 11 often means fibromyalgia.

Fibromyalgia tends to affect women between the ages of 20 and 50, although people of both sexes and all ages get it. It may be present all the time or it may run in 3- or 4-day cycles. Symptoms are treated with antidepressants, painkillers, and muscle relaxants. Frequent exercise also may help relieve pain.

For more help: Fibromyalgia Network, 800-853-2929, M–F 8–4 PST. Call for names of doctors, a list of support groups in your area, and a newsletter.

WHAT YOU CAN DO NOW

➤ Take over-the-counter painkillers, such as ibuprofen, for muscle aches and headaches (see **pain relief** box, page 315).

➤ Stay active, but don't become overtired.

➤ Join a support group for people with chronic pain or depression.

WHEN TO CALL THE DOCTOR

➤ If you have fatigue that won't go away and other symptoms of CFS.

➤ If you feel new symptoms after you have been diagnosed.

HOW TO PREVENT IT

There is no known way to prevent chronic fatigue syndrome.

FOR MORE HELP

Key Websites: *www.SavonHealth.com*. For more information on chronic fatigue syndrome: *www.SavonCFS.com*.

Organizations: American Chronic Pain Association, P.O. Box 850, Rocklin, CA 95677. 916-632-0922, 24-hour line; *www.theacpa.org*. Call for information and a list of support groups run by and for people who have chronic pain.

■ Centers for Disease Control and Prevention, 1600 Clifton Rd., Atlanta, GA 30333. Voice Information System, 888-232-3228, 24-hour recording; *www.cdc.gov/ncidod/diseases/cfs/cfshome.htm*. Offers data on current research on and treatments for chronic fatigue syndrome.

■ Chronic Fatigue and Immune Dysfunction Syndrome Association of America, P.O. Box 220398, Charlotte, NC 28222. 800-442-3437, 24-hour recording, or 704-365-2343, M–Th 9–5, F 9–1 EST; *www.cfids.org*. Sends information, a newsletter, notices of forums for patients, and a list of local support groups.

■ National Institute of Allergy and Infectious Diseases Communications Department, National Institutes of Health, 301-496-5717, M–F 8:30–5 EST; *www.niaid.nih.gov/publications*. Staff members answer questions by phone. At Website, click on *Chronic Fatigue Syndrome*.

Books: *Alternative Medicine Guide: Chronic Fatigue, Fibromyalgia & Environmental Illness*, by Burton Goldberg. Physicians discuss the techniques and natural substances that helped their patients. Future Medicine, 1998, $18.95.

■ *Osler's Web*, by Hillary Johnson. Explores the history of chronic fatigue syndrome, and charges the medical world with ignoring the ailment. Crown, 1997, $15.95.

■ *Running on Empty*, 2nd edition, by Katrina Berne, Ph.D. Discusses how to cope with chronic fatigue syndrome. Hunter House, 1995, $14.95.

Diabetes
www.SavonDiabetes.com

SIGNS AND SYMPTOMS

- Extreme thirst and hunger.
- Need to urinate often, sometimes every hour.
- Weight loss for no known reason.
- Blurred vision.
- Lasting tiredness.
- In women: frequent yeast and bladder infections, sometimes missed menstrual periods.

Diabetes mellitus affects about 16 million people in the United States, yet perhaps only 2 out of 3 of them know they have it. *Mellitus,* from the Latin for "sweetened with honey," refers to having too much unused sugar in the blood.

People who have the most common type, which tends to show up in older adults, often think their symptoms are a result of aging or being overweight. As a result, they don't get the treatment they need. Untreated diabetes can cause severe problems, including stroke and heart attack, blindness, kidney trouble, nerve damage, and loss of limbs due to circulatory problems.

The two main types of diabetes are type 1 and type 2. Type 1 most often starts in childhood when the pancreas fails to make insulin, a hormone that converts sugar in the muscles to energy. People with type 1 diabetes need daily insulin shots.

About 90 percent of diabetes is type 2: The muscles can't use insulin even though the body may be making enough of it. People with type 2 may not need insulin shots.

Type 2 used to be called adult-onset diabetes because it mostly comes on after age 40. You're at risk if someone else in your family has type 2 diabetes. A high-fat diet, lack of exercise, and being overweight also raise the risk.

Some women get a kind of high blood sugar called gestational diabetes when they are pregnant. In most cases, it goes away once the baby is born.

Danger in the Medicine Cabinet

Some drugs can affect blood sugar levels, which people with diabetes need to track closely.

➤ Aspirin can lower blood sugar if taken in large amounts over a long period of time.
➤ Phenylephrine, epinephrine, and ephedrine—found in some asthma and cold medicines and even herbal teas—can raise blood sugar and blood pressure.
➤ Fish oil, which some people take to lower their cholesterol, may raise blood sugar.
➤ Caffeine, found in coffee, sodas, appetite suppressants, some headache drugs, "pep" pills, and diuretics, may also raise blood sugar.

While neither type 1 nor type 2 diabetes can be cured, you can manage either one quite well by watching your blood sugar levels and combining medicine, exercise, and a healthful diet.

WHAT YOU CAN DO NOW

➤ If you know you have diabetes, follow your doctor's advice about diet, exercise, and tracking your blood sugar levels.
➤ Keep a log to help manage your diabetes. For a month, record your blood sugar level many times each day, always at the same times (use a home glucose monitor). Also record when and what you eat at each meal; the type of exercise you do and for how long; and your times of low and high energy. Take this record to your doctor.
➤ Practice good foot care. Check your feet often for cuts and sores. Call your doctor if you think you have an infection.
➤ Get eye exams often.
➤ Eat a low-fat, low-cholesterol diet to keep your blood sugar and weight in check.
➤ Exercise often to help balance your blood sugar, control your weight, and cut your risk of heart disease. Ask your doctor how

GENERAL PROBLEMS

that works, and about the right way to balance your blood sugar with medicines.

➤ Wear a medical alert tag. Make sure the tag includes the type of diabetes you have.

➤ Stay in touch with your doctor and schedule visits with him or her often.

➤ If your blood sugar level drops too low, you may notice symptoms of hypoglycemia: confusion, dizziness, or weakness; sweating; shaking; hunger; headache; and blurred vision. As soon as you can, eat one of these: 4 ounces of fruit juice or a sugared drink; some candy, such as 6 or 7 jelly beans or 3 large marshmallows; 1 cup of skim milk; or half a tube of Glutose (80-gram size). If you don't feel better in a few minutes, eat one more portion. (Don't eat chocolate for quick sugar—the fat in it slows the rate at which sugar gets into your bloodstream.)

➤ If your blood sugar level rises too high, you may have hyperglycemia. Symptoms include blurred vision, thirst, hunger, and the need to urinate. Test your blood sugar level with your monitor. If it is much higher than your normal reading, call your doctor promptly.

WHEN TO CALL THE DOCTOR

Call 911 or go to an emergency room **right away:**

➤ If your stomach hurts, you are breathing quickly and urinating very often, you are tired and nauseated, and your breath is very sweet. You may have ketoacidosis, a sometimes fatal ailment.

➤ If you are extremely thirsty, tired, weak, and confused. You may have very high blood sugar levels that could lead to coma.

➤ If you are with a person known to have diabetes who loses consciousness.

Call for a prompt appointment:

➤ If you have symptoms of diabetes, or if your child does.

➤ If you have diabetes and you get the flu. Flu and some other illnesses can make your blood sugar levels go out of control.

➤ If you have any problems with your vision.

➤ If you notice swelling that is not normal, particularly in the legs.

➤ If you have painful urination or feel the urge to urinate often.

HOW TO PREVENT IT

There is no way to prevent type 1 diabetes. To prevent type 2 diabetes:

➤ Keep your weight within the healthy range for your age, height, and build.

➤ Exercise often. This is vital for preventing diabetes or for managing it once it occurs.

➤ Eat a high-fiber, low-fat diet, and don't eat large meals or skip meals.

➤ If you are over 40 and overweight, or have a family history of diabetes, get screened for diabetes every 1 to 3 years.

FOR MORE HELP

Key WebSites: *www.SavonHealth.com*. For more information about diabetes: *www.SavonDiabetes.com*.

Organizations: American Diabetes Association, 1701 N. Beauregard St., Alexandria, VA 22311. 800-342-2383, 8:30–8 EST; *www.diabetes.org*. Offers facts on how to manage diabetes and other brochures, and helps you find local diabetes groups.

■ Juvenile Diabetes Foundation, 120 Wall St., 19th Floor, New York, NY 10005-4001. 800-533-2873, M–F 9–5 EST; *www.jdf.org*. Lists local chapters that have free materials, and gives names of doctors near you.

■ National Diabetes Information Clearinghouse, 1 Information Way, Bethesda, MD 20892-3560. 301-654-3327, M–F 8:30–5 EST; *www.niddk.nih.gov/health/diabetes/diabetes.htm* for an online brochure on diabetes. Offers free printed information.

Books: *American Diabetes Association Complete Guide to Diabetes: The Ultimate Home Reference*, 2nd edition. Offers a wide range of information on how to manage diabetes, in an easy-to-read format. American Diabetes Association, 2000, $23.95.

■ *101 Nutrition Tips for People With Diabetes*, by Patti B. Geil, M.S., R.D. Gives advice on nutrition, weight loss, meal planning, and medication. American Diabetes Association, 1999, $15.

■ *The Type 2 Diabetic Woman*, by M. Sara Rosenthal. Focuses on how to work with your doctor, make lifestyle changes, and prevent long-term complications. Lowell House, 1999, $17.95.

Five Kinds of Viral Hepatitis

Type of hepatitis	How transmitted	People at risk	Incidence in United States	Risks	Vaccine available
A	Food, water, feces, sex.	Those exposed to poor sanitation.	50% of acute hepatitis cases.	Few long-term effects.	Yes.
B	IV drug use, blood, sex, body fluids.	IV drug users, people with multiple sex partners, health workers.	33% of acute hepatitis cases.	Can be chronic; increases risk of liver cancer.	Yes.
C	IV drug use, blood, sex.	Same as B.	15% of acute hepatitis cases.	High risk of chronic liver disease, cancer.	No.
D	Found only with B.	Same as B.	Not common.	May become chronic.	B vaccine prevents D as well.
E	Food, feces, water.	Travelers to Asia, India, and Africa.	Very rare.	High death rate for pregnant women.	No.

Hepatitis
www.SavonHepatitis.com

SIGNS AND SYMPTOMS

Note: Some forms of hepatitis produce no symptoms.
First symptoms are flulike:
- Fever and fatigue.
- Nausea, vomiting, loss of appetite.
- Pain in upper right side of the abdomen.

Other, less common symptoms:
- Dark urine; pale stools.
- Jaundice—yellowed eyes and skin.

Hepatitis means "inflammation of the liver." Certain viruses that target the liver are most often the cause. But it can be brought on—or made worse—by other diseases, poisons, and long-term alcohol or drug abuse.

Viral hepatitis, a worldwide health problem, is highly contagious. Symptoms can be mild or can lead to liver failure and death. It comes in 2 basic forms—oral and blood-borne—with several subtypes:

Oral—hepatitis types A and E. These are spread through feces, tainted food and water, or sex. They are common in places with poor water and toilet facilities. Hepatitis E, rare in the United States, is found mostly in Asia, India, and Africa, but A is common in the United States—1 in 3 Americans has had it.

These types come on quickly and may feel like a mild flu or make you very sick. Nearly everyone with A gets better and is then immune to it. The vaccine for A is advised for those who travel or live in areas with poor sanitation. Hepatitis E, for which there is no vaccine, can be fatal to pregnant women.

Blood-borne—hepatitis types B, C, and D. These are spread through body fluids in much the same way as HIV (the human immunodeficiency virus that causes AIDS) is—by intravenous needles, blood, and sexual contact. A person may have few or no symptoms when he or she is first infected, but these types of hepatitis can lead to lifelong problems or death. Most people who have blood-borne hepatitis remain able to pass the illness along for the rest of their lives, even if they have no symptoms.

Hundreds of millions of people worldwide carry hepatitis. Many get better, but several who get hepatitis B and more than 70 percent who get C have chronic illness. C is the leading reason for liver transplants in the United States. Hepatitis D infects only those who have B and makes it worse.

WHAT YOU CAN DO NOW

➤ Don't drink alcohol. Alcohol can damage a *healthy* liver; it's far worse for a sick one.
➤ Rest as much as you need to.
➤ Eat frequent small meals.
➤ Drink at least 8 glasses of water each day.
➤ Don't take aspirin or acetaminophen. Ask your doctor about **pain relief** (see box on page 315).
➤ Urge those close to you to be vaccinated. Tell sex partners you have hepatitis, and practice **safe sex** (see box on page 224).
➤ If you have chronic B or C, join a support group.

WHEN TO CALL THE DOCTOR

➤ If you have any of the less common symptoms listed on page 279.
➤ If you have been exposed to hepatitis.
➤ If you have had hepatitis and you start to have symptoms again.

HOW TO PREVENT IT

➤ Drink little or no alcohol: for men, no more than 2 drinks per day; for women, no more than 1. (A drink is a 12-ounce beer, a 5-ounce glass of wine, or a 1.5-ounce shot of hard liquor.)
➤ If you have a drinking problem or are an alcoholic, get help right away (see **alcohol abuse,** page 204).
➤ Hepatitis A and E:

■ Get a vaccination for hepatitis A if you plan to travel to a place where it is widespread or that has poor water or toilet facilities. It takes 2 to 4 weeks for the vaccine to take effect, but you can get faster-acting short-term shots.
■ While in areas with poor sanitation, drink only boiled or bottled fluids. Don't eat unpeeled or uncooked foods or shellfish, and don't use ice cubes.
■ Wash your hands with soap and water after using the toilet and before touching food.
■ If you are infected with A or E, don't prepare or touch other people's food. Take extra care to wash hands, clothing, and bedding.
➤ Hepatitis B, C, and D:
■ Get a vaccination for B if you have more than 1 sex partner, work in a health field, travel widely, or live with anyone who has B or who is from Asia (where it is widespread). Hepatitis B vaccine is now given at birth. It also protects against type D.
■ Use the same safeguards as for HIV: Practice safe sex. Don't share IV needles, manicuring tools, razors, toothbrushes, or other items that can collect or hold blood.
■ Insist on sterile needles for acupuncture, body or ear piercing, or tattoos.
■ If you are infected, take care not to spread hepatitis to others through your blood or body fluids. Tell sex partners about your illness, and practice safe sex.

FOR MORE HELP

Key Websites: *www.SavonHealth.com.* for more information on hepatitis: *www.SavonHepatitis.com.*

Organizations: American Liver Foundation, 75 Maiden Ln., Suite 603, New York, NY 10038. 800-223-0179, M–Th 9–7, F 9–5 EST; *www.liverfoundation.org.* Staff answers questions and sends brochures on hepatitis prevention and treatment.

■ Hepatitis B Foundation, 700 E. Butler Ave., Doylestown, PA 18901-2697. 215-489-4900, M–F 9–5 EST; *www.hepb.org.* Staff answers questions, suggests hepatitis support groups, and for a $35 donation sends a quarterly newsletter and directory of liver specialists.

■ Hepatitis Foundation International, 30 Sunrise Terr., Cedar Grove, NJ 07009-1423. 800-891-0707 or 973-239-1035 M–F 9–5 EST; *www.hepfi.org*. Counselors answer questions and mail information.

Website: HepNet, The Hepatitis Information Network, *www.hepnet.com*. Provides online reports on all types of hepatitis, answers to common questions, and links to other Websites.

Infections
www.SavonInfections.com

SIGNS AND SYMPTOMS

Main symptoms:
■ Fever higher than 100 degrees (oral thermometer reading) and/or chills and sweating.
■ Headache.
■ Muscle aches or soreness.
■ Fatigue.
■ Swollen lymph nodes (sometimes).
Intestinal infection:
■ Diarrhea.
■ Nausea and vomiting.
■ Abdominal cramps or gas pains.
■ Dehydration.
Respiratory infection:
■ Coughing and sneezing.
■ Sinus or chest pain, sore throat, congestion, and excess mucus.
■ Watery eyes.
Bladder infection:
■ Burning pain when you urinate; need to urinate often.
■ Bloody urine.
Infection of the mouth, ears, or eyes:
■ Pain or irritation in the affected area.
■ Swelling, tenderness, and/or redness that is not normal.
Joint infection:
■ Tenderness, redness, or pain and swelling in the joints, often in only one part of the body.

Germs get into our bodies in many ways: through torn skin, during sex, or from air, food, and water. Whether a germ is a bacterium, virus, or fungus, it tries to survive once it's inside your body. Viruses invade living cells and multiply. They may weaken the body's defenses for a time against more dire bacterial infections.

You feel sick in part because of your body's response. When your body senses an attack, your immune system releases antibodies and white blood cells to fight off the invaders. The white blood cells make chemical triggers; these cause the fevers that often come with infection. Some germs release toxins and steal nutrients from healthy cells. This assault also makes you feel sick.

In most cases, all your immune system needs to fight infection is for you to rest and maintain a healthy diet. For more stubborn infections, germ-destroying drugs will help. Sometimes, your body will recall an earlier bout with an ailment such as measles, mumps, or chicken pox. If your body meets the same germ again, it is quite often able to ward off a new attack. This is what gives you immunity. Vaccines also can offer immunity to some infections.

For infected wounds, see **cuts, scrapes, and wounds,** page 28.

WHAT YOU CAN DO NOW

➤ If you are in good health, let a low fever run its course. A fever under 104 degrees (oral thermometer reading) in adults, 102 (oral) in children, and 100.4 (rectal) in infants under 3 months is seldom risky and may speed recovery from infection.
➤ Give your body a chance to get better. Rest, drink lots of water, and eat well. Don't drink alcohol or smoke.

WHEN TO CALL THE DOCTOR

Call for advice and an appointment:
➤ If you are over 65 and in poor health, and have symptoms of an infection.
➤ If your temperature rises to 104, or goes over 101 with joint pain; if a child's rises to 102 (oral) or an infant's to 100.4 (rectal).
➤ If you have symptoms of severe infection, such as problems speaking, seeing, swallowing, breathing, or moving.
➤ If your skin has been broken by a human or animal bite.
➤ If your throat is sore, or if you're vomiting or have diarrhea that doesn't go away after

(continued on page 284)

GENERAL PROBLEMS

Sudden Weight Gain or Loss

Your weight changes slightly from day to day even when you eat normal amounts of food. Dieting or overeating can, of course, cause greater weight changes. But not all changes come from gains or losses of fat. You might lose several pounds of fluid in a single day from sweating if you're doing hard work. Changes in hormone levels during the menstrual cycle, or eating a lot of salty food, can make your body hold fluids (often signaled by puffy hands and ankles) and may cause you to gain several pounds in a short time. Many medicines can cause loss of appetite and loss of weight. So can depression. But weight gain or loss for no known reason can be a sign of a hidden disease—such as those listed here. If you gain or lose more than 10 to 15 pounds in a month and you don't know why, call your doctor for advice and an appointment.

WEIGHT GAIN

SYMPTOMS	WHAT IT MIGHT BE	WHAT YOU CAN DO
Rapid weight gain with swelling in legs, ankles, and midriff; fatigue; yellowed skin; easy bruising and bleeding; impotence; dark urine; black or bloody stools; blood in vomit.	Cirrhosis—liver damage. May be caused by alcohol abuse, hepatitis (see page 279), or a disease passed on in your genes.	If you vomit blood, call 911 or go to emergency room **right away.** Otherwise, call doctor for prompt appointment.
Weight gain with swelling in legs, ankles, and midriff; shortness of breath; fatigue; need to urinate often; loss of appetite.	Congestive heart failure (see page 109). ■ Kidney disease.	If you have severe chest pain or shortness of breath, call 911 or go to emergency room **right away.** Otherwise, call doctor for prompt appointment.
Slow weight gain with swollen face, fat on torso and upper back; fatigue; acne; reddish skin; trouble sleeping. In men: impotence, breast growth. In women: facial hair, periods that slow or stop.	Cushing's syndrome—adrenal glands make too much of a stress hormone that affects connective tissue. Most often caused by taking corticosteroids for rheumatoid arthritis, asthma, or other illnesses.	Call doctor for advice.
Slow weight gain, fatigue, dry skin, goiter (swelling in neck).	Underactive thyroid gland (see thyroid problems, page 288).	Call doctor for advice.

Sudden Weight Gain or Loss

WEIGHT LOSS

SYMPTOMS	WHAT IT MIGHT BE	WHAT YOU CAN DO
Rapid weight loss, fatigue, extreme thirst, frequent urination, infections in vagina.	Diabetes (see page 277).	Call doctor for advice and appointment.
Rapid weight loss despite increased appetite, anxiety, sweating, rapid heartbeat, goiter (swelling in neck).	Overactive thyroid gland (see thyroid problems, page 288).	Call doctor for prompt appointment.
Weight loss, fatigue, vomiting, diarrhea, darkened skin, hair loss, feeling cold, big mood changes (confusion, aggression, or depression).	Addison's disease—adrenal glands make too little of the hormones that control metabolism and responses to stress. Very rare.	Call doctor for prompt appointment.
Slow weight loss, fevers, night sweats, swollen lymph nodes, repeat infections, fatigue, diarrhea, sores.	HIV infection. ■ AIDS.	Call doctor for advice and testing appointment.
Weight loss with changes or lumps in skin, bleeding that is not normal, digestive problems, changes in bowel or bladder habits.	Cancer—unchecked growth of cells. Symptoms vary with type of cancer.	Call doctor for advice and appointment.
Weight loss and diarrhea; fatigue; gas and stomach pains; bulky, frothy, foul-smelling stools.	Malabsorption—intestines fail to absorb one or more nutrients from food.	Call doctor for advice and appointment if symptoms last longer than a few days.
Extreme weight loss from not eating, compulsive exercising, menstrual periods that slow or stop, depression (in anorexia). Extreme weight loss from binge eating and vomiting (in bulimia).	Eating disorder.	See eating disorders, page 216.

GENERAL PROBLEMS

(continued from page 281)
a few days.

➤ If you have symptoms of a bladder infection, such as painful urination.

HOW TO PREVENT IT

➤ Keep your immune system strong:
- Eat well. Drink plenty of fluids.
- Exercise often.
- Get enough sleep.
- Don't smoke or use drugs.
- If you drink alcohol, do so lightly—no more than 2 drinks a day for men and 1 for women. (A drink is a 12-ounce beer, a 5-ounce glass of wine, or a 1.5-ounce jigger of hard liquor.)
- Take steps to reduce stress in your life; stress weakens the immune system. Try meditation, yoga, or deep breathing.

➤ Get a flu shot before each flu season.

➤ Ask your doctor about getting immunized against pneumonia.

➤ Have your children vaccinated against childhood diseases (see **children's immunization** chart, page 250).

➤ Wash your hands very often with plain soap and warm water, and avoid putting your fingers in your mouth or rubbing your eyes.

➤ Practice **safe sex** (see box on page 224).

➤ Women who have their periods should change tampons at least every 6 hours to keep harmful bacteria from growing (see **toxic shock syndrome,** page 243).

➤ Watch out for changes in your body—from swelling around nicks and cuts to a runny nose or genital discharge. Attend to symptoms right away.

Lupus
www.SavonLupus.com

SIGNS AND SYMPTOMS

- Butterfly-shaped rash across the nose and cheeks.
- Aching, swollen joints.
- Fever over 100 degrees.
- Long-lasting fatigue.
- Sores in the nose, mouth, or throat.
- Unusual bleeding or bruising.
- Numbness in the fingers and toes.
- Swollen abdomen and ankles (sometimes).
- Dark urine.
- Chest pain when breathing deeply.
- Sensitivity to sunlight; a rash that results after time spent in the sun.
- Mental or personality changes, including depression.

When you have lupus, your body's immune system attacks proteins in your tissues as if they were invaders. This war in your body causes swelling and pain, most often in the joints. It may also inflame the kidneys, skin, and lining of the lungs, heart, and brain, and it may damage white blood cells. When it is severe and untreated, lupus can lead to kidney failure. A person with lupus may also become depressed.

The disease is chronic—it can last for the rest of your life, with symptoms that come and go—but it may lie low for a long time between flare-ups or even subside completely.

Why the body attacks itself in this way is unknown. It is known that lupus can be triggered by infections, ultraviolet or fluorescent light, and certain drugs, such as some used to treat high blood pressure.

Lupus most often strikes people between 35 and 45, women almost 10 times more often than men. It's most common among African Americans, and it runs in families.

The long-term outlook for people with lupus has improved in recent years. Now 80 to 90 percent can expect to have long and healthy lives with early treatment, including drugs to ease symptoms, as well as changes in diet, exercise, and mental outlook.

WHAT YOU CAN DO NOW

➤ Get lots of rest if you're tired. Take naps when you're having a flare-up.

➤ When the disease is low-level and not causing you pain, and you feel well, start an exercise program. Swimming is one good way for people with lupus to keep their muscles in shape.

➤ Put warm compresses on achy joints.

➤ For pain, take aspirin or ibuprofen—with meals to avoid stomach upset (see **pain relief,** page 315).

➤ Sunlight alone can cause a flare-up in some people. Avoid the sun during the middle of the day. Half an hour before leaving home each day, apply a sunscreen with an SPF of at least 15.

➤ Eat well—stick to a diet that's low in fat and salt, high in complex carbohydrates and calcium.

➤ Wear gloves to protect your hands from anything that may cause pain.

➤ Avoid alcohol, tobacco, and caffeine.

WHEN TO CALL THE DOCTOR

Call for emergency advice (if you can't get any, call 911 or go to an emergency room):

➤ If you have symptoms of kidney disease: frequent urination; swollen ankles; shortness of breath; nausea and vomiting; chest and bone pain; itching, bruising, or bleeding; confusion; loss of consciousness.

Call for advice:

➤ If you have symptoms of lupus.

➤ If you know that you have lupus and your symptoms get worse or change.

FOR MORE HELP

Key Websites: *www.SavonHealth.com*. For more information about lupus: *www.SavonLupus.com*.

Organizations: Lupus Foundation of America, 1300 Piccard Dr., Suite 200, Rockville, MD 20850-4303. 800-558-0121, 24-hour recording; *www.lupus.org*. Sends a packet with brochures on lupus and a list of chapters with support groups near you.

■ National Institute of Arthritis and Musculoskeletal and Skin Diseases Information Clearinghouse, 1 AMS Circle, Bethesda, MD 20892-3675. 301-495-4484 or 877-22-NIAMS, M–F 8:30–5 EST; *www. nih.gov/niams*. Request a packet of recent articles on lupus or a free copy of the patient information book *Lupus*.

Website: Hamline University Lupus Home Page, *www.hamline.edu/lupus/index.html*. Offers reports on lupus and lists conferences

and other sources of help.

Books: *The Lupus Book: A Guide for Patients and Their Families,* by Daniel J. Wallace, M.D. Explains lupus and how to cope with it. Oxford University Press, 2000, $25.

■ *The Lupus Handbook for Women,* by Robin Dibner, M.D., and Carol Colman. Fireside, 1994, $11.

Lyme Disease
www.SavonLymeDisease.com

SIGNS AND SYMPTOMS

■ Rash in a bull's-eye shape, often with pale center, from a tick bite 2 days to a month before. The rash may last 2 to 4 weeks or longer. (Some people don't see a rash.)

■ Within a month, aching joints and muscles, weakness, fever, chills, sore throat, headache.

■ After a few weeks or a few months, paralysis of the face, stiff neck, sensitivity to light, uneven heartbeats, and fainting.

■ Joint pain and swelling.

Lyme disease, a bacterial infection spread by tick bites, can be a long illness. More than 10,000 people get it each year.

The ticks pick up the bacteria from mice, deer, and other animals. The tick, often as small as a poppy seed, must remain attached to a person for 36 to 48 hours to transmit the bacteria, which can then invade the skin, nervous system, heart, and joints.

Lyme disease can be hard to diagnose. Its symptoms seem like those of other illnesses, and the blood test can't always be counted on (a new, more accurate blood test is being studied). If untreated, the infection can lead to nerve problems, a type of arthritis, and heart troubles such as uneven heartbeat.

The good news is that the illness can be prevented, responds well to treatment in the early stages, and sometimes goes away by itself. There is a vaccine, too, which should be considered for adults who live in tick-infested areas. Treatments include antibiotics and, if arthritis develops, corticosteroids for inflamed and painful joints.

GENERAL PROBLEMS

WHAT YOU CAN DO NOW

After a walk in the woods or through dense grass, check your clothing and skin for ticks. If you find one on you:

➤ Pull it out right away. Using tweezers, grab it as near to your skin as you can. Then pull up with slow, even pressure to remove the entire tick. Don't squeeze or twist the tick; this may spread bacteria into your skin or blood (see **tick bites,** page 45).

➤ Drop the tick in a jar of rubbing alcohol to save it for tests.

➤ Clean the bite with alcohol. Wash your hands in soap and water.

➤ Don't try to dislodge a tick with kerosene, petroleum jelly, or a lighted cigarette or match. None of these methods works.

WHEN TO CALL THE DOCTOR

➤ If you've been in tick country or you've been bitten by a tick, and you have symptoms of Lyme disease.

➤ If your symptoms return after treatment.

HOW TO PREVENT IT

➤ Wear light-colored clothes in grassy or wooded areas to make ticks easy to spot. Wear shoes (not sandals), long pants, and long-sleeved shirts. Pull your socks up over your pant legs.

➤ Use an insect spray with DEET on clothing. Use just a little on skin.

➤ Check your skin, hair, and clothing for ticks after an outing; check your pets, too.

➤ Fit your pet with a tick-repellent collar.

➤ Clear away brush near your home that might attract ticks. Stack your firewood away from the house (woodpiles attract mice, which carry ticks).

➤ Ask your doctor about a vaccine.

FOR MORE HELP

Key Websites: *www.SavonHealth.com*. For more information on lyme disease: *www.SavonLymeDisease.com*.

Organizations: American Lyme Disease Foundation, 293 Route 100, Somers, NY 10589.

800-876-5963, 24-hour recording, or 914-277-6970, M–F 9–5 EST; *www.aldf.com*. Offers a list of doctors and free brochures on Lyme disease and tick control.

■ Arthritis Foundation, 1330 W. Peachtree St., Atlanta, GA 30309. 800-283-7800, 24-hour recording; *www.arthritis.org*. Offers a free brochure on Lyme disease and a list of local arthritis support groups.

Book: *Coping With Lyme Disease*, by Denise Lang and Joseph Territo, M.D. Gives advice on how to live with Lyme disease, explores treatments, and lists support groups. Henry Holt, 1997, $14.95.

Sleep Disorders

www.SavonSleepDisorders.com

SIGNS AND SYMPTOMS

Insomnia:
■ Trouble falling asleep.
■ Waking often during the night.
■ Early waking.
■ Being sleepy often during the day.
■ Trouble staying focused.

Obstructive sleep apnea:
■ Loud bursts of snoring and gasping that jerk the sleeper (as well as anyone sleeping nearby) awake.
■ Morning headaches.
■ Daytime sleepiness with trouble staying focused.
■ Short temper, bad moods.

Narcolepsy:
■ Falling asleep all of a sudden and with no control in the daytime.
■ Sudden loss of muscle control triggered by strong emotion or fatigue.
■ Vivid dreams or visions when falling asleep or waking up.
■ Fatigue.

Restless legs syndrome:
■ Creepy, crawly, or painful feelings in the legs, most often when trying to fall asleep or during sleep.
■ Constant urge to move feet and legs.
■ Jerking of legs (and sometimes arms) that you can't control.

Sleep disorders range from mild insomnia to severe sleep apnea. They affect as many as 70 million Americans.

Short-term insomnia is chiefly caused by stress, emotional upset, hormone fluctuations, or a change in schedule. Long-term trouble with sleep may be a sign of a medical problem, such as **thyroid problems** (see page 288), **chronic bronchitis** or **emphysema** (see page 91), **Parkinson's disease** (see page 57), **Alzheimer's disease** (see page 48), **alcohol abuse** (see page 204), or **drug abuse** (see page 213). Another major cause is **depression** (see page 211). Treating the basic ailment, and creating restful bedtime routines, can often help.

Obstructive sleep apnea is most common among overweight men who sleep on their backs. The muscles in the throat sag, briefly closing off the airway. The effort to catch a breath wakes the sleeper. This process goes on all night long. People with sleep apnea don't get enough deep sleep and feel tired during the day. Obstructive sleep apnea can cause serious health problems over time, including heart disease. People deprived of sleep may become depressed or have other personality changes.

People with **narcolepsy** may fall deeply asleep almost anywhere, anytime. Not much is known about the ailment, but it seems to run in families. It can be treated with prescribed stimulants and antidepressants.

People with **restless legs syndrome** are bothered by odd feelings, most often in the legs, at night when they are still awake or trying to fall asleep, or even after they've been asleep for a while. Those with this ailment may feel tired the next day, especially if they can't get back to sleep or if they get out of bed and walk around to relieve discomfort. No one knows what causes restless legs syndrome, but it, too, seems to run in families.

WHAT YOU CAN DO NOW

Insomnia:
- ➤ Follow a calming bedtime routine: Drink warm milk, listen to soothing music, or read a book.
- ➤ Use your bed only for sleep and sex, not for working or watching TV.
- ➤ Don't thrash. If you can't fall asleep, get up and read until you feel sleepy.

Catching Up to Jet Lag

When you change time zones quickly, your sleeping patterns are out of sync with the local time. Jet lag can leave you drowsy and confused.

If you will be staying more than 2 days in a new place, you can avoid many of the symptoms. (It's hard to adjust on trips of 2 days or less.) Here's what to do:
- ➤ A few days to a week before leaving, adjust your schedule to the new time zone. Get up and go to bed as if you were already there.
- ➤ If you arrive in the daytime, spend some time outdoors. The sunlight helps reset your inner clock.
- ➤ Avoid alcohol, caffeine, rich and sweet foods, and too much talking before bed. All can keep you awake.
- ➤ Bring earplugs and a blindfold to block out noises and lights when you're sleeping.
- ➤ Wake up at the right local time, even if your day's plans don't require it.

- ➤ If you have chronic insomnia, try sleep restriction: At first, allow yourself only 4 hours of sleep a night. Once you are able to sleep through 4 hours, slowly add 15 to 30 minutes until you reach your goal. Be sure to get up at the same time every day.

Obstructive sleep apnea:
- ➤ Sew a tennis ball into the back of your pajamas so you don't sleep on your back.
- ➤ For mild snoring, try an over-the-counter nasal strip, which widens your nostrils and eases breathing.
- ➤ Ask your dentist about a retainerlike device that moves your tongue and lower jaw forward. Or ask your doctor about a special device called CPAP (continuous positive airway pressure) that pumps air to you through a mask. Surgery is also an option.

Narcolepsy:
- ➤ Schedule one or more daytime naps at regular times.

Restless legs:

➤ Your doctor can prescribe a drug that may relieve the twitching and discomfort.

WHEN TO CALL THE DOCTOR

➤ If you notice symptoms of obstructive sleep apnea or narcolepsy, especially if you feel sleepy all the time.
➤ If you have had insomnia for more than 2 weeks.
➤ If you are taking prescription drugs. Some can cause insomnia.

HOW TO PREVENT IT

➤ Avoid drinks with caffeine for at least 6 hours before bedtime.
➤ Don't drink alcohol or smoke for at least 2 hours before bedtime.
➤ Exercise often, but not within 3 hours of bedtime.
➤ If you have sleep apnea and are overweight, lose the extra pounds.
➤ Make sure your bedroom is quiet and dark and has plenty of air.
➤ Don't take a nap in the late afternoon or early evening.
➤ Get up each day at the same time, no matter when you go to sleep.

WHAT YOU CAN DO NOW

Insomnia:

➤ Research shows the scent of lavender helps people sleep. Try a lotion or room spray.
➤ Valerian seems to ease mild insomnia. Take 300 to 400 milligrams before bedtime (look for products with 0.8 percent valerian extract). Results may take a week.
➤ Kava may help. Try a supplement with 30 to 50 percent kavalactones; take 150 to 300 mg an hour before bedtime.

FOR MORE HELP

Key Websites: *www.SavonHealth.com*. For more information on sleep disorders: *www.SavonSleepDisorders.com*.

Organizations: Narcolepsy Network, 10921 Reed Hartman Way, Suite 119, Cincinnati, OH 45242. 513-891-3522, M–F 8–2 EST;

www.narcolepsynetwork.org. Offers brochures and names of support groups.

■ National Sleep Foundation, 1522 K St. NW, Suite 500, Washington, DC 20005. 202-347-3471, M–F 9–5:30 EST; *www. sleepfoundation.org*. Write for free brochures on sleep disorders.

■ Restless Legs Syndrome Foundation, P.O. Box 7050, Dept. WWW, Rochester, MN 55902-2985. 507-287-6465, M–F 9–5 CST; *www.rls.org*. Send a 55-cent-stamped self-addressed envelope for a brochure on RLS.

Websites: National Center on Sleep Disorders Research, *www.nhlbi.nih.gov/about/ncsdr/index.htm*. Has a "Test Your Sleep I.Q." quiz, and lists publications and resources.

■ The Sleep Medicine Home Page, *www.cloud9.net:80/~thorpy*. Offers links to research centers and support groups.

■ The Sleep Well, *www.stanford.edu/~dement*. Offers tips for good sleep and a test to determine if you're sleep-deprived.

Books: *Say Good Night to Insomnia*, by Gregg D. Jacobs, Ph.D. Describes how to end insomnia in 6 weeks. Owl Books, 1999, $13.

■ *The Complete Idiot's Guide to Getting a Good Night's Sleep*, by Martin Moore-Ede, M.D., Ph.D., and Suzanne LeVerte. Covers simple ways to manage sleep disorders. Macmillan, 1998, $16.95.

Thyroid Problems
www.SavonThyroid.com

SIGNS AND SYMPTOMS

Hyperthyroidism:

■ Losing weight even though you want to eat more than ever.
■ Trembling hands.
■ Higher-than-normal blood pressure, faster heartbeat, anxiety, sweating.
■ Bulging, watery eyes.
■ Frequent bowel movements.
■ Lighter and less frequent menstrual periods.
■ Sometimes a goiter—swelling in the front of the neck.

Hypothyroidism:
- Low energy, slowed thinking.
- Weight gain for no reason.
- Feeling cold too easily; hands and fingers numb or tingling.
- Dry, thick, flaky skin and hair loss.
- Constipation.
- Heavier, longer menstrual periods.
- Sometimes a goiter—swelling in the front of the neck.

Thyroiditis:
- Pain in the front of the neck, either mild or sharp.
- Pain when swallowing or turning the head.
- Fever.

Your thyroid gland makes hormones that control how fast your body absorbs food and turns it into energy.

People with **hyperthyroidism** have a thyroid that makes too large a supply of hormones. One result is that some of their body's processes speed up. Graves' disease, the most common form, can be brought on by severe stress. Hyperthyroidism is 5 times more likely to strike women than it is men, and occurs most often in people 20 to 40.

People with **hypothyroidism** have a shortage of the hormones. Most people with this ailment—mainly women over 65—don't know they have it. Hypothyroidism can be caused by some drugs, or it can follow treatment for hyperthyroidism.

In **thyroiditis,** the body's own immune system attacks the thyroid, causing it to produce too much or too little of the hormones. Thyroiditis can follow a viral illness or pregnancy.

Most of these conditions can give rise to a goiter, which is a swelling of the thyroid gland. The goiter goes away with treatment.

Most thyroid problems can be treated. Some hyperthyroidism responds to drugs; sometimes doctors cut back hormones either with radioactive iodine or by removing part of the gland. Hypothyroidism is treated with hormone supplements. Thyroiditis often goes away on its own or after treatment with medications, including hormones.

WHAT YOU CAN DO NOW

➤ If you suspect you have a thyroid problem but aren't sure, think about whether you're taking an over-the-counter cold medicine or getting a lot of caffeine—for instance, drinking 10 cups of coffee a day. Either one can cause some of the symptoms of hyperthyroidism. If you stop the medicine or caffeine and still have symptoms, call your doctor.

➤ For thyroiditis, try aspirin and other over-the-counter pain relievers to ease pain (see **pain relief,** page 315).

WHEN TO CALL THE DOCTOR

➤ If you feel nervous, tremble (especially in your hands), lose weight, and have a rapid pulse. You could have an overactive thyroid gland.

➤ If you often feel cold, drowsy, and low on energy, and you gain weight. You could have an underactive thyroid gland.

➤ If you have symptoms of thyroiditis.

➤ If someone in your family has had a thyroid problem, tell your doctor when you have your next checkup.

HOW TO PREVENT IT

There is no known way to prevent thyroid problems.

FOR MORE HELP

Key Websites: *www.SavonHealth.com*. For more information on thyroid problems: *www.SavonThyroid.com*.

Organization: Thyroid Foundation of America, Ruth Sleeper Hall–RSL 350, 40 Parkman St., Boston, MA 02114-2698. 800-832-8321, 24-hour recording; *www.tsh.org*. Send a 55-cent-stamped self-addressed envelope with your questions.

Book: *Thyroid Disease: The Facts,* by R.I.S. Bayliss and M.G. Tunbridge. Covers thyroid disorders and lists support groups. Oxford University Press, 1999, $19.95.

GENERAL PROBLEMS

Staying Healthy

THE BIG QUESTION about taking good care of yourself is this: Who's in charge? Who makes the daily decisions about your health and well-being? The answer, of course, is you. Not that it's easy to do all you're supposed to do to stay healthy. How many of us really get up and move around briskly for half an hour at least 5 days a week? Who wants to give up ice cream forever?

One reason it's hard to follow the experts' advice is that you may not feel the lifesaving results for a long time. And while there's nothing wrong with trying to defend yourself against heart attacks, diabetes, and other ailments, there is more to life— there is also living well. This section of *The Sav-on Self-Care Advisor* gives you a blueprint for living long *and* well:

Eight Ways to Feel Your Best lays out a clear, complete plan of action for lifelong good health, based on the latest research.

Know Your Health Plan outlines what to expect from health insurance, if you have it, and what your plan expects from you.

How to Choose a Physician and **How to Choose a Natural Healer** suggest what to look for in a health care provider.

Helping Your Doctor Help You offers tactics for making sure that you and your doctor are full partners in your health care.

Your Personal Health Record shows how to set up a family health tree and keep track of the things you should know about.

Medicines: Playing It Safe shows, at a glance, common medications you shouldn't mix.

You'll probably see a number of good things you're doing now. And whatever else you choose to add from this feast of expert advice will only improve your chances of feeling your best.

Eight Ways to Feel Your Best

You get the most out of life when you're healthy, fit, and full of energy. It's easier to pull off than you might think. For all its complexity, the human body needs little special care. Of course, there are some obvious don'ts: Don't live on potato chips. Don't drink and drive. Don't let a plugged-in hair dryer drop into the tub while you bathe. But the key to feeling your best is to take charge of what you do every day—how much you move, what you eat, how you deal with stress. Experts can always argue over details (butter or margarine? mammograms starting at 40 or 50?), but the basics are well known and simple, and even the experts agree on them. When you follow these 8 proven steps, you not only enhance your prospects of a long and healthy life, you also add spring to your step.

1. **GET SOME EXERCISE.**

2. **MAINTAIN A HEALTHY WEIGHT.**

3. **EAT WELL.**

4. **PUT OUT THE SMOKE.**

5. **BE CAREFUL OUT THERE.**

6. **STAY INVOLVED.**

7. **RELAX.**

8. **TAKE CARE OF YOUR TEETH.**

Get Some Exercise

Our bodies were made to move—to walk and run, to climb and carry. Movement builds bones and muscles and keeps us feeling our best. Among the rewards of exercise:

More energy and a stronger heart. When you raise your heart rate often, you improve your body's ability to deliver oxygen to cells. This not only determines how much pep you have day to day, it also cuts your risk of heart disease.

A stronger immune system. In one study, women who began a program of brisk walking 45 minutes a day, 5 days a week, cut their risk of colds and flu in half. In another,

women who had been active through their 20s and 30s, 4 hours weekly, had a 60 percent lower risk of breast cancer than women of the same age who hadn't been active. Regular exercise may help fend off other types of cancer as well.

Less stress. Hundreds of studies have shown that regular doses of steady, rhythmic exercise—walking, running, or swimming, for example—cut anxiety. And after 10 weeks of workouts, these studies show, the calmer feeling starts to last from one day to the next. These same activities can also help boost your mood and ease bouts of the blues.

Greater strength. Any kind of exercise can maintain and even build muscle mass. Strength training combined with weight-bearing exercise, such as aerobics, climbing stairs (the real kind, not the low-impact stair steppers in gyms), jumping rope, or racket sports, is also an ideal bone-saving routine. Walking won't *build* bone, but it may slow bone loss. This is important for women at risk for thinning bones (osteoporosis).

One study found that men and women in their 80s doubled their strength after 10 weeks of workouts. Many got better at climbing stairs, and a few even replaced their walkers with canes.

Weight control. The more calories you burn with exercise, the fewer you store as fat. And as you replace fat with new muscle, you ratchet up the calories your body burns even while you're just sitting around. (Muscle burns more calories to maintain itself than fat does.)

A sharper mind. An active life preserves blood supply to the brain and boosts the brain chemicals we need to learn and remember. Active older people, for example, score better on tests of thinking skills than inactive older people.

But how much exercise, and what *kinds*, offer these glowing benefits? If you're out of shape, even a little bit helps—neighborhood strolls, walking the dog, weeding in the garden, taking the stairs instead of the elevator. The chart below can help you figure out how to build such life-giving spurts into your day-to-day life.

But for the *most* rewards, you'll need to do more. (See the next page for more details on how much exercise you need in order to get which benefits.) Start with a program of at least 3 20-minute workouts a week, then build from there. Work hard enough to get your heart beating faster and to feel your breathing quicken. Brisk walking, swimming, jogging, bicycling, and stair stepping are good choices. For added stress-reducing benefits, repeat a calming word or phrase, or even a prayer, as you go.

Twice-a-week strength training sessions might be the best exercise of all, say some experts. That's because they not only build new muscle, they also help you develop the balance, endurance, and confidence you need to keep active into old age. Work all the major muscle groups—in your back, chest, shoulders, arms, abdomen, hips, and thighs—either by using the weight machines you'll find in most gyms or by lifting hand and ankle weights at home. Do 2 sets of 10 to 12 repetitions of each exercise. How much weight is enough? Use about half the weight you can lift just once.

How to Extend Your Life—Without Workouts

You know the slightly winded feeling you get when you're rushing to catch a train or scrubbing a tough stain on the floor? That feeling means you're exercising hard enough to enjoy real health benefits—in numerical terms, burning 4.5 or more calories a minute if you weigh about 130 pounds or 6 calories a minute if you weigh about 180. (The heavier you are, the more calories an activity burns.)

Burn about 200 calories a day beyond your normal output by doing things like weeding or biking to work: You'll cut your risk of disease and live longer—without ever going near the gym. Not all household tasks qualify, though. Changing bed linens or putting on makeup, for instance, burns but 2.5 calories a minute; doing the dishes, just 2.3. Walking around the office (3.5) won't cut it either. The important thing is to get your heart rate up and breathe a little harder. When you vacuum, it won't count unless you're a whirling dervish. When you walk the dog, make sure the dog is trotting after *you*.

Here are the calories burned by
20 common activities.

CALORIES BURNED (10 MINUTES)*	WOMEN	MEN
Walking fast	45	60
Painting	45	60
Weeding	45	60
Passionate sex	45	60
Washing a car	45	60
Playing tag with a child	50	67
Cleaning gutters	50	67
Pushing a lawn mower	55	73
Square-dancing	55	73
Scrubbing floors	55	73
Hiking off-trail	60	80
Biking to work	60	80
Shoveling snow	60	80
Moving furniture	60	80
Walking up stairs	70	93
Cross-country skiing	80	106
Backpacking	80	106
Carrying a 2-year-old up stairs	80	106
Running to catch a plane	115	153
Running up stairs	150	200

Figures are for a 132-pound woman and a 176-pound man.

STAYING HEALTHY

Exercise: What You Get for What You Do

How much exercise do you need? It all depends on what you want. To cut the risk of heart disease, stroke, diabetes, and perhaps even some types of cancer, you barely need to work up a sweat. But if you want to do more—for instance, trim a few pounds and tighten up your torso—get ready to push harder. Here's what the latest studies say exercise has to offer—and what it takes to get there.

A LONGER LIFE

Every hour you're active, the experts say, adds one and a half hours to your life. But to ward off most of the major killers and perhaps osteoporosis, you don't have to kill yourself.

What it takes: Move around enough each day to burn at least 200 calories beyond your usual output—all told, about 30 minutes—by walking, gardening, climbing stairs, playing with the kids, lifting groceries, or getting "formal" exercise. Don't worry about how hard you're working; what matters is making exercise a part of your daily life.

What to expect: Nothing right away. The payoff—reduced risk of heart attack and many chronic diseases—doesn't come until later in life. Don't expect to see extra pounds melt away quickly. Over time you may slim down, but it will happen gradually.

BETTER HEALTH NOW

When you commit yourself to working out, you get more benefits more quickly—a boost in energy, a more robust immune system, a more relaxed outlook, lower blood pressure, and lower cholesterol levels.

What it takes: To notice quick health gains, you need to get your heart thumping hard enough so you're winded for at least 20 minutes at a stretch 3 times a week. Brisk walking, aerobics classes, fast dancing, running, swimming, or any other aerobic exercise will do the job.

What to expect: Fewer colds and bouts of flu. A better ratio of good to bad cholesterol. For people with high blood pressure, an average drop of 10 points. Most important, you'll look better and feel better, and you'll feel better about yourself.

READY-FOR-ANYTHING FITNESS

More vigorous exercise will help you maintain strength and vitality well into old age.

What it takes: Twenty minutes to an hour of walking, running, swimming, biking, or other aerobic activity 3 to 5 times a week. You need to drive your heart rate up to at least 60 percent of its maximum (220 minus your age). Add to that a twice-weekly program of floor exercises or strength training, plus stretching or yoga, to put your arms, abdomen, and legs through their paces.

What to expect: Greater strength, balance, flexibility, and endurance. Improved sports performance with fewer injuries and less soreness. The beginnings of a better body. And, for those who stay this fit for their whole lives, a slower decline in the immune system—the body's defense against invaders—which could help ward off infection and even cancer.

A SLEEKER PHYSIQUE

A weight-loss program that works must include both exercise and healthy eating. But if the formula sounds simple—cut the calories you take in and increase the calories you burn—in truth, it's hard to do.

What it takes: Set a goal of 60 minutes total of brisk walking, running, swimming, biking, or other exercise 5 days a week. The more calories you burn, the better, so go for things you can stick with. Then, to tighten muscles, put your body through a full round of floor exercises, weight lifting, and stretching 3 times a week.

What to expect: Exercise builds muscle, which is denser than fat. That's why you may gain weight at first, even as you lose inches off your waist. But by adding muscle, you'll speed up your metabolism, making weight loss easier. Keep at it and eat right, and weight loss will follow.

Maintain a Healthy Weight

In the past 20 years, we've become a *lot* fatter. In fact, according to a recent government report, more than half the adults in the United States are now overweight. (For how you're doing, see the chart on the next page.) That extra weight does more than keep a person from being active—it can also kill. When you weigh too much, you have a much higher risk of heart disease, high blood pressure, stroke, diabetes, gallbladder disease, and some cancers.

But how do you determine *your* healthy weight? And what's the best way to stay at that weight for life? Here's what the experts advise.

Be realistic. Many diets fail because people shoot for a fantasy weight they can't maintain. To know whether your weight-loss goal makes sense for you, ask yourself: What is the least I've weighed as an adult for at least a year? What weight was I able to reach and stay at during previous diets without feeling a lot of hunger pangs? Those weights are good places to start when you set your goal for weight loss. And remember: Losing as little as 5 percent of your current weight will help you feel and look better.

Start by exercising. In one study, 90 percent of people who lost weight and kept it off made a habit of staying active. A brisk half-hour walk burns about 150 calories—roughly as much as you'd get in a scoop of ice cream. Exercise is vital when you're dieting. That's because cutting back on calories tends to decrease muscle mass; the exercise will help you *increase* it.

Cut calories. When you take in fewer calories than you burn, you can't help dropping some weight. The best way to cut calories, oddly, is to eat *more* of some kinds of food—such as fresh fruit, vegetables, and grains. These are full of the nutrients we need for good health, yet they carry less than half the calories in the same amounts of fatty foods. An example: Half a cup of tomato sauce weighs in at 35 calories. Exactly the same amount of cheese sauce, which is high in fat, packs 230 calories. (See page 297 for tips on how to choose tasty, healthful, slimming foods in place of foods that make you fat.)

Don't deprive yourself. Instead of giving up all the fat-filled foods you love, just eat less of them. Treat yourself to 1 cookie instead of 4—and savor every bite.

Give yourself time. Any program that promises fast weight loss is almost certain to fail. When you set out to lose weight, think in terms of a year or more. The more gradually you lose weight, the more likely you are to keep it off. Remember: The healthful changes in your exercise and eating habits will make you look and feel better in ways that don't show up on the bathroom scale. So stick with them even if the pounds are slow to budge.

How to Keep Yourself From Quitting

Starting an exercise program is easy. Staying with it is the challenge. Here are some simple tips from the fitness experts:

Slow down. When they start off, many exercisers walk, run, or swim too hard (or, with strength training, they heft too much weight). Then they quit after a few workouts because they dread the pain. Sure, you should feel tired after a workout, but an hour later you should feel full of energy. If not, you're doing too much, too soon.

Find a partner. Working out with someone doubles the chance that you'll stick with it.

Write up a contract. Set sensible goals for yourself and write them down. Tell friends and family members so that they can support you.

Chart your progress. Keep a training log. Reward yourself along the way when you meet clear-cut goals, such as pedaling that extra mile or lifting twice a week for a month straight.

Be patient. The first 3 to 6 months on a new exercise program are the hardest. If you make it to 6 months, the experts say, odds are good you'll still be working out a year later.

Eat Well: Tips for Creating Healthy Meals

The only way to keep your health, Mark Twain once quipped, is to "eat what you don't want, drink what you don't like, and do what you'd druther not." For once, Twain was wrong. That's because the hallmark of healthful eating is in fact good taste and variety. Even the best diets have room for sweets, meats, and other treats when you:

Eat plenty of fruits, vegetables, and grains. High in fiber, plant-based foods fill you up with nutrients without loading you down with fat and cholesterol. And the fiber in fruits, vegetables, and grains helps speed toxins out of the body. Plants also contain a wealth of active compounds, called phyto-chemicals—*phyto* for plant—that boost the body's disease-fighting defenses. The more of these foods you eat, the better your health.

Watch the fats. All of us know we should eat less saturated fat, the kind found in fatty meats, whole milk, ice cream, and cheese. This fat raises cholesterol levels and increas-es the risk of heart disease and stroke. So do trans fats, which are found mostly in solid or semisolid (hydrogenated) vegetable oils such as margarine and shortening.

To cut some of the fat in your diet, reach for nonfat or low-fat milk. If you eat meat, help yourself to 3-ounce portions (the size of a deck of cards) of lean beef, pork, poul-try, or fish. On your pasta, try a light tomato sauce instead of a heavy cream sauce. Instead of a rich dessert, reach for a piece of fruit. If you use margarine, go for soft spreads, and when cooking, use liquid vegetable oils in-stead of shortening. At the grocery store, check package labels and steer clear of foods containing hydrogenated or partially hydro-genated vegetable oil.

Go easy on smoked, salt-cured, and charbroiled foods. All contain high levels of nitrates, which have been linked to sever-al forms of cancer. Enjoy them only now and then, if at all.

Drink lightly, if at all. A little alcohol—1 drink a day for women, 2 a day for men—may have some health benefits. Moderate drinkers have less risk of heart disease. But if you don't drink now, that's no reason to start. You'd be much better off eating less saturated fat, for example, than adding al-cohol to your diet.

What's 1 drink? A jigger of hard liquor (1.5 ounces), a glass of wine (5 ounces), or a bottle of beer (12 ounces).

Is Your Weight Healthy?

The weight chart below will help you get an idea of where you stand. But don't take it as the final word. You should also think about:

Your fitness level. If you land in the moderately overweight zone, your weight is less likely to be a health risk—*if* you're in good shape.

Your family history. Overweight peo-ple with a family history of heart disease, high blood pressure, or diabetes should make weight loss a top priority.

Your body type. People with a "pear" shape (fat in the thighs, hips, and but-tocks) seem to have a far lower risk of weight-related diseases than those with an "apple" shape (fat around the ab-domen), so they can worry less about be-ing moderately overweight.

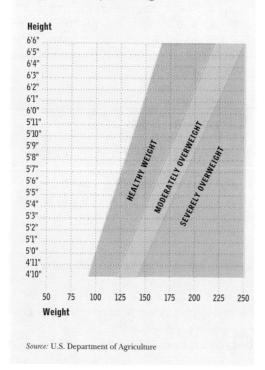

Source: U.S. Department of Agriculture

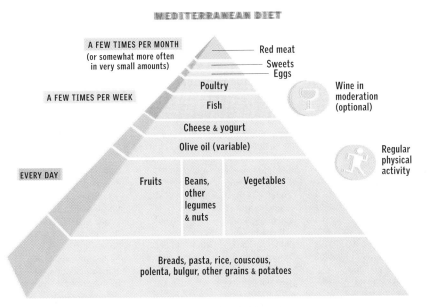

Copyright © 1994 Oldways Preservation & Exchange Trust

For the ideal mix of foods, some experts favor a change from the well-known U.S. Department of Agriculture Food Pyramid. It's the Traditional Healthy Mediterranean Diet Pyramid, developed in 1994 by researchers at the Harvard School of Public Health. Based on the eating habits of southern Italy and Greece—where people tend to live long, healthy lives—it calls for big helpings of starches and other complex carbohydrates every day in the form of pasta, bread and grains, fresh fruits, beans, and other vegetables, along with protein from small portions of cheese or yogurt. Modest amounts of fish and poultry are okay, but they're not for every day. Red meat is only a once-in-a-while treat.

Easy Exchanges: Trusty Low-Fat Substitutes

Cutting back on fat doesn't mean going hungry. The swap chart below offers some low-fat alternatives to common foods. (Portions are average serving sizes.)

INSTEAD OF	FAT GRAMS	GO FOR	FAT GRAMS
Corn muffin	5	English muffin and jam	1
Granola	12	Nonfat yogurt sprinkled with granola	2
Bacon and eggs	37	Pancakes with syrup	6
Tuna salad sandwich	16	Turkey breast sandwich with mustard	7
Cheeseburger	30	Bagel with lox and low-fat cream cheese	10
French fries	20	Oven-fried potatoes	8
Cream-of-chicken soup	18	Chicken noodle soup	6
Potato chips	18	Pretzels	2
Bean dip	4	Salsa	0
Alfredo sauce	10	Tomato sauce	1
Sautéed vegetables	14	Steamed vegetables	0
Ranch-style dressing	18	Vinaigrette	8
Ice cream	18	Sorbet	0
Apple pie	16	Fig bars (4)	4

STAYING HEALTHY

The Nutrition Top Ten

Here's a handy chart to fill you in on the richest food sources of vitamins C, A, and E, folic acid, iron, calcium, and fiber. This chart lists the top ten foods for each item. The RDA (recommended dietary allowance) figures show you the minimum to aim for daily.

VITAMIN C
RDA: 60 MILLIGRAMS

	mg
Red bell peppers, raw, chopped, 1 cup	283.0
Green bell peppers, raw, chopped, 1 cup	133.0
Brussels sprouts, raw, 6	96.0
Strawberries, halves, 1 cup	86.2
Broccoli, raw, chopped, 1 cup	82.0
Oranges, 1 medium	69.7
Kiwifruit, no skin, 1 medium	57.0
Red cabbage, raw, chopped 1 cup	50.7
Edible-pod peas, raw, 10 pods	20.4
Parsley, 5 sprigs	6.7

VITAMIN A
RDA: 4,000–5,000 INTERNATIONAL UNITS

	IU
Sweet potatoes, boiled, mashed, 1 cup	55,937.1
Pumpkin, canned, without salt, 1 cup	54,037.2
Carrots, raw, chopped 1 cup	36,005.1
Butternut squash, 1 whole	14,352.1
Apricots, dried, 1 cup stewed halves	10,973.4
Red bell peppers, raw, chopped, 1 cup	8,493.0
Cantaloupe, diced, 1 cup	5,029.4
Red chile peppers, raw, 1	4,837.5
Spinach, raw, 1 cup	2,014.5
Broccoli, chopped, 1 cup	1,357.0

VITAMIN E
RDA: 30 INTERNATIONAL UNITS

	IU
Wheat germ oil, 1 tbs	39.0
Sunflower seeds, dry-roasted, without salt, 1 oz	21.0
Wheat germ, toasted, 1/4 cup	5.1
Peanut butter, 2 tbs	4.8
Palm oil, 1 tbs	4.5
Almonds, 10	4.3
Butter, with salt, 1 pat	1.2
Margarine, without salt, 1 tsp	0.9
Peanuts, dry-roasted, without salt, 10	0.8
Asparagus, cooked, 8 medium spears	0.5

FOLIC ACID
RDA: 400 MICROGRAMS*

	mcg
Lentils, cooked, 1 cup	358.0
Pinto beans, cooked, 1 cup	294.0
Wheat germ, toasted, 1/4 cup	99.5
Green peas, raw, 1 cup	94.3
Spinach, raw, 1 cup	58.3
Fortified breakfast cereal, 1 cup	44.0
Romaine lettuce, shredded, 1/2 cup	38.0
Peanut butter, 2 tbs	23.7
Peanuts, dry-roasted, without salt, 10	14.5
Hummus (garbanzo puree), 1 tbs	11.6

CALCIUM
RDA: 1,000 MILLIGRAMS**

	mg
Mozzarella cheese, part skim, 1 cup	965.3
Tofu, firm, 1/4 block	553.2
Plain low-fat yogurt, 1 cup	447.4
Salmon, canned, with bones, 6 oz	407.0
Ricotta cheese, part skim, 1/2 cup	337.3
Skim milk, 1 cup	302.3
Orange juice, with added calcium, 1 cup	300.0
Parmesan cheese, 1 tbs	68.8
Collard greens, raw, 1 cup	52.0
Almonds, 10	29.8

IRON
RDA: 10–15 MILLIGRAMS

	mg
Oysters, 10	26.0
Clams, 10	20.0
Chicken liver, 1 cup	11.9
Tofu, firm, 1/4 block	8.5
Lean beef, tenderloin, 8 oz	6.3
Apricots, dried, 1 cup stewed halves	4.2
Cashews, dry-roasted, without salt, 1/2 cup	4.1
Fortified breakfast cereal, 1 cup	3.8
Spinach, raw, 1 cup	0.8
Parsley, 5 sprigs	0.3

FIBER
SUGGESTED DAILY TOTAL: 25–30 GRAMS

	grams
High-fiber breakfast cereal, 3/4 cup	15.3
Pinto beans, cooked, 1 cup	14.7
Granola, 1 cup	12.8
Bran flakes, 3/4 cup	4.6
Wheat germ, toasted, 1/4 cup	3.6
Mixed nuts, dry-roasted, without salt, 1 oz	2.6
Whole wheat bread, 1 slice	1.9
Rye crisp cracker, 1	1.7
Wheat bran bread, 1 slice	1.4
Popcorn, air-popped, 1 cup	1.2

TOP TEN MOST NUTRITIOUS VEGETABLES

Broccoli

Spinach

Brussels sprouts

Lima beans

Peas

Asparagus

Artichokes

Cauliflower

Sweet potatoes

Carrots

*600 mcg for pregnant women
**1,500 mg for women after menopause

Some fortified breakfast cereals designed to provide most or all of the RDAs have been omitted from this ranking.

Sources: U.S. Department of Agriculture *Handbook 8.* Food composition data from the Food and Nutrition Information Center, National Agricultural Library, Agricultural Research Service—Website: *www.nalusda.gov/fnic.*

Food and Nutrition Board, National Academy of Sciences—*National Research Council Recommended Dietary Allowances, revised 1989.*

Put Out the Smoke

Smoking kills. Period. Cigarettes cause heart disease, lung cancer, and a host of other life-threatening ailments. If you don't smoke, don't start. If you do, quit.

Nicotine is one of the most addictive drugs around, so many people find they have to try over and over before they quit smoking for good. Even if you've tried and failed, don't give up. There are many ways to kick the habit, ranging from nicotine patches to support groups. And the body quickly mends itself once you do quit. Within 2 days after you stop, carbon monoxide levels in the blood return to normal. Within 3 months, lung function improves by as much as 30 percent. After a year, your risk of heart disease will be half that of a smoker's.

Be Careful Out There

Accidents are the top reason Americans land in the emergency room. In fact, for people under the age of 45, accident—not disease—is the leading cause of death. More than half of all these deaths involve motor vehicles or firearms. Guns kill more than 32,000 Americans every year and wound hundreds of thousands more—and the numbers keep climbing. Half a million people a year are hurt riding bicycles. Nearly 20 million a year have an accident at home that sends them to a doctor or limits what they can do for at least half a day. And many people get sunburns, which can lead to skin cancer.

To increase safety on the road:

➤ Always wear seat belts in the car.
➤ Use child safety seats for kids under 4.

Vitamin & Mineral Basics

Pills can't replace a healthy diet. But if you don't always eat as well as you should, vitamin and mineral supplements can help ensure that you get all the nutrients you need.

Be careful about getting too much of some vitamins. Vitamin A is toxic in doses above 50,000 international units (IU). Supplements are usually safe to about 10,000 IU daily. Taken during pregnancy, high doses can cause birth defects. Vitamin B6 in high doses (100 milligrams a day for several months) can cause nerve damage. Very high doses of vitamin D (5,000 IU every day) can cause kidney and heart problems.

A few tips:

Skip fancy pills loaded with vitamins C and E. Instead, choose a basic formula that provides the recommended dietary allowance (RDA) of a broad range of vitamins and minerals.

If you want extra vitamins C and E, buy them separately. For C, take 25 to 500 milligrams (mg) once a day. For E, choose a capsule with 100 to 400 IU—a lot more than the RDA.

Folic acid cuts the risk of birth defects in the spine, so pregnant women should eat foods rich in it—whole-grain breads, leafy green vegetables, beans, and cereals. Many doctors suggest taking 600 micrograms (mcg) daily before and during pregnancy.

Calcium can protect against osteoporosis (thinning of the bones). Milk, yogurt, and leafy green vegetables have plenty. But if you don't feel you're getting enough in your food, take a supplement. Choose one that contains vitamin D if you don't eat dairy products (you need some D to help use calcium). Common antacids are also good calcium sources. Your body can most easily absorb calcium from supplements if you take less than 500 mg at a time and spread the doses throughout the day. Take no more than 1,500 mg of calcium a day, since too much can cause nausea, constipation, or perhaps even kidney stones in some people.

For iron, the RDA of around 15 mg for women and 10 mg for men is plenty. Pregnant women—especially those who eat little red meat—are often advised to take 30 mg to 60 mg supplements. But don't go higher than that. More than 100 mg a day can cause heart and liver problems.

STAYING HEALTHY

Sun Lovers: Are You in the Dark?

Close to 1 million Americans will find out they have skin cancer this year (see color illustrations, page 172). The next step isn't pretty. At best, the cut-away tumor will leave a scar. At worst, it'll turn out to be melanoma, which kills 7,000 people a year. But most skin cancers can be avoided. All you have to do is protect your skin from sunlight. Did you know, for instance, that men get lip cancer far more often than women? It may be that ordinary lipstick protects the lips as well as light-duty sunscreen does. Still, what gives true protection? Do your sunscreen habits measure up? Take this quiz: Are these statements true or false?

1 A light tan is fine, as long as I don't get a sunburn.　TRUE or FALSE

2 A T-shirt will protect my shoulders from sun damage.　TRUE or FALSE

3 I'm safe driving around with my windows rolled up.　TRUE or FALSE

4 I'm more likely to get too much sun when I'm swimming than when I'm sunbathing.　TRUE or FALSE

5 Growing my hair long is the best way to protect my ears and scalp.　TRUE or FALSE

6 For best blockage, I should put on sunscreen just before I go outside.　TRUE or FALSE

7 The higher my sunscreen's sun protection factor (SPF) rating, the better protected I am.　TRUE or FALSE

1. False. Some always-tan people—those who work outside for at least 40 hours a week—do have lower rates of melanoma. That could be because tan skin protects against the sunburns linked to the cancer. But if you don't work as a park ranger, you raise your odds for getting skin cancer each time you burn or tan. That's because the damage that causes most cancers adds up; ultraviolet light causes cells in the skin to reproduce faster, at the same time holding down the body's immune response to this growth. After decades, the result can be a reddish patch, shiny bump, or open sore—a tumor.

2. True. A boldly colored T-shirt might have a sun protection factor, or SPF, of 15. That means someone who might burn in 15 minutes is protected for 15 times as long—about 4 hours—before starting to color. But one study did find that very light-colored or loosely knit shirts let through too much light to be effective: A plain white T-shirt has an SPF of 9 at most (and much less if it's wet). Hold a layer of fabric up to a window. If you can see outlines through it, think about changing your shirt.

3. True. Glass windows block the most harmful ultraviolet rays, UVB. But if your car has a sunroof, you're being exposed to UVA rays, which shine through horizontal (but not slanted) panes of glass.

4. False. Whether you're playing in the water or lounging on a beach chair, the exposure to the sun is the same. But you should use a waterproof sunblock and put on more after your dip.

5. False. A full head of hair—it doesn't matter which color—does shield the scalp and ears from sun damage. (Cancer on the tops of the ears is a special risk for people with short hair.) But the best defense isn't hair, which can leave many parts of your head exposed. It's a wide-brimmed hat.

6. False. Put on sunscreen (SPF 15 or higher) 30 minutes before leaving the house. That's how long it takes for sunscreen to bond to the outer layer of your skin. Reapply sunscreen every 2 hours, even if it's waterproof.

7. True. For most people, SPF 15 lotion or moisturizer blocks the sun. But watch your skin. If you see signs of sunburn despite being covered with SPF 15, switch to a stronger sunscreen—say, SPF 30. And use plenty. It takes at least 2 tablespoons to cover most bodies, but according to one study, beach-goers put on just a third that much.

➤ Wear a helmet when you ride a bike or in-line skates (it should meet the ANSI or Snell standard) or motorcycle (the U.S. Department of Transportation—DOT—standard).

➤ Never drink and drive—or ride with anyone who has been drinking.

➤ Keep a flashlight in the car for emergencies and for walking through unlit parking areas after dark.

To accident-proof your home or office:

➤ Install smoke detectors.

➤ Keep a fire extinguisher in the kitchen.

➤ Plan escape routes in case of fire.

➤ Buy anti-scald devices for showerheads or faucets, or keep your water heater set at 120 degrees or lower to protect children from scalding.

➤ Store drugs and toxic chemicals out of the reach of children.

➤ Post poison control and other emergency numbers near the phone.

To prevent falls:

➤ Have a sturdy stepladder handy for reaching high shelves.

➤ Install nonslip pads and mats in showers and bathtubs.

➤ Don't use loose throw rugs.

➤ Be sure stairways are well lighted.

➤ Use night-lights in bathrooms and halls.

➤ Never leave objects on stairs.

To protect yourself outdoors:

➤ Wear a sunscreen with an SPF of at least 15, and a wide-brimmed hat, long-sleeved shirt, and long pants when in the sun. Better yet, stick to the shade between 10 AM and 2 PM.

➤ Use bug spray with no more than 30 percent DEET to keep ticks and mosquitoes at bay.

Should You Reach Out?

There's no magic recipe for social support that works for everyone. A loner might need just one close confidant, while a "people person" may feel lost without an army of friends. This quiz is based on one given by Carnegie Mellon psychologist Sheldon Cohen to gauge whether a person has the right mix of connections to stay healthy. Circle true or false.

1 If I needed a loan of $100, there is someone I could get it from.   TRUE OR FALSE

2 There is someone who takes pride in my accomplishments.   TRUE OR FALSE

3 I often meet or talk with family or friends.   TRUE OR FALSE

4 Most people I know think highly of me.   TRUE OR FALSE

5 I feel there is no one with whom I can share my most private worries and fears.   TRUE OR FALSE

6 If I needed an early morning ride to the airport, there's no one I would feel comfortable asking to take me.   TRUE OR FALSE

7 Most of my friends are more successful at making changes in their lives than I am.   TRUE OR FALSE

8 I would have a hard time finding someone to go with me on a day trip to the beach or country.   TRUE OR FALSE

For your score, add your number of true answers to questions 1 to 4 to the false answers you gave to questions 5 through 8.

If that score is 4 or higher, you have enough support to protect your health, even if your safety net has a few holes. During tough times people need connections to draw on or the confidence to ask for help; you have one or both.

If your score is 3 or lower, you may need to reach out. If you're not a group person, make an effort to become close to a trusted relative, friend, or neighbor. If closeness isn't your strength, join a social or religious group or sign up for a class.

STAYING HEALTHY

Is Stress Putting Your Health at Risk?

Each of us reacts in unique ways to life's challenges. Faced with a long line at the bank, most of us will get heated up for a few seconds before we shrug and move on. But for others—the 1 in 5 of us whom the experts call hot reactors—such moments are an assault on good health. That's why rating your stress requires you both to tally your life's stressors (part one) and to figure out whether you are prone to stress (part two).

Part One
THE STRESS IN YOUR LIFE

How often are the following stressful situations a part of your daily life?

1 Never   2 Rarely   3 Sometimes
4 Often   5 All the time

I work long hours 1 2 3 4 5

There are signs my job
isn't secure 1 2 3 4 5

Doing a good job goes
unnoticed 1 2 3 4 5

It takes all my energy just to
make it through the day 1 2 3 4 5

There are severe
arguments at home 1 2 3 4 5

A family member is
seriously ill 1 2 3 4 5

I'm having problems
with child care 1 2 3 4 5

I don't have enough
time for fun 1 2 3 4 5

I'm on a diet 1 2 3 4 5

My family/friends count on
me to solve their problems . . 1 2 3 4 5

I'm expected to keep up a
certain standard of living 1 2 3 4 5

My neighborhood is
crowded or dangerous 1 2 3 4 5

My home is a mess 1 2 3 4 5

I can't pay my bills on time . . 1 2 3 4 5

I'm not saving money 1 2 3 4 5

Your total score . . . .

Below 38: You have a lower-stress life.
38 and above: You have a high-stress life.

Part Two
YOUR STRESS SUSCEPTIBILITY

Think how you would react in these situations.

You've been waiting 20 minutes for a table in a crowded restaurant, and the host seats a party that arrived after you. You feel anger rise as your face gets hot and your heart beats faster.   TRUE OR FALSE

Your sister calls out of the blue and starts to tell you how much you mean to her. Uncomfortable, you change the subject without telling her what you feel.   TRUE OR FALSE

You come home to find the kitchen looking like a disaster area and your spouse lounging in front of the TV. You tense up and can't seem to shake your anger.   TRUE OR FALSE

Faced with a public speaking event, you get keyed up and lose sleep for a day or more, fretting about how you'll do.   TRUE OR FALSE

On Thursday your repair shop promises to fix your car in time for a weekend trip. As the hours go by, you become more and more worried that something will go wrong and your trip will be ruined.   TRUE OR FALSE

Two or Fewer True: You're a cool reactor, someone who tends to roll with the punches when a situation is out of your control.

Three or More True: Sorry, you're a hot reactor, someone who responds to mild stress with a "fight-or-flight" adrenaline rush that drives up blood pressure and can lead to a host of problems such as heart rhythm troubles, accelerated clotting (which can cause strokes and heart attacks), and damaged blood vessel linings. Some hot reactors can seem cool on the outside, but inside their bodies are silently killing them.

What Your Scores Mean

Combine the results from parts one and two to get your total stress rating.

Lower-Stress Life		Cool Reactor

Whatever your problems, stress isn't one of them. Even when stressful events do occur—and they will for all of us—your health is not likely to suffer.

Lower-Stress Life		Hot Reactor

You're not under stress—at least for now. Though you tend to overreact to problems, you've wisely managed your life to avoid the big stressors. Before you honk at the guy who cuts you off in rush hour traffic, keep in mind that getting angry can destroy thousands of heart muscle cells within minutes.

High-Stress Life		Cool Reactor

You're under stress, but only you know if it's hurting. Even if you normally thrive with a full plate of challenges, now you might be biting off more than you can chew. Note any increase in headaches, backaches, or insomnia; that's your body telling you to lighten your load. If your job is the main source of stress, think about reducing your hours. If that's not possible, find a way to make your job more enjoyable, and stress will become manageable.

High-Stress Life		Hot Reactor

You're in the danger zone. Make an extra effort to exercise, get enough sleep, and keep your family and friends close. It's too bad, but even being physically fit does little to protect you if your body is always in stress mode. To survive, you may need to make major changes—walking away from a life-destroying job or relationship, perhaps—and you may need to work out a whole new approach to life's hourly obstacles. Such effort will pay off. In one experiment, 77 percent of hot reactors were able to cool down—lower their blood pressure and cholesterol levels—by training themselves to stay calm.

Stay Involved

How would you describe the healthiest person you know? Perhaps as someone who is alert and curious. Excited about new possibilities. Good at love and friendship. Passionate about life's simple pleasures. Well, experts couldn't agree more. They've found that healthy people tend to stay enthusiastic about life as they age. They suggest you:

Be an optimist. Studies show that people who most often look on the bright side remain healthier than pessimists, perhaps because their immune systems are stronger.

Join a group. Even among retired people, those who remain active in volunteer work or church and social groups have better health and sharper minds than those who shut themselves in.

Challenge yourself. The more you challenge yourself, the more vital your mind remains. Studies show that learning something new increases the links between brain cells and makes the brain more robust.

Cherish your friends and loved ones. In one study, single people who didn't feel they had anyone to share their feelings with were 3 times more likely to die over the next 5 years than those who had someone close to talk to. Indeed, social isolation can be as bad for your health as smoking or high cholesterol.

Stay active. A lifetime of exercise helps preserve blood supply to the brain, because it keeps the heart, lungs, and blood vessels in top shape. Exercise also seems to boost chemicals in the brain that strengthen memory and help us think. The bottom line: Active and fit older people not only live longer, they also have faster reaction times and score better on tests of thinking power than do inactive older people.

Relax

These days, most of us lead busy, crowded lives. And most of the time we cope smoothly with the pressures we face. But sometimes life's strains and letdowns become too much and our bodies react. Blood pressure rises, heart rate quickens, and the stress hormone adrenaline surges through the bloodstream.

STAYING HEALTHY

How Well Do You Know Your Teeth?

Of course we're supposed to brush every day. But how many of us know why? Take this test to find out if you're truly treating your teeth well.

1   You can catch gum disease from
   a. kissing   b. sharing a toothbrush   c. both   d. neither

2   Toothbrushing prevents
   a. detached gums   b. root decay   c. stained teeth   d. none of these

3   You're least likely to get cavities from eating
   a. raisins   b. pure sugar   c. an English muffin

4   Who's most at risk of getting gum disease?
   a. pregnant women   b. menopausal women   c. teetotalers

5   If you can't brush your teeth after a meal, what's the best thing to do?
   a. eat a banana   b. chew gum   c. use a toothpick

6   Thorough toothbrushing takes at least
   a. 1 minute   b. 2 minutes   c. 4 minutes

7   Which will relieve toothache pain fastest?
   a. aspirin   b. clove oil   c. salt water

ANSWERS

1. c By age 35, 3 in 4 Americans have at least the beginnings of gum disease, an infection below the gum line caused by certain kinds of bacteria in dental plaque. But sometimes bacteria passed in the saliva of a person with gum disease can bring on the condition in someone who doesn't even have plaque. So if your partner isn't taking care of his or her teeth, take the problem seriously. Your own gums may be at risk.

2. d Toothbrushing removes plaque and prevents cavities above the gum line, but not below. When plaque isn't cleaned out, germs get at your roots and even at the bone anchoring the teeth. Gum disease is the nation's leading cause of tooth loss. To prevent it, you have to floss.

3. b Sugary foods, such as candy and chocolate, are cleared from the mouth more quickly than starchy foods are. Raisins are a special case because they stick like glue between the teeth.

4. a Nearly all pregnant women get some signs of gum disease, because hormone changes during pregnancy increase swelling, bleeding, and tiny infections in the gums. There's an old saw: Lose a tooth for every child. To keep it from coming true, brush after every meal, floss daily, and see a dentist at the beginning of your pregnancy.

5. b We make more saliva when we chew gum, and saliva's chemicals neutralize tooth-decaying acids. Pop in a piece when you finish a meal. Sugarless gum works much better than regular, and gum containing xylitol works best of all, reducing tooth decay by as much as 85 percent. (The sweetener keeps bacteria from multiplying.) This gum is sold mostly in health food stores.

6. b To make this task seem less daunting, divide your mouth into 10 sections. (Include a section each for the roof of your mouth, your tongue, and the insides of your right and left cheeks, all places where bacteria gather.) Then count to 20 alligators as you brush each section. The average American spends about 30 seconds brushing.

7. b If your dentist can't see you right away for a painful tooth, saturate a cotton ball in oil of clove (sold at many pharmacies) and put it on the aching tooth. The pain-killing oil should ease the ache in a couple of seconds.

Stress can lead to everything from colds, headaches, and back pain to allergies, asthma, arthritis, infertility, insomnia, depression, and heart disease. (For more information, see **stress,** page 218.)

Luckily, you can do a lot to reduce stress and cut your risk of health problems. In one study, students who used simple relaxation techniques at exam time were much less likely to show a slump in their immune systems than other students. Here are several simple ways to calm frazzled nerves:

Take a 15-minute breather. When things get hectic, go for a walk, listen to music you like, browse through a magazine, or soak in a hot bath. Any pleasant "time-out" from the day's pressures can calm you down.

Practice relaxation techniques, such as deep breathing, meditation, or simply sitting with your eyes closed. They all can reverse the symptoms of stress. Studies have shown that meditation lowers levels of a chemical linked to tension. Meditation also protects the body from the harmful effects of adrenaline—exactly what the leading blood-pressure-lowering drugs do. Here are 2 easy exercises to help you banish stress:

➤ Watch your breath: 10 minutes. Sit or lie down in a quiet place. Breathe normally through your nose. Focus on each breath as it flows in and out. Don't try to control it—just watch. When your attention wanders, bring it gently back to your breathing. Repeat as often as you like.

➤ Meditate: 20 minutes. Find a quiet place. Sit in a chair with your feet on the floor and your hands in your lap. Close your eyes and in your mind say a simple word or phrase. Try the word *one*. When any thoughts come to mind, ignore them and return to the word. Make it the focus of your attention, but don't force it or work at it—let it come as though you are hearing it, not thinking it. As you relax, you may drift briefly into sleep. Don't worry, just al-

low yourself to let go. Practice this once a day (twice is better) for lasting results. If you don't have 20 minutes, try 10.

Use your imagination. Positive mental images can have a strong calming effect on the body. If you feel your stress level spiking, close your eyes and take 5 minutes to picture yourself in a quiet, peaceful, pleasant setting—say, you and a friend on a clean, sunny beach lapped by gentle waves.

Move around. Doing a favorite form of exercise—one that leaves you slightly winded—will ease your anxiety and help you feel more in control of your life.

Laugh it off. Laughter really *is* one of the best medicines. A good laugh eases tension and boosts levels of anti-stress brain chemicals. Read a book that makes you laugh, or sit down to watch a favorite comedy show or film. Another good bet: Meet some friends for a lighthearted conversation.

Take Care of Your Teeth

Cavities used to be the big deal in dental care. While people still get them, the new frontier is gum disease—a bacterial infection that works below the gum line to ravage the bone and ligaments holding your teeth in place. So, as they say, "Clean only the teeth you want to keep." Here's what to do:

Brush *and* floss at least twice a day, in the morning and before bed. It doesn't matter whether you floss first or brush first—just be thorough. (See **tips on tooth and gum care,** page 82.) The nighttime cleaning amounts to a preemptive strike—knocking down the bacteria before you lie there all night asleep, letting the fluids in your mouth stagnate. The morning cleaning knocks them down again when their numbers have peaked.

Dentists want you to have your teeth cleaned at least once every 6 months to keep ahead of any damage that might creep in despite your best efforts.

STAYING HEALTHY

SO . . .

If you can follow all 8 steps, great. If you can't, try 7, or 6.
The point is not just to live longer, though you very well might.
The real reward is feeling better and enjoying life.

Know Your Health Plan

When choosing a health plan, make sure you understand the coverage each plan offers, especially if you have a specific health concern or if you expect a change in your health care needs, such as pregnancy. Many health plans have a telephone number you can call to ask about coverage. Once you've joined a plan, read your member handbook so you know your plan's benefits and limits, as well as how to get the services or information that you need. Here's what you should know about your health plan and some questions you'll want your plan to answer.

Benefits. Most plans cover the same basic medical services, such as checkups and hospitalization. But coverage for things such as counseling, complementary treatments, and even prescription drugs can vary. What does—and doesn't—your plan cover? Look for the "Explanation of Benefits" in your handbook to find out.

Costs. Does your plan have copayments or deductibles? A copayment is a fixed amount you pay for each visit, prescription, or test. A deductible is a fixed amount you pay before your plan begins covering the cost of care.

Your primary care physician. Does your plan require you to select a primary care physician? If so, how do you choose? Are you required to pick from a list of physicians approved by your plan, or can you choose any doctor you wish? Can your plan give you information about physicians? If you want to change your doctor, how do you do so? Is there a limit on how many times you can switch?

Scheduling an appointment. Find out how to make an appointment. Some plans have a central number you call. In other plans, you call your doctor's office directly. Is there a customer service office that can help if you have problems?

Emergencies or urgent care. Most health plans define an emergency as a life- or limb-threatening problem that requires care right away. An "urgent" problem is slightly less serious; it needs prompt treatment but isn't life-threatening. What are your plan's rules for the use of emergency or urgent care? Do you need approval from your primary care physician first? If you go to an emergency or urgent care center for a problem that does not call for immediate care, will your plan still cover treatment?

Referrals and second opinions. Does your plan require you to go through your primary care physician before you can see a specialist, or can you see a specialist directly? Are there rules for second opinions? Not all plans will pay for one.

Hospital care. You may never need to go to the hospital, but it's a good idea to know ahead of time about your health plan's rules for hospitalization. Find out what hospitals are part of your plan. Are there limits on how long you can stay in the hospital?

Help and information. Does your plan have an advice line to call if you have questions or concerns about your health? Are there customer service representatives who can help if you have questions, complaints, or trouble getting the care you expect? Find out how to reach your plan's advice line or customer service office. What days and times are representatives available? What problems can they help you with? Keep the phone numbers handy.

Your Rights & Responsibilities

You and your providers are partners in your health care. There are some important things you can expect from your providers, and some things they can expect from you.

YOU HAVE THE RIGHT TO:

Be informed. Your health plan will give you information about how the plan works, including the services it covers and what you need to do to receive care. If you're part of a managed care system, you may also get a list of approved providers. Your doctor will talk with you about your health, and you have the right to be told if you have a health problem. If you're going to receive treatment for it, your doctor will discuss the risks and benefits of that treatment. You also have the right to read your medical record, and the right to be spoken to in language you understand.

Make decisions. You and your doctor are a team, and you have the right to take part in all treatment decisions and to help design a treatment plan. You also have the right to refuse treatment (though this may not be possible in an emergency).

Plan for future care. You can plan for times when you may not be able to make decisions about the type of care you want. You do this by choosing a family member or friend you trust to make those choices for you. You can name your representative in a durable power of attorney for health care, a living will, or some other advance directive.

Expect privacy. Your medical records are private. Your health plan will not release them to anyone except you, unless required to do so by law. If you need your records, your provider must give you copies.

Make complaints and report grievances. If you're having a problem with your care or if you can't get answers to any questions, you can bring these concerns to your health plan, which has procedures in place for member complaints or grievances.

Be treated with respect. You need to feel comfortable asking questions and talking with your providers. You have the right to be heard, and your providers should treat you with respect. It is a two-way street, though—you need to be courteous as well.

YOU HAVE THE RESPONSIBILITY TO:

Take good care of yourself. Health care begins with the way you take care of yourself. Be sure to exercise, to eat sensibly, and not to smoke. If you drink alcohol, drink moderately. Also, remember to get screenings such as blood pressure checks as often as your doctor advises. (See *Staying Healthy,* page 291.)

Use self-care when you can. There's a lot you can do for yourself when you have a minor illness or injury, such as a cold or a strained muscle. (Refer to *Problems and Solutions,* beginning on page 47, to find out more.) Be sure to call your plan's advice line or your doctor's office whenever you have questions. Use the emergency room or urgent care center only for true emergencies or urgent problems (see *Lifesaving Skills and First Aid,* page 11).

Stay in touch. Let your providers know about your medical history, any medications you are taking or have allergies to, and any worries you have about a possible treatment. Also, remember to tell your doctor about any major life changes that may be affecting your health, such as a job change, the birth of a child, or a divorce. If you're receiving treatment for a health problem or an injury, let your providers know right away of any change in how you feel.

Follow your treatment plan. Once you and your doctor agree on a course of treatment, follow it all the way through. Take medications on schedule, and make all needed follow-up appointments. If you think the treatment isn't working, talk to your doctor about it.

STAYING HEALTHY

How to Choose a Physician

Some health plans ask you to choose a primary care physician from among the plan's own list of approved providers. But even if your plan is one that doesn't, it's a good idea to have a primary care physician. You may not need a doctor now, but if you ever do, you'll want one whom you trust and who knows you and your medical history. He or she will be the one provider with the whole picture of your health needs and your desires about care.

Most primary care physicians specialize in pediatrics, internal medicine, family practice, or obstetrics and gynecology. Some have training in other fields, such as cardiology, but have chosen to practice in primary care. All primary care physicians have expertise in disease prevention and detection, and many have had training in health education as well.

If you need care from any other specialist, your primary care physician can make the referral, then help coordinate the care you receive.

Be sure you and your physician are a good match. The two of you will be partners in your care, and it won't matter how skilled your physician is if you don't communicate well with each other. Here are some tips for finding the right primary care provider.

Decide What You Want

Start by listing what you want in the way of care. The items on that list will help you focus your search for just the right provider. Some things to consider:

Your health care needs. If you have a particular health problem—or a family history that puts you at risk for one—you may prefer a primary care physician who has special training or experience in that area. For example, if you know you're at risk for heart disease, you may want a primary care physician who has training in the prevention of heart problems. If you're older, you may want a physician with an interest in the health care needs of seniors.

Personal and professional qualities. You can't predict whether the chemistry of a relationship will be right—you'll need to meet face-to-face with your doctor to find out for sure if you two are a good fit. But it will help if you go into your first few appointments knowing clearly what qualities you prefer. For example, is the doctor's clinical skill more important to you than personal warmth? Do you want a doctor who is willing to talk over treatment plans—or one who will take charge and make decisions for you? Does it matter to you whether your physician is a man or a woman, or close to you in age?

Convenience. If transportation is difficult for you, or lack of time is a problem, look for a physician whose office is near your home or workplace. Find out about office hours: Do you prefer your physician to be available for office visits in the evening or on weekends? Does it matter to you who covers for your physician when he or she is on vacation?

Use Your Health Plan as a Resource

Most plans have a customer service office that can help you find a physician who's right for you: representatives can often tell you about a doctor's specialties, experience, spoken languages, and office hours, and who covers for the physician when he or she is out of town. Some plans, and even some hospitals, also provide "health match" services that link members with providers based on details from member surveys and physician profiles.

Ask Around

Get recommendations from friends, relatives, neighbors, and coworkers. If you know any nurses or other health care professionals, talk with them as well. Nurses work with physicians every day, so they may have a good idea which physicians are most effective, personable, and available.

Make Good Use of Your First Appointment

Once you've selected a physician, make an appointment, even if you feel fine. This first meeting will give you and the doctor a chance to get to know one another. It's important for another reason: If you suddenly need urgent or emergency care, but the physician you've selected doesn't know you—other than as a name on a patient list—or your health history, he or she may refuse to treat you or to authorize care on your behalf.

Keep in mind that most emergencies don't happen during regular office hours. Your health plan may not pay for a plain get-acquainted appointment, but it will pay for a basic physical exam.

Before you go, write out a list of any concerns or questions you have about your health, along with the details of your health history, your family health history, and any medications you're taking (see **helping your doctor help you,** page 312). Remember that for your partnership to work, the physician needs to know about any health problems or concerns you have. You and your doctor will discuss your medical history at this first meeting; the doctor may check your blood pressure, height, and weight, and may recommend other screenings, such as those for high blood sugar or cholesterol.

During this appointment, notice whether the physician takes time to answer your questions. Is the doctor easy to understand, or does he or she use a lot of medical terms without explaining them? Do you feel at ease? Is the doctor a good listener?

After this appointment, you'll have a better idea whether you and the doctor are a good match. If you don't think so, it's okay to try another physician.

Some Specialists You May Meet

Allergist: treats allergies and asthma.

Cardiologist: treats diseases of the heart, arteries, and veins.

Dermatologist: treats skin problems.

Endocrinologist: treats disorders such as diabetes and thyroid problems.

Family practitioner: specializes in a combination of internal medicine, pediatrics, psychiatry, and obstetrics and gynecology.

Gastroenterologist: treats diseases of the stomach and intestines.

Internist: specializes in the treatment of problems of the internal organs.

Neurologist: treats diseases of the nervous system and related disorders.

Obstetrician/Gynecologist (OB/GYN): treats women during pregnancy and childbirth; also deals with disorders of the female reproductive tract.

Ophthalmologist: treats vision problems and diseases of the eye.

Orthopedist: treats diseases and injuries of the extremities, spine, and related structures, such as the ligaments.

Otolaryngologist: specializes in diseases of the ear, nose, and throat.

Pediatrician: specializes in the development and medical problems of children from birth through adolescence.

Psychiatrist: treats mental problems.

Rheumatologist: treats inflammation and pain in the joints, muscles, and bones.

Urologist: treats diseases of the genitourinary tract.

STAYING HEALTHY

How to Choose a Natural Healer

For all the strong feelings people have about doctors, we rarely wonder whether they're qualified. Those diplomas and certificates lined up on the office wall provide reassurance that the physicians have gone to the right schools and passed all their licensing exams.

But what happens when you're in the office of an acupuncturist, say, and those familiar seals of approval aren't there? Searching for a trustworthy alternative healer can be like wandering in a wilderness empty of landmarks.

Fortunately, there are some signposts that can guide you to a competent healer. Here's what to look for—and what you should avoid—when choosing a practitioner from any of the 3 most popular complementary disciplines.

Acupuncture

Of the roughly 10,000 acupuncturists practicing in the United States, 3,000 are physicians. You might think that a medical doctor who can do acupuncture should be your first choice. Yet some nonphysicians who work with acupuncture needles full time might be a better choice because they have more experience and know-how.

What to look for: A nonphysician who is licensed or certified in acupuncture, or a doctor with plenty of experience in it. If you're considering a nonphysician and you live in a state that requires an acupuncture license (about half do), make sure that your practitioner has one. If acupuncturists are not licensed by your state, pick someone approved by the National Certification Commission for Acupuncture and Oriental Medicine.

Finding a good physician-acupuncturist is a little trickier because most states allow doctors to practice acupuncture without a special license or other proof of training. One way you can assure competence is by selecting one of the 1,800 members of the American Academy of Medical Acupuncture.

What to avoid: Acupuncture performed by chiropractors who are not certified by the National Certification Commission for Acupuncture and Oriental Medicine. In states that don't license acupuncturists (and even in some that do), chiropractors have stepped in to fill the void. In Colorado, for instance, chiropractors can be licensed to practice acupuncture after completing only 100 hours of course work, well below the requirements for certified acupuncturists.

Chiropractic

Chiropractors are licensed in all states and the District of Columbia. The most common path to licensure is 2 to 4 years of preprofessional school, then four years of full-time study in chiropractic college and the passing of a national board exam.

Practitioners fall into 2 groups. The "straights," who make up about 15 percent of the 56,000 chiropractors nationwide, believe that most diseases are caused by misalignments of the spine that impinge on nerves. They claim that an "adjustment"—a snap that brings a vertebral joint to the limit of its range of motion—corrects the misalignment. Straights, despite a lack of scientific support, believe that spinal adjustments can cure almost any illness.

"Mixers" also rely on adjustments, but do them mostly to relieve back and neck pain and headaches, all ailments for which chiropractic treatment has proved effective.

What to look for: A chiropractor who is willing to work closely with your doctor. Mixers are more likely to do this than straights. Ask, "Are you willing to trade information about treatments with my regular doctor?" You want a chiropractor who sees himself or herself as a member of the health care team.

Also, because there are plenty of chiropractors to choose among, stick with those who have at least 3 years of experience.

What to avoid: Practitioners who are too commercial. Some chiropractors try to get patients to sign up for 25 to 40 visits. But chiropractic is not a long-term treatment, some experts say. If you don't get better after 10 to 12 sessions, this therapy is probably not going to help.

Naturopathy

Currently licensed in 19 states and Puerto Rico, naturopaths are the general practitioners of the alternative world. In the states with the most liberal licensing laws, which include Oregon and Washington, they can prescribe some drugs, such as antibiotics, and even perform minor outpatient surgeries such as mole removal. But their primary tools are "natural" ones: herbs, vitamin and mineral supplements, advice on stress management and diet, and homeopathic preparations.

What to look for: A licensed naturopath in states where that's possible. Elsewhere, make sure the practitioner you choose is a graduate of one of the 3 accredited colleges of naturopathy (Bastyr University in Kenmore, Washington; the National College of Naturopathic Medicine in Portland, Oregon; and the Southwest College of Naturo-

pathic Medicine in Tempe, Arizona), and has passed the national board examination. These schools require 2 years of health sciences and 2 more of hands-on training.

What to avoid: Although licensed naturopaths receive some education in both acupuncture and chiropractic, they aren't the right sources for these therapies unless they've had advanced training in them. And steer clear of graduates of correspondence schools. Their training is minimal, and they are ineligible for licensure.

Looking for a Credentialed Provider?

➤ National Certification Commission for Acupuncture and Oriental Medicine, 703-548-9004, M–F 9–5 EST; *www.nccaom.org*. Go to the Website or call to learn if an acupuncturist is certified.

➤ American Academy of Medical Acupuncture, 800-521-2262, 24-hour recording; *www.medicalacupuncture.org*. Go to the Web site or call to find a physician trained in acupuncture.

➤ American Chiropractic Association, 800-986-4636, M–F 8:30–5:30 EST; *www.amerchiro.org*. Go to the Web site or call for a referral to a chiropractor.

➤ American Association of Naturopathic Physicians, 206-298-0125, 24-hour recording; *www.naturopathic.org*. Go to the Website for a list of members near you.

Herb Safety

Herbal supplements in the United States don't have to meet government quality-control standards or regulations, so it can be hard to know which brands to trust. Here are some tips about buying herbal remedies.

➤ Don't assume that "natural" means "safe." You could be putting yourself at risk for a possible interaction with any prescription or over-the-counter medications you're already taking (see **drug combinations to avoid,** page 323).

➤ Look for products made by major

drug companies. They have been jumping on the alternative bandwagon by adding herbal supplements to their vitamin lines. Their experience could result in more trustworthy products.

➤ Choose products with a National Formulary seal, a quality marker available for herbs. The seal indicates that the supplement was made according to the guidelines set by the U.S. Pharmacopeia, an organization that establishes standards for drug safety and quality.

STAYING HEALTHY

Helping Your Doctor Help You

To get the best care from your health professionals, you'll need to meet them halfway. Here's how: ■ **Learn how to stay well.** It may seem obvious, but the better you take care of yourself, the less likely you are to get sick in the first place—and the more quickly you'll get well if you do get sick. ■ **Know as much as you can.** Learn about your body and how it works. If you start feeling sick, pay close attention to your symptoms. If you have an illness, study up on it. When it comes to your health, knowledge really is power. ■ **Be active on your own behalf.** When you visit the doctor, take an interest, listen closely, and ask questions. Here are 10 ways to help your doctor help you, plus tips on how to find out what you need to know.

Talk first about what worries you most. Don't save your biggest concern for last—or you may not have time to ask about it. But be realistic, too. If you have a number of health concerns, your doctor may not be able to deal with them all in one visit.

Be specific. Saying "I feel hot and I've had a sharp pain in the right side of my stomach since last night" is much more helpful than saying "I feel rotten." Be sure to bring up all the changes you've noticed in your health or how you feel, even if you don't think they're very important.

Tell the truth. Be honest about what you eat, how much you exercise, and whether you smoke, drink alcohol, or use drugs. Your doctor needs to know.

Tell your doctor what medications you're taking—include all prescription and over-the-counter drugs. You should also tell your doctor about any alternative or family remedies you've been using—going to a chiropractor, for instance, or taking big doses of vitamins. Even if you feel uneasy talking about sexual habits or problems, be sure to mention them, too.

Bring up any big life changes or stresses you may be under, such as the recent death of a loved one or working a double shift—and even good news, such as getting married.

Ask questions. Some physicians welcome questions from patients and some don't. But many doctors say they are surprised by how few questions patients have, given that the patient's health is at stake.

Clear up things you don't understand during your visit. If you're the least bit puzzled, ask your doctor to explain carefully. Ask for other sources of information.

If you're being treated for an illness or injury, ask your doctor what to expect, and find out what you can do to keep the problem from coming back.

If your doctor can't answer all your questions in one visit, ask for time to talk at the next appointment. Or find out when to call, if you can get the answer by phone. If you feel a question is crucial, request—politely but firmly—an answer before you leave.

Ask for translations. If your doctor speaks in terms you can't follow, ask for a simpler approach. If information comes at you too fast, ask the doctor to slow down. To make sure you understand, say, "Now, let me see if I've got that straight," and then repeat what the doctor just told you.

Find out more about referrals and tests. If your primary care physician sends you to a specialist, find out why. Be sure you understand the diagnosis or suspected diagnosis, and what your doctor wants the specialist to do. Is the specialist supposed to confirm a diagnosis, conduct tests, or take over your case? Make sure your records are sent to the specialist, or take copies with you to the first appointment. Ask your primary care physician to stay involved.

If you're scheduled for a test, make sure you know the following:

➤ **Why it's necessary.**

➤ **How accurate and reliable it is.**

➤ **How you should prepare for it.**

➤ **What to expect during the test.**

➤ **How the results will affect treatment.**

➤ **When and how you'll get the results.**

➤ **Whether it's covered by your health plan.**

➤ **Whether your health plan has to okay it.**

➤ **How much it will cost you.**

➤ **What the recovery time, if any, will be.**

If you learn you have something serious, you might face hard choices about treatment. Ask your doctor to explain all your options. Make sure you find out about the benefits and risks of each choice—as well as the pros and cons of doing nothing. You can also ask about other sources of information or how to get a second opinion. Once you are fully informed, you and your doctor can pick the best course.

Speak up. If you would like a medication to relieve your symptoms, say so. If you're worried you can't afford a certain drug and think a generic version might be cheaper, ask. If you want a certain test, say so. If you don't speak up, you may leave frustrated— and still worried. If you need reassurance, be open about it—your doctor might be able to help you regain peace of mind. Don't forget: You have to say what's bothering you. Doctors are often rushed, and medical schools don't teach mind reading.

If you can't follow a doctor's orders, say so. There may be times when you just don't think you can do what your doctor advises— whether it's getting more sleep, cutting down on work, exercising every day, giving up your favorite dessert, or taking a certain medication. Maybe your schedule's too irregular or you just tend to forget. Don't leave your doctor's office feeling discouraged, thinking you'll just ignore it all. Instead, explain your concerns to your doctor; together, you and your doctor may be able to come up with some ideas for other treatment plans that will work for you.

Be willing to negotiate. For instance, if your doctor suggests a drug or treatment that has side effects that you would find hard to accept, try saying, "That's going to be hard for me to live with. Is there another option I could try?"

Bring along your own ideas. If you read or hear about a treatment or medicine you'd like to try, bring the information along. Ask your doctor if it's something that could work for you. That way you can make informed choices about your own care.

Don't leave what you've learned at the office. It can be tough to recall everything the doctor tells you, especially when you're nervous. You may want to take notes or use a tape recorder. Or have a trusted friend or relative come with you to take notes and help clarify information.

Before you leave the doctor's office, know what you should do once you get home. Be sure you have all the prescriptions for any drugs you need, and be sure you know how you should take them, how you should handle any side effects, and whether you need to make changes in your diet or activities. Ask your doctor to write down the key points. Also, find out about any warning signs to watch for, and whom to call and when to call if you do run into any problems. Last, ask your doctor whether you'll need a follow-up visit.

STAYING HEALTHY

Reminders for Recovery

When you're ill, you and your doctor will come up with a treatment plan. But you won't get all the benefits from that plan unless you do your share of the work. Here are some ways to speed recovery:

Find out how long your recovery should take. If you know what to expect—how long it might be before you can walk comfortably again, for example—you will have a better idea about when to check in with the doctor. If you're taking longer to heal than you were told to expect, call and say so.

Stay in touch. Call for an appointment right away if your illness takes a turn for the worse or if you get new symptoms.

Take your medications exactly as prescribed, even if you begin to feel better. This is especially important if you're taking antibiotics, which kill bacteria. If you stop taking antibiotics too early, your infection may linger and perhaps even get worse because some germs have survived. Be sure to call your doctor at once to report any new or extreme side effects. (See **medicines: playing it safe**, page 322.)

Find a care partner. If you are sick and feeling overwhelmed, ask for help from a friend, neighbor, or relative. He or she can help you stay on top of your medications, drive you to the doctor's office, and give you support. If you're facing a long illness, loneliness can be one of your worst enemies. Surround yourself with people who are cheerful and helpful. Ask your doctor whether there is a support group for people in a similar situation.

View your health as a long-term project. Getting well and staying well isn't just a matter of taking a drug and then neglecting yourself. It's best to make good self-care a part of your life—for the rest of your life.

For More Help

A wealth of information is waiting for anyone who wants to seek it out. For a specific health concern, see the For More Help listing at the end of most entries in this book.

Here are some other sources:

Your health plan or local hospital. Many health plans and hospitals have resource centers stocked with pamphlets, books, and videos on a range of health topics—from losing weight to coping with Alzheimer's disease. Many also offer health education classes, lectures, and support groups.

Libraries and computer networks. Both public and college libraries have health sections. Some libraries also provide access to free computer databases of health information, such as MEDLINE, which can help you find health information.

The National Network of Libraries of Medicine is a referral service that will connect you to a medical library in your area. Call 800-338-7657, M–F 8–5 PST. Website: *www.nnlm.nlm.nih.gov.*

Planetree, Inc., has a useful network of consumer health libraries. For the location of the center nearest you and for information about its services, call the national office at 203-732-1365, M–F 7:30–5 EST. Website: *www.planetree.org.*

The National Institutes of Health offers information on allergies and infectious diseases (including AIDS), mental health, aging, cancer, diabetes, digestive diseases, and more. For more information on specific topics, call 301-496-4000, 24-hour line. Website: *www.nih.gov.*

The National Health Information Center. If you have specific health or medical questions, the staff members can direct you to national organizations. You can also order publications from the NHIC list for a fee. Call 800-336-4797, M–F 9–5 EST. Website: *nhic-nt.health.org.*

Support groups. National organizations often have local support groups. Two major ones, the **American Cancer Society** and the **American Heart Association,** list local chapters in the phone book. If you can't find them, call the national office of the American Cancer Society at 800-227-2345, 24-hour line; or the American Heart Association at 800-242-8721 (hours vary). Look in the yellow pages under "social service organizations" for more support groups.

Pain Relief: The Big Four

In this era of high-tech medicine, over-the-counter pain relievers still rank as wonder drugs. They ease pain, reduce fever, and are almost always harmless when used as they should be. You can get them just about everywhere as generics, identical to name brands.

Of course, you should use any drug with care (check the **drug combinations to avoid** chart, page 323).

Some cautions:

➤ A pregnant woman should ask her doctor before taking any medicine.

➤ Don't take any of these together, or along with other painkillers.

➤ Ask your doctor before taking any of these with other drugs. Be sure to read the labels.

➤ Ask your doctor before taking any of these with an anticoagulant or with an antacid or acid blocker. Some combinations can cause bleeding.

Acetaminophen (common brand name: Tylenol). For fever and pain but not for inflammation. It's the only one of the 4 that doesn't prolong bleeding and that can be taken with acid blockers (such as Pepcid or Tagamet) or antacids (Mylanta, Maalox). It's advised for anyone having dental work or other treatment that causes bleeding, and for those with ulcers, frequent nosebleeds, or other bleeding problems. It's safest for children and teenagers because it is not linked to **Reye's syndrome** (see box on page 95). **Cautions:** Taking larger-than-advised doses for several weeks or with alcohol can cause liver damage. Daily use for several months may damage the kidneys.

Aspirin (common brand names: Bayer, Bufferin, Anacin). For fever, pain, and inflammation. Many take an aspirin every day to guard against heart attack, stroke, and colon cancer. **Cautions:** Aspirin can cause stomach upset—

take it with meals or try buffered or coated types. Don't take it with stomach-acid drugs.

More than the other 3, aspirin makes blood less able to clot: As a result, it makes bleeding harder to stop. Don't take it if you have ulcers or other bleeding problems, or for about 5 days before oral or other surgery. (If you take aspirin every day, ask your doctor if it's okay to quit.) Aspirin can also trigger asthma attacks. It's linked to **Reye's syndrome** (see box on page 95): Never give aspirin to a child or teenager who might have an illness caused by a virus.

Ibuprofen (common brand names: Advil, Motrin, Nuprin). For pain, inflammation, and fever. Very good for menstrual and other cramps, arthritis, and muscle aches. **Cautions:** Ibuprofen can cause bleeding in people with ulcers if taken for more than 2 weeks or with stomach-acid drugs. Like aspirin, it can cause stomach upset (take it with meals or milk) and may trigger asthma attacks. Don't take ibuprofen if you've had an allergic reaction to any other painkiller. Also, ibuprofen may cause fluid buildup. Daily use for several months can cause kidney problems.

Naproxen sodium (common brand name: Aleve). For fever, minor aches and pains, muscle pain, arthritis, and menstrual cramps. Naproxen works longer than the other 3 painkillers. For chronic pain, that's important, but for most pain naproxen may be more than you need. **Cautions:** Follow dose limits carefully. Don't give it to children under age 12. Don't use it in the last 3 months of pregnancy. Don't take naproxen if you've had an allergic reaction with any other painkiller. Naproxen can cause mild heartburn, or stomach upset or bleeding (drink an 8-ounce glass of water with each dose).

Your Personal Health Record

You can do a lot to improve your chances of staying well: ■ **Learn all you can about your family's health history.** ■ **Do regular self-exams.** ■ **See your doctor for regular checkups.** ■ **Keep your shots up to date.** It costs a lot less to prevent an illness than to treat it—and it hurts less, too. Not only that, the earlier you detect any problem, the easier it will be to treat. Below are the basic things you should know about keeping track of your health:

A Family Tree

To get a clear look at your family's health history, make a family health tree—a genogram.

A genogram shows at a glance the names of family members, how they are related, their dates of birth, their health problems, and the dates and causes of their deaths. Making a genogram lets you see patterns in your family's health history. It's a tool you and your doctor can use to judge your risks for some of the many ailments believed to run in families—including heart disease, some birth defects, diabetes, alcoholism, depression, and schizophrenia.

If you know your risks, you can usually decrease them by changing your health habits or by spotting an ailment early so that it can be treated.

➤ To make your own genogram, start with yourself and work back through time. Use circles for women, squares for men.
➤ Write in your name, date of birth, and any serious health problems or operations you've had.
➤ To the side of your own information, add the names of your sisters and brothers. Include notes about their health.
➤ Add your parents and any aunts or uncles on the 2 branches above you. Above them, list your 4 grandparents. Include dates of birth. Add as much information as you can about their health. Include chronic ailments such as ulcers, migraines, or allergies, as well as major surgeries.
➤ For anyone who has died, write down the date of death and the cause of death, if you know it. For example:

John Smith: b. 4-1-1890 d. 7-8-1952
Asthma, hypertension at 38, heart disease at 45. Died of heart attack.

You may need to call some of your relatives or check family records to find out all you need to know. Official records may also help. To find death certificates, call or write to the Division of Statistics in the state where the relative died. Some hospitals and doctors keep archives of medical records. To get copies, you'll need a letter of consent from the person's closest living relative and a copy of the death certificate.

The National Genealogical Society offers several publications that explain ways to track down family health records. For more information, call 800-473-0060 or write to the society at 4527 17th St. N., Arlington, VA 22207. Website: *www.ngsgenealogy.org.*

The Family History Library of the Church of Jesus Christ of Latter-day Saints houses the world's largest collection of genealogical records (church members are only a fraction of the database). The staff can answer brief questions and refer you to sources for more information. For the nearest branch, call 801-240-2364 or 800-346-6044, or write to the library at 35 N. West Temple St., Salt Lake City, UT 84150. Website: *www.family-search.org.*

The sample on the next page can help you get started. Copy the form and make a chart for yourself. If you have children, make a chart for their other parent; then combine that chart with yours to make a single 2-parent chart for your children. If your family is large, you will need to extend the chart. Update the genogram every year or so.

(continued on page 319)

Your Family Tree

Use this form or a copy to create your own family health history, or genogram. You and your doctor will find it valuable.

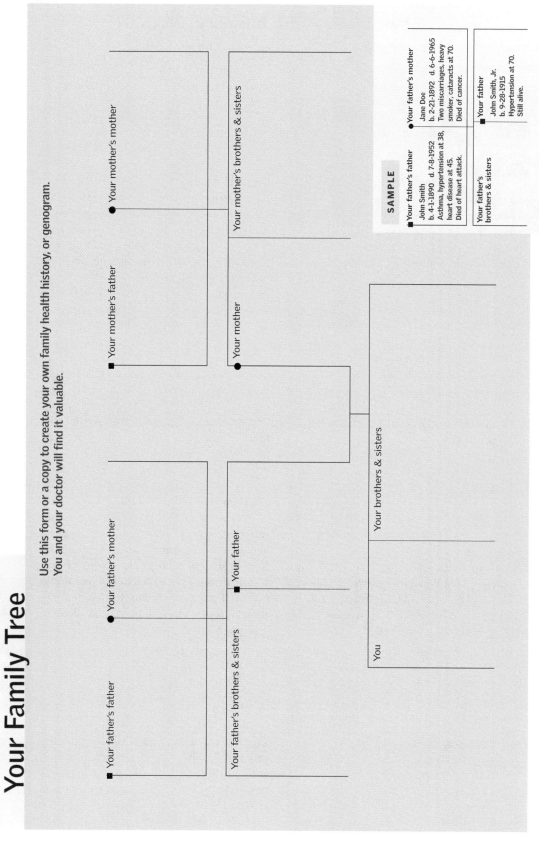

Your father's father

Your father's mother

Your father's brothers & sisters

Your father

You

Your mother's father

Your mother's mother

Your mother's brothers & sisters

Your mother

Your brothers & sisters

SAMPLE

■ **Your father's father**
John Smith
b. 4-1-1890   d. 7-8-1952
Asthma, hypertension at 38, heart disease at 45.
Died of heart attack.

● **Your father's mother**
Jane Doe
b. 2-21-1892   d. 6-6-1965
Two miscarriages, heavy smoker, cataracts at 70.
Died of cancer.

Your father's brothers & sisters

■ **Your father**
John Smith, Jr.
b. 9-28-1915
Hypertension at 70.
Still alive.

STAYING HEALTHY

Preventable Perils: Are You at Risk?

Many inherited tendencies—to alcoholism or obesity, for example—can be made worse by family habits such as having cocktail hour every night or eating fried foods. Whatever your habits, use this rule of thumb: The more close relatives who suffered one of the conditions listed below—and the younger they were at the time—the likelier you are to develop the same illness. Here's how to size up your risk, along with some suggestions on how you can improve your odds.

Heart Disease

If your father or grandfather had a heart attack or bypass surgery before age 55 or your mother or grandmother before 65, your risk of having heart disease goes way up. If it runs in your family: Get plenty of exercise, cut back on fatty foods, keep off any extra pounds, and do what you can to ease stress (see **artery disease,** page 104, and **eight ways to feel your best,** page 292).

High Blood Pressure

A family history of high blood pressure increases your risk. This condition can cause a host of health problems, including stroke and heart attack. If high blood pressure runs in your family: Get a blood pressure check as often as your doctor recommends. Also, follow the same habits of good health you would to prevent heart disease (see **high blood pressure,** page 111).

Diabetes

If you have one parent with type 1 diabetes, you have a 4 to 6 percent chance of getting it yourself. If one parent has type 2, your risk is 7 to 14 percent. African Americans, Mexican Americans, and Pima Indians are at highest risk. Left untreated, diabetes can cause a number of health problems, including blindness and heart disease. If it runs in your family: Exercise regularly, lose weight if you are overweight, and eat a low-fat, high-fiber diet. Have your blood glucose level checked as often as your doctor recommends (see **diabetes,** page 277).

Breast Cancer

Five to 10 percent of breast cancers are inherited. If your mother, sister, or daughter has had breast cancer, then your risk is higher. If breast cancer runs in your family: Talk with your doctor about how soon you should begin getting mammograms. If many members of your family developed the disease at a young age, your doctor may suggest that you get tested for the presence of errors in certain genes that have been linked to a higher risk of breast and ovarian cancer.

Colon Cancer

Ten to 15 percent of all colon cancers are inherited. If it runs in your family: Ask your doctor whether you should get a sigmoidoscopy. Regular, low doses of aspirin may offer some protection, as does a low-fat diet that includes plenty of fruits, vegetables, and whole grains.

Alcoholism

Children of alcoholics are 4 times more likely than others to become alcoholics. If it runs in your family: You need to be very careful about your drinking. If you've ever found it hard to keep your use of alcohol under control, or anyone close to you thinks your drinking has become a problem, you may want to seek help (see **alcohol abuse and alcoholism,** page 204).

Depression

Not everyone with a family history of the problem will develop depression, but stress is believed to trigger its onset. If it runs in your family: Your doctor is more likely to suggest early intervention with antidepressants if you become depressed and your family history includes suicide attempts or major depressions requiring hospitalization (see **depression,** page 211).

(continued from page 316)

Self-Exams

Most doctors advise these self-exams:

Skin checkup (once a month). Look yourself over—more often if you have fair skin or a lot of moles, or if you spend a lot of time in the sun. Examine yourself fully. Use a mirror for hard-to-see places, or ask a partner to look. Keep an eye out for scaliness, oozing, or bleeding, or changes in freckles or moles. Report any changes to your doctor. (See **simple steps to save your skin,** page 178, and **skin cancer,** page 179.) Once a year, get a professional exam.

Weighing in. Keep your weight at a healthy level (see page 295). It's vital for good health. Know what you should weigh for your height (see page 296 for healthy weight ranges). Your weight can vary throughout the day, so whenever you weigh yourself, always try to do it at the same time—in the morning upon rising, for example. If your clothes start to feel too tight or too loose, step on a scale. Tell your doctor about any unusual weight gain or loss. (Also see **sudden weight gain or loss** chart, page 282.)

For Women

Breast self-exam (once a month). Check your breasts at the same time each month. You'll have a good chance of finding any lump that may need a doctor's attention. (For how to do it, see page 239.) Tell your doctor right away about any changes.

For Men

Testicular exam (once a month). Though testicular cancer amounts to only 1 percent of all cancers, it is the leading cancer in men age 20 to 35. Finding it early can lead to a complete cure. Every month, roll each testicle between your thumb and forefinger, feeling for lumps. It's best to do the exam after a warm shower or bath, when any lumps or changes are easier to feel. Report any new lump or swelling to your doctor right away.

Tests

The following tests require a visit to a doctor or clinic. Depending on your age and physical condition, your doctor may advise you to have checkups more often or less often.

For Women & Men

BLOOD PRESSURE

The test. A blood-pressure cuff around your arm measures the force of blood pressing against your artery walls. The longer high blood pressure goes undetected and untreated, the higher your risk of heart attack, stroke, and liver and kidney damage.

When to get it. Once a year for most adults; more often if your doctor advises it. If your blood pressure is higher than it should be (see **high blood pressure,** page 111), your doctor may suggest lifestyle changes or medication to bring it down.

Who's at risk. African Americans; anyone who is overweight; anyone who has heart disease or a family history of hypertension.

Test tips. Stress, some medications, and even the time of day can affect your results. So can simply going to the doctor. In fact, as many as 25 percent of people whose pressure is a little high turn out to have "white coat hypertension" brought on by just being in a doctor's office.

CHOLESTEROL

The tests. A basic blood test measures total cholesterol. A reading of less than 200 (milligrams of cholesterol per deciliter of blood) is good. A reading of 200 to 239 is borderline. A higher reading means you may have a greater than normal risk of heart disease and stroke. Your total cholesterol tells only part of the story, however. You should pay attention to the various *types* of cholesterol in your blood. One form—low density lipoprotein, or LDL—has been nicknamed bad cholesterol because it can clog your arteries. There is also good cholesterol—high density lipoprotein, or HDL—which actually helps prevent artery disease (see **artery disease,** page 104, and **eat well,** page 296). Your level of HDL should be at least 40; an HDL reading above 60 gives good protection. Your LDL level should be less than 130.

STAYING HEALTHY

When to get them. There's some debate over timing. The National Cholesterol Education Program recommends a basic blood test at least once every 5 years for most adults. The United States Preventive Services Task Force recommends regular screening only for men ages 35 to 65 and women ages 45 to 65. Discuss your risks with your doctor to decide when you should get screened.

Who's at risk. Smokers; anyone with high blood pressure or diabetes, or who is sedentary or overweight; anyone who has a family history of heart disease; postmenopausal women who aren't taking estrogen.

Test tips. You'll need to fast for 9 to 12 hours before getting the HDL/LDL/triglyceride test. For a total cholesterol test, you don't need to fast.

COLORECTAL CANCER

The tests. During a digital rectal exam (DRE), a doctor inserts a rubber-gloved finger into the rectum to check for rectal growths and, in men, signs of prostate problems. During a sigmoidoscopy, the doctor guides a flexible, lighted tube into the rectum and lower intestine, looking for signs of colon cancer or for polyps that may become cancer. A fecal blood test detects blood in the stool, a common sign of colon cancer.

When to get them. Every routine physical should include a digital rectal exam. If your risk for colorectal cancer is average, you should have an occult blood test every year beginning at age 50, and a sigmoidoscopy every 3 to 5 years starting at age 50 or earlier. If you have a high risk, talk with your doctor about getting checked more often.

Who's at risk. Anyone with a history of inflammatory bowel disease or precancerous intestinal polyps; anyone with a family history of colorectal cancer.

Test tips. For 72 hours before the fecal occult blood test, eat foods with lots of fiber and avoid red meat, aspirin, foods containing large amounts of vitamin C, and certain fruits and vegetables—get a list from your doctor—all of which can throw off the test results. Before a sigmoidoscopy, the colon needs to be emptied by means of laxatives or an enema.

GLAUCOMA

The test. To detect glaucoma, your eye doctor will measure the pressure inside your eye—intraocular pressure (IOP)—with a device called a tonometer.

When to get it. Get an eye exam with a glaucoma test every 3 to 5 years after age 39, or every 1 to 2 years if you're at risk.

Who's at risk. Anyone age 45 or older who hasn't had regular eye exams; anyone with a family history of glaucoma or who has diabetes or high blood pressure; anyone who is nearsighted or who regularly uses certain drugs, including steroids or cortisone; anyone who has ever had a serious eye injury; anyone of African or Asian descent.

For Women

BREAST CANCER

The tests. Even if you do monthly breast exams yourself, get regular exams from your doctor as well. During a clinical breast exam, a doctor or nurse carefully feels all areas of your breasts, looking for any suspicious lumps. A mammogram is an X-ray of your breasts that a radiologist will examine for cancer in the early stages, when lumps may be too small to feel.

When to get them. Get a clinical breast exam every 3 years if you are in your 20s or 30s, then every year from age 40 on. Beginning at age 50, get a mammogram every year. If you're at risk for breast cancer, talk with your doctor about starting at age 40.

Who's at risk. Any woman whose mother, sister, grandmother, or daughter had breast cancer before reaching menopause.

Test tips. Because having your breasts squeezed between the mammography plates can be uncomfortable, avoid scheduling the test for the week before your period, when your breasts are more likely to be tender. Take an over-the-counter pain reliever an hour before the exam.

CERVICAL CANCER

The test. For a Pap smear, a health care worker gently scrapes cells from the cervix and sends them to a lab to be examined for changes that can signal problems.

When to get it. After you turn 18 or become sexually active, you should have a Pap smear every year—after you have 3 normal tests in a row, possibly less often.

Who's at risk. Smokers; women with more than one sexual partner; women who have HIV or human papilloma virus.

Test tips. A Pap smear is more accurate when done 12 to 14 days after the first day of menstruation.

OSTEOPOROSIS

The test. The most accurate tests use X-rays to measure bone density in the hips and spine—areas most vulnerable to fracture. Knowing your bone density may help you decide whether to start hormone replacement therapy or bone-building drugs when you reach menopause.

When to get it. Women age 45 or older who are at risk for thinning bones should be screened every year; all women age 65 or older should be screened at least every 2 years. Most experts agree that screening should be done only if a woman plans to make treatment decisions based in part on the test results.

Who's at risk. Women who are underweight, who smoke, or who drink heavily; women with a history of unexplained fractures or a family history of osteoporosis; postmenopausal women who don't take estrogen; women who take corticosteroids.

For Men

PROSTATE CANCER

The tests. During a digital rectal exam, the doctor feels the prostate to see if it is enlarged or unusually hard. A blood test for a protein made in the prostate—prostate-specific antigen (PSA)—can sometimes pick up early signs of prostate cancer.

When to get them. Get a DRE every time you have a checkup, or at least once a year beginning at age 50. Start at age 40 if you're at risk. There's a lot of debate about when, or even if, you should get the PSA test. PSA levels alone do not signal the presence or absence of cancer, and some doctors warn that a positive test can cause needless worry

and unnecessary biopsies. You may decide, based on your risks, that the PSA test is not right for you.

Who's at risk. African American men, or anyone whose father or brother had or has prostate cancer.

Test tips. It may help to refrain from ejaculating within 48 hours of a PSA test, since ejaculation can raise your PSA levels.

Immunizations

Immunizations are a shot of prevention against many health problems, including polio, hepatitis, diphtheria, tetanus, and whooping cough.

They work by exposing the body to a killed or weakened form of a virus or other infectious agent. This prompts the body's immune system to strengthen its own defenses. Most doctors advise the following:

Children & Teenagers

For information, see **children's immunizations** chart, page 250.

Adults

Tetanus-diphtheria (Td) booster. Once every 10 years.

Influenza vaccine. Yearly for people age 65 and over and for those at high risk for flu, including adults with diabetes, kidney disease, cancer, chronic heart and respiratory conditions, or anemia; people with weakened immune systems; and adults who work with people at risk.

Pneumococcal vaccine. Once in a lifetime (or more, depending on your doctor's advice) for adults at high risk of pneumonia, including those who have had organ transplants, those age 65 and older, and those with diabetes, alcoholism, cirrhosis (liver damage), congestive heart failure, kidney failure, chronic pulmonary disease, or weakened immune systems.

Hepatitis B vaccine. A single series, once in a lifetime, for those at high risk, including health care workers, people who have contact with dirty needles, and people with hemophilia who have frequent blood transfusions (see **hepatitis,** page 279).

STAYING HEALTHY

Medicines: Playing It Safe

If you're like most people, you've taken prescription drugs. And occasionally, you've probably taken more than one kind at the same time. Most likely you also take over-the-counter drugs now and then—painkillers, for instance, and allergy medicines—or herbal remedies. Yet many drugs, whether over-the-counter or prescription, can have serious side effects when they bump up against each other. Other drugs are dangerous when combined with alcohol, nicotine, herbal remedies, caffeine, some vitamins or minerals, or certain foods. Also, some drugs cancel out each other's usefulness if you take them together. (Older people are at higher risk for harmful reactions to drug combinations because their systems don't handle drugs as well as younger people's, and because they often take more than one prescription medicine at a time.) To protect yourself, follow these medication safety tips:

➤ Tell *each* doctor you see about all the medications you are taking—both prescription and over-the-counter.

➤ Mention vitamins as well, and whether you drink alcohol or use tobacco.

➤ If you're taking a number of medications, bring the containers with you to show the doctor; have them recorded in your file.

➤ Be sure all your doctor's directions about a drug make sense to you. Always read the label and follow the instructions exactly.

➤ Also, ask your doctor or pharmacist:

■ Does it matter what time I take the medication? If so, should I take it with food or an hour or two before or after eating?

■ Should I avoid any foods, prescription medicines, or over-the-counter drugs while taking this? Should I avoid vitamins, herbal products, and other supplements? Is it safe to drink alcohol while I'm taking it? Will it affect my driving? What about caffeine, tobacco, or exposure to sunlight?

■ What side effects, if any, might I have?

■ What should I do if they occur?

➤ Your pharmacist is an excellent source of information. Fill all your prescriptions at the same pharmacy. That way your pharmacist will have a computerized record of your medications and can alert you to any problems.

➤ Always take the full course of medication prescribed for you. But call your doctor at once if you notice any new or strange symptoms. These include confusion, depression, insomnia, rashes, or memory loss. Dizziness as you get up, vomiting, diarrhea, constipation, or abdominal pain also may be side effects of certain drugs.

➤ Store medications as the label directs; some, for instance, should be refrigerated.

➤ Don't share medications.

➤ Don't buy a medicine if the packaging is broken or looks as though someone has tampered with it.

➤ Always take medications in good light—never in the dark. You need to see what you're swallowing or applying.

➤ Throw out leftover medicine if the package date shows it has expired. That makes it less likely that you—or someone else—will take it by mistake.

Drug Combinations to Avoid

This chart lists some potentially dangerous drug combinations. Some drugs react badly with each other; others shouldn't be combined with alcohol, certain foods, herbal remedies, or vitamins. This is by no means a complete list of all harmful drug interactions. (For other sources of information, see For More Help, page 314.) Nor is the chart meant to replace medical advice. Be sure to tell your health care providers about every prescription and over-the-counter medicine you're taking. Never start or stop taking any medication without talking to your doctor first.

IF YOU'RE TAKING	DON'T MIX WITH	WHAT CAN HAPPEN	RECOMMENDATION
Antibiotics— ciprofloxacin (Cipro), other quinolones.	Antacids (Mylanta, Maalox, others), iron and calcium supplements.	The antibiotic will not work as well.	Don't combine these drugs without asking your doctor.
Antibiotics— ciprofloxacin (Cipro), erythromycin, others.	Theophylline (Theo-Dur, Slo-bid, Bronk-aid, others), used to treat asthma.	High levels of theophylline in blood. Symptoms include nausea, vomiting, palpitations, seizures.	Make sure your doctor knows you are taking both. Ask for advice about checking theophylline levels in your blood.
Antibiotics— metronidazole (Flagyl, Femizole, others).	Alcohol (beer, wine, hard liquor); warfarin (Coumadin).	Low blood pressure, vomiting, confusion, rapid heartbeat, increased risk of bleeding.	Don't combine these antibiotics with alcohol, or with warfarin without asking your doctor or pharmacist.
Antibiotics— quinolones, including ciprofloxacin (Cipro) and norfloxacin (Noroxin).	Iron, including supplements and iron-laden tonics.	The antibiotic may not work as well.	Check with your doctor or pharmacist before combining these antibiotics with iron.
Antibiotics— tetracycline, quinolones (Cipro, Noroxin, others).	Calcium in dairy products, supplements, and antacids (such as Tums); or aluminum and magnesium antacids (such as Mylanta or Maalox).	Lower absorption of tetracycline or quinolones, so they don't work as well.	Wait 2 hours after eating dairy products to take medication. Do not take antacids with these medications without your doctor's approval.
Anticoagulants (oral)—including warfarin (Panwarfin, Coumadin, others), used to help prevent blood clots.	Aspirin, ibuprofen (Advil, Motrin), naproxen (Aleve), acetaminophen (Tylenol), ketoprofen (Actron, Orudis KT); stomach-acid blockers (Tagamet, Zantac, Pepcid).	Bleeding, particularly in stomach. Symptoms include black stools, blood in urine, bleeding gums.	Ask your doctor or pharmacist before taking *any* other drug—including over-the-counter drugs.
Anticoagulants (oral)—including warfarin (Panwarfin, Coumadin, others).	Vitamin K–rich foods and drinks (broccoli, cabbage, lentils, soybeans, others); antacids (Mylanta, Maalox).	Reduce effect of anticoagulant.	Check with your doctor about combining drug with foods rich in vitamin K, or with any other drugs.

(continued)

Drug Combinations to Avoid (continued)

IF YOU'RE TAKING	DON'T MIX WITH	WHAT CAN HAPPEN	RECOMMENDATION
Anticoagulants—(oral)—including warfarin (Panwarfin, Coumadin, others).	Herbal remedies (garlic, ginkgo biloba).	May increase the effect of anticoagulant and possibly increase the risk of bleeding.	Talk with your doctor or pharmacist; it's best not to combine these drugs with herbal remedies.
Antidepressants—selective serotonin-reuptake inhibitors, such as Fluoxetine (Prozac), sertraline (Zoloft), paroxetine (Paxil), citalopram (Celexa).	Monoamine oxidase (MAO) inhibitors (Nardil, Parnate, others used to treat depression); Eldepryl, used for Parkinson's disease; and herbal remedies (Saint-John's-wort).	Confusion, muscle twitches, sweating, shivering, agitation; in very rare cases, can be fatal. Saint-John's-wort interaction remains to be determined.	Discuss with your doctor. Don't take these antidepressants with an MAO inhibitor or herbal remedy, or for 2 weeks after quitting an MAO. Wait up to 5 weeks after going off these drugs to start an MAO.
Antidepressants—monoamine oxidase (MAO) inhibitors (Nardil, Parnate, others).	Over-the-counter cold medicines, decongestants, or diet pills with phenylpropanolamine (Allerest, Dexatrim, others); phenylephrine (Dristan, others); and pseudoephedrine (Sudafed, others).	Rapid heartbeat, light-headedness, headache, sudden rise in blood pressure; could lead to a fatal stroke.	Don't take these cold medicines with an MAO inhibitor, or for 2 weeks after quitting an MAO.
Antidepressants—MAO inhibitors (Nardil, Parnate, others).	Alcoholic drinks containing tyramine (including red wines). Also foods with tyramine (aged cheeses; liver; yeast concentrates; broad beans; salted, smoked, or pickled fish; others).	May cause a dramatic rise in blood pressure, dizziness, nausea; in rare cases, bleeding around brain and death.	Avoid alcoholic drinks and foods rich in tyramine if you're taking an MAO inhibitor.
Antidepressants—tricyclic medications (Elavil, Sinequan, others).	Antidepressants—MAO inhibitors (Nardil, Parnate, others).	Confusion, fever, dizziness, seizures, overexcitement, coma.	These drugs should be combined only if prescribed to be taken together.
Calcium channel blockers—(Plendil, Procardia, Adalat, others). Used to treat high blood pressure and angina.	Grapefruit juice (contains flavonoids, including naringenin).	Hazardous increase in the level of medication in blood. Symptoms include headaches and light-headedness.	Do not take these drugs with grapefruit juice.
Gastrointestinal drugs—acid blockers (Tagamet, Zantac, Pepcid) and antacids (Mylanta, Maalox, others) for heartburn and ulcers.	NSAIDs (aspirin, ibuprofen, naproxen); anticoagulants; some heart, antifungal, antibiotic, or other drugs.	Taken with NSAIDs, can mask ulcer symptoms. May change effects of many other drugs.	Read drug warnings carefully or ask your doctor or pharmacist before you mix these with other drugs.

Drug Combinations to Avoid

IF YOU'RE TAKING	DON'T MIX WITH	WHAT CAN HAPPEN	RECOMMENDATION
Gastrointestinal drugs—cisapride (Propulsid), for nighttime heartburn.	Antifungal drugs and some antibiotics.	Irregular heartbeat, heart attack.	Don't combine these drugs. Ask your doctor or pharmacist.
Heart drugs—digoxin (Lanoxin).	Antacids (Mylanta, Maalox).	Heart drug may not work as well.	Don't combine these drugs.
Heart drugs—digoxin (Lanoxin).	Quinidine, diuretics, verapamil, and herbal remedies (Saint-John's-wort, ma-huang).	Abnormal heartbeat, nausea, loss of appetite, vision changes.	Ask your doctor or pharmacist before mixing this with other drugs or herbal remedies.
Heart drugs—nitrates (Isordil, Nitro-Dur, nitroglycerin, Sorbitrate).	Sildenafil (Viagra).	Can lower blood pressure to dangerous levels; can be fatal.	Don't combine these drugs.
Hormonal drugs—estrogen-containing birth control pills (Demulen, Ortho Novum, others).	Tobacco (all forms) and nicotine patches, gum, or other products.	Increased risk of stroke, heart attack, blood clots.	Never smoke or use other nicotine products if you take birth control pills.
Hormonal drugs—estrogen-containing birth control pills (Demulen, Ortho Novum, others).	Some antibiotics (including ampicillin, penicillin, rifampin, tetracycline); barbiturates; tranquilizers.	Birth control pills may not work well while you take these and other drugs.	Talk to your doctor about using other birth control methods while taking any medications.
Pain relievers—NSAID-type, including aspirin, ibuprofen (Advil), naproxen (Aleve), others.	Anticoagulants; antacids and acid blockers; alcoholic drinks.	Irritation of stomach lining; greater risk of ulcers and bleeding.	Consult your doctor about mixing these drugs.
Pain relievers—acetaminophen (Tylenol, Panadol, others).	Alcohol (beer, wine, hard liquor); anticoagulants.	Possibility of liver damage; stomach bleeding.	Consult your doctor or pharmacist about mixing these drugs, and ask how much alcohol is safe.
Tranquilizers and sleeping pills—benzodiazepines, including diazepam (Valium), triazolam (Halcion).	Alcohol (beer, wine, hard liquor); herbal remedies (kava, valerian).	With high amounts, dizziness, severe drowsiness, impaired reactions (in driving, operating machinery), coma.	Don't take these drugs with alcohol or herbal remedies.

FOR MORE HELP

Organization: United States Pharmacopeia, 12601 Twinbrook Pkwy., Rockville, MD 20852. 800-227-8772, M–F 7:30–5 EST; *www.usp.org.* Call to order free booklets on understanding your medications, using medicines properly, recognizing drug tampering, and preventing medication errors.

Website: Healthtouch, *www.healthtouch.com.* Click on the drug information tool to find useful facts about the medication you're taking.

STAYING HEALTHY

Index

Note: Page numbers in **bold** refer to the main discussion of a topic and to charts. Page numbers in *italic* refer to illustrations. Drugs named in the text are listed under *Drugs* on page 332.

A

ABCD test for moles, *173*, 179
ABCs of emergency care, **12**
Abdominal injuries, emergency care, **25**
Abdominal muscles, *171*
  exercise to strengthen, **127**
Abdominal pain
  chart, **117–118**
  after blow to abdomen, 25
  after heat exposure, 38
  during pregnancy, 240
  in upper area, 124, 136
  lasting more than four hours, 24
  moving to lower right, 24
  while lifting or bending, 127
  with bloody stools, 131
  with blurry vision, muscle weakness or paralysis, 34
  with burning, sour taste, 124
  with dizziness, trouble seeing, odd-smelling breath, 40
  with drooling, confusion, sweating, dizziness, 34
  with itchy rash (after eating), 84
  with menstrual changes, 233, 234
  with rectal bleeding, 131, 132
  with watery diarrhea, rapid weight loss, 131
  See also Gas and gas pain; Nausea and vomiting
Abscess
  breast, 237
  lung, 76
  tooth, 76, 77
Absence seizures, 58
Accidents
  life-saving skills for, **11–23**

ways to avoid, 17, 261, 299, 301
Acetaminophen, 95, **315**
Achilles tendon, *171*
  tendinitis, 199, **202**
Acid indigestion. *See* Heartburn
Acne, **142,** 241
Acoustic nerve, *73*
Acquired immune deficiency syndrome. *See* AIDS
ADD (attention deficit disorder), **210**
Addiction
  alcohol, 204
  drug, 213
Addison's disease, 283
Adenoids, **103**
ADHD (attention deficit hyperactivity disorder), 210
Adrenal gland disorders, 283
Aggressive or violent feelings, behavior, 208, 213–215
Agitation
  with carbon monoxide poisoning, 205
  with drug abuse, 214–215
AIDS, 274, 283
  safe sex and, 224
  test for, 221
Airplane ear, **68**
Airway, Breathing, Circulation (ABCs), of emergency care, **12**
Airway clearance, 12
  if person is vomiting, 22
  if you are choking and alone, 19
  in choking adult or child, 18–19
  in choking infant, 20
  in drowning, 30
  in head, neck, or back injuries, 37
Alcohol abuse, **204**
  triggering seizures, 41, 58

Alcohol drinking
  drug combinations to avoid chart, **323–325**
  what is moderate, 296
Alcoholism, **204,** 318
  complementary care for, 207
Allergic conjunctivitis, 63
Allergic purpura, 247
Allergic shock, **22,** 84, 143, 205
Allergies, **84**
  airplane flying and, 68
  anaphylactic shock (shock from allergy), **22,** 87, 205
  causing conjunctivitis, 63
  drug, 22, **84**
  food, **84,** 133
  severe, emergency care, **22**
  using humidifiers if you have, 92
Allergist, 309
Alveoli, *164*
Alzheimer's disease, **48**
Amenorrhea, 234
Anaphylactic shock (shock from allergy), **22,** 87, 205
Anemia, **272**
  bleeding ulcers and, 135
  heavy menstrual flow and, 234
  itching and, 149
Aneurysm, aortic, 105
Angina, 27, 104, 105
Angioedema, 155
Animal allergies, 84, 87
Animal bites, **24**
Ankles
  pain chart, **199**
  bones, *170*
  fractures, emergency care, **35**
  purple rash on, 247
  scaly, dry reddish rash on, 150
  sprains or strains of, **44**
  swelling of, 282

Ankylosing spondylitis, 192
Anorexia, **216,** 283
Antacids, drug combinations to avoid chart, **323–325**
Antibiotics
  drug combinations to avoid chart, **323–325**
  fungal infections from, 154, 253
  overuse of, **254**
Anticoagulants, drug combinations to avoid chart, **323–325**
Antidepressants, drug combinations to avoid chart, **323–325**
Antifungal drugs, drug combinations to avoid chart, **323–325**
Antihistamines
  for allergic reactions, 22
  for colds, 94
Anti-inflammatories, drug combinations to avoid chart, **323–325**
Antioxidants
  to help prevent cataracts, 63
  See also Diet
Antitussives, 94
Anus
  rectal bleeding and itching chart, **131–132**
  hemorrhoids, 115, 116, **126,** 132, 241
  itchy bumps around, 222
  muscle tear, 131, 132
  painful swelling in or around, 126
Anxiety, **208**
  complementary care for, 209
Aortic aneurysm, 105
Aortic valve, *168*
Aplastic anemia, 272
Appendicitis, **24**
  blood poisoning from, 29
  pain referred from, *176*
  vs. gas, 124
  vs. heartburn, 125
Appendix, *174*
Appetite loss
  in children, 56, 255
  in infants, 50, 71, 255
  with abdominal pain, 118
  See also Nausea and vomiting
Armpits, dry scaly rash, then greasy patches on, 249
Arms
  blistered, crusty patches on, 149
  broken or injured, **35**
  pain
    shooting, with tingling or numbness, 188
    worse with activity, 198

sudden numbness, with trouble seeing, 44
  See also Shoulder pain
Arterial pressure points, 13
Arteries, *169*
Artery disease, **104,** *169*
  See also Heart and circulation problems
  complementary care for, 109
Arthritis, **182**
  complementary care for, 185
Aspirin, **315**
  blood sugar and, 277
  in heart attack emergency care, 37–38
  Reye's syndrome from, **95**
Asthma, **88,** *164*
  drug combinations to avoid chart, **323–325**
  emergency care for, **42**
  using humidifiers if you have, 92
Atherosclerosis, *169*
  See also Artery disease
Athlete's foot, **153**
Atopic dermatitis (eczema), **152**
  in children, 248
Attention deficit disorder (ADD), **210**
Attention deficit hyperactivity disorder (ADHD), 210
Atrium, left, *168*
Atrium, right, *168*
Auras, seizure, 58

B

Babies. *See* Infants; Newborns
Baby measles (roseola), **265**
Back injuries, **36**
Back pain
  chart, **192–193**
  during pregnancy, 192, 240
  in sharp waves starting below ribs, moving to groin, 136
  low, *166,* **190**
  of strains or sprains, 44, 190
  shooting pain if head bent forward, 56
  stress-related, 218
  with pregnancy, 192
  with prostate problems, 228
Bad breath, **76**
  from sinus problems, 98
  odd-smelling, in poisoning, 40
Bad taste in mouth, 76, 77, 78, 80
Bad temper, sudden.
  See Mood changes

Balance problems.
  See Loss of balance
Balanitis, 230
Bald patches on scalp, after round itchy rash, 248
Balloon angioplasty, 107
Barotrauma (airplane ear), **68**
Basal cell carcinoma, 172, 179
Basal cells, skin, *172*
Bed-wetting, **246**
Bee stings
  allergic reaction to, **25**
  emergency care, **25**
  removing the stinger, 25
Behavior and health
  alcohol abuse, alcoholism, **204**
  drug abuse, **213**
  in children, 210, 260
  smoking, 92, 299
  See also Emotions
Belching
  with upper abdominal pain, 106, 123, 127, 134
  See also Gas and gas pain
Benign paroxysmal positional vertigo, 50
Biceps muscle, *171*
Bicuspid (mitral) valve, *168*
Binge eating, purging (bulimia), **216,** 283
Bipolar affective disorder, 212
Birth control
  choosing among methods, **220, 223–224**
  emergency, 224
  health risks, 220, 223–224
  menstrual irregularities and, 234
Bites and stings
  allergic reactions to, **22**
  animal, **24**
  bee or wasp, **25**
  emergency care, **22**
  mosquitoes, encephalitis and, 56
  snake, **42**
  spider or scorpion, **43**
  tick, **45**
Black widow spider bites, **43**
Blackheads, 142
Blackouts, 204, 213
Bladder, *138, 174, 175*
  exercises for control of, 141
  training, for children, 246
Bladder problems
  cancer, 137
  control
    after spinal injury, 183
    loss of, 140
    low back pain and, 190
    with prostate problems, 228
    with seizures, 41, 58

incontinence, **140**
infection (cystitis), 137, 138, 281
 bed-wetting as sign of, 246
 with diabetes, 277
pain referred from, *176*
See also Urinary problems
Blank or fixed stare, 41, 57, 58
Bleeding
after head injury, **13,** 29, 36, 49
cuts, scrapes, or wounds, **28**
emergencies, **13**
from ears, 29, **30**
from eyes, 29, **32**
from fractures, **35**
from mouth, **22**
from nose, 29, **40**
from tooth socket, 45
gums, 76, 77, 78
internal, **22**
in throat, 40
pressure points to stop, 13
rectal, **131–132**
shock from severe, **22**
that won't stop, **13**
unusual or unexplained, 283, 284
vaginal
 after blow to abdomen, 25
 in shock, 22
with object still stuck in wound, 13
Blepharitis, 62
Blind spots, with trouble looking at lights, 275
Blindness
shingles and, 177
sudden, 61
Blinking
extreme, after eye injury, 32
lack of, or odd, 57, 58, 59
Blisters, **145**
after burns, 26, 145
after spider bite or scorpion sting, 43
after sunburn, 178
fever, **79**
following red itchy spots on face, torso, 248, 249
itchy rash with (children), 248, 258
on buttocks, 144, 149
on genitals, 221, 230
on hands or legs, 149
on nose, 177
on or around lips, 79
or crusty round patches, 149
painful rashes of, on one side of body, 160
that ooze, crust over, 149

Bloating
after eating dairy foods, 118
premenstrual, 241
See also Gas and gas pain
Blood clots, 169
aspirin and, 37, 38, 315
birth control pills and, 220
in deep vein of leg, 194
in lungs, 85
Blood in stools
with abdominal pain, 118
with anemia, 272
with menstrual problems, 233
with pasty skin, pale gums, brittle nails, 272
with rapid weight gain, yellowish skin, 282
with rectal bleeding, 131, 132
See also Bowel movements
Blood in urine, 137
with menstrual problems, 233
See also Urinary problems
Blood infection (septicemia), **29**
Blood loss
causing shock, **22**
See also Bleeding
Blood poisoning, **29,** 273
Blood pressure
dizziness from drop in, 50
normal range for, 111
tests of, 319
See also High blood pressure
Blood sugar
high or low, 277, 278
medications that affect, **277**
Bloodshot eye, 32, 62
with headache, 54
Bloody nose, emergency care, **40**
Bluish fingernails, 37, 89
Blurred vision. *See* Vision problems
Body lice, **157**
Body temperature
below normal, 29, 39
how to take a child's, **255**
See also Fever
Body weight
sudden or unexplained gain/loss chart, **282–283**
chart of healthy, **296**
gain in. *See* Weight gain
how to maintain a healthy, 295
loss of. *See* Weight loss
See also Health and fitness basics; Overweight
Boil-like lumps, 142
Boils, **146**
in ear canal, 70

Bone loss
hormone replacement to prevent, 235
osteoporosis, *167,* **196**
Bones (skeletal system), *170*
broken, emergency care, **35**
osteoporosis, *167,* 193, **196**
spinal. *See under* Spinal
spurs, *165,* 182
Botulism, 34
Bowel blockage, 121
Bowel movements
constipation, **116**
diarrhea, **119**
folk remedy for constipation, 119
foul-smelling, with weight loss, 124, 283
impacted, 119
increase in, with weight loss, trembling hands, 288–289
none, after three days, 116
painful, with blood on toilet paper, 126, 131, 132
pale, 279
thin, with abdominal pain, 118, 121
what is "normal" number of, 116
See also Blood in stools; Rectal bleeding and itching
Brain disorders
Alzheimer's disease, **48**
encephalitis, **55**
hemorrhage (bleeding in brain), 49
meningitis, **55**
Parkinson's disease, **57**
tumor, 50, 53
Breast cancer, 318, 237, 239
birth control pills and, 220
exams by doctor, 320
hormone replacement and, 235
self-exam, **239**
signs of, 237, 239
Breast feeding
and nipple soreness, 237
children's diarrhea and, 120
menstrual periods and, 234
Breast pain or lumps
chart, **237–238**
during pregnancy, 241
premenstrual, 241
Breastbone (sternum), *170*
Breath, bad. *See* Bad breath
Breathing problems
chart, **85–86**
after blow to abdomen, 25
after chemical burns, 26
after heat exposure, 38
during light activity or rest, 109

emergency care
ABCs of, **12**
for shortness of breath, **42**
rescue breathing and CPR,
14–17
humidifiers and, 92
in allergies, **84**
in asthma, **88**, *164*
in bronchitis, **90**, **91**
in colds, **93**
in emphysema, **91**
in flu, **95**
in pneumonia, **97**
with crushing chest pain, 37
with droopy eyelids, trouble
swallowing, 34
with fatigue, pale skin, 50
with muscle weakness or
paralysis, 34
with nagging awareness of
heartbeat, 112
with red skin, intense itching,
swelling face or tongue, 23
with trouble seeing, odd-
smelling breath, 40
See also Choking; Lung problems
Brittle fingernails, 272
Broken blood vessel in eye, 62
Broken bones. *See* Fractures and
dislocations
Broken nose, 40
Bronchial tubes, *164*
Bronchitis
acute, **90**
chronic, **91**
Brown recluse spider bite, **43**
Bruises
abnormal or unexplained,
206, 284
after fractures or dislocations,
35–36
first aid for, **147**
in sprains or strains, 44
on eye, 32
RICE treatment for, **198**
Brushing your teeth, **82**
Bruxism (tooth grinding), 80,
83, 201
Bulge, in abdomen or groin,
118, 127
Bulging eyes, 288
Bulimia, **216**, 283
Bunions, **185**, 199
Burns
blisters from, 26, 145–146
blood poisoning from, 29
chemical, **26**
emergency care, **26**
of electric shock, **31**
on skin, as sign of poisoning, 40

what not to do, 27
Burping, 118, 124
See also Gas and gas pain
Bursitis, **187**
Buttocks
blistered, crusty patches on, 149
burning skin, blistery rash
on, 144
pain in, with back problems, 190,
192, 193
purple rash on, 247
Buzzing in ears, **74**

C

Caffeine
blood sugar raised by, 277
heart palpitations and, 112
ringing in ears and, 74
withdrawal headache, 54
Calcium
basics of, 299
richest food sources of, 298
supplements, 197
Calcium channel blockers, drug
combinations to avoid chart,
323–325
Calluses and corns, **148**, 199
Calories
burned by common
activities, **293**
how to cut, 296–297
Cancer
bladder, 137
breast, 220, 235, 237
self-exam, how to do, 239
cervical, 220, 222
colon, 116, 131
endometrial, 235
esophageal, 101
eyelid, 67
mouth (oral), 77, 102
ovarian, 233
pancreatic, 118
penile, 230
pneumonia and, 97
prostate, 230
skin, *172*, *173*, **300**
ABCD test for moles, *173*, 179
self-exam, 178, 319
stomach, 272
testicular, 227
weight loss in, 283
Cancer prevention. *See* Health and
fitness basics
Canker sores, **78**
Carbon monoxide poisoning,
40, 205

Carbuncles, 146
Carcinoma, 179
Cardiologist, 309
Cardiomyopathy, 110
Cardiopulmonary resuscitation.
See CPR
Carpal tunnel syndrome (CTS),
188
complementary care for, 190
Carpal (wrist) bones, *170*
Cartilage
chest, 106
joint, *165*
knee, 200, *201*
Cataracts, **60**, 62, 161, *162*
retinal detachment and, 61
surgery, *161*
Cavities, 80, 304, 305
tips on tooth care, **82**
Cerebral embolism, 113
Cerebral hemorrhage, 113
Cerebral thrombosis, 113
Cervical acceleration/deceleration
injury (whiplash), 184
Cervical cancer
birth control pills and, 220
genital warts and, 222
Cervical cap (contraceptive),
220, 223
Cervical spondylosis, 183, 186
Cervix, *175*
Chelation therapy, 261
Chemical food poisoning, **34**,
133, 134
Chemicals
burns from, **26**
in eyes, **33**
Chest compressions in
emergency CPR
cautions with, 15
for adults, children over eight,
14–15
for children ages one to eight, **17**
for infants, **16**
Chest pain
chart, **105–106**
after bending over or lying
down, 124
crushing, with trouble
breathing, 37
dull with weakness and
fatigue, 109
emergency care, **27**
in upper chest, worsened by
coughing fits, 90
sharp, shortness of breath, cold
moist hands, rapid pulse, 85
sharp, with sudden shortness of
breath, cough, 85

sharp, worsens with deep
  breathing, 86
with high fever, chills, 97
See also Breathing problems
Chicken pox, **249**
  aspirin caution with, 95
  encephalitis and, 56
  shingles and, 160
  sore throat and, 100
  vaccine, 250, 251
Childbirth
  emergency, **27–28**
  heavy menstrual flow after, 234
Children's health
  rashes chart, **247–249**
  adenoids, enlarged, 103
  airplane flying and, 68
  aspirin caution, **95**
  bed-wetting, **246**
  chicken pox, **249**
  choking, emergency care, **18–20**
  colic, **251**
  constipation, 116
  croup, **252**
  diaper rash, **253**
  diarrhea, **120**
  ear infections, 71
  emergency CPR
    ages one to eight, **17**
    infants to age one, **20**
    over eight years, **18–19**
  encephalitis, **55–56**
  fever, **255**
  fever seizures, **256**
  fifth disease, **257**
  German measles, **257**
  hand, foot, mouth disease, **258**
  immunization schedule, **250**
  impetigo, **259**
  lead poisoning, **260**
  leukemia, 247
  measles, **262**
  meningitis, **55**, **263**
  mental health, resources for, 271
  mumps, **264**
  nausea and vomiting, **133**
  pertussis (whooping cough), **269**
  pinworms, 131
  resources for parents and
    caretakers, **271**
  Reye's syndrome, **95**
  rheumatic fever, **265**
  roseola, **265**
  rubella (German measles), **257**
  safety, **17**, **261**
  scarlet fever, **266**
  seizures (fever), **256**
  slapped cheek (fifth) disease, **257**
  sore throat, **100**
  strep throat, **267**

teething, **268**
temperature taking, **255**
tonsillitis, **102**
vomiting and nausea, **133**
whooping cough, **269**
See also Infants
Chills and fever
  fever chart, **273–274**
  after tick bite, 45
  after wound or infection, 29, 281
  with dizziness, trouble seeing,
    odd-smelling breath, 40
  with ear infection, 71
  See also Fever
Chlamydia, 221
Chlorine gas poisoning, 40
Chocolate, blood sugar raised
  by, 278
Choking, **18–20**
  after head injury, 37
  from nosebleeds, 40
  Heimlich maneuver, **18**
  how to avoid, 17, 19
  if you are alone, 19
  infant, 16
Cholesterol
  high, complementary care
    for, 109
  hormone therapy and, 235
  in arteries, *169*
  tests of, 319
Chronic fatigue syndrome (CFS),
  219, **275**
Chronic obstructive pulmonary
  disease (COPD), **91**
Chronic pain, RICE treatment
  for, 198
Cigarettes, 299
Circulation, how to check for a
  pulse, 12
Circulation problems. *See* Heart
  and circulation problems
  See also Artery disease
Cirrhosis, 282
Clavicle (collarbone), *170*
Clicking noise, when opening
  mouth, 54, 70, 78, 201
Clitoris, *175*
Clots, blood. *See* Blood clots
Clumsiness
  with weakness, after cold expo-
    sure, 39
  See also Loss of coordination
Cluster headaches, **52**, **54**
Coccyx (tailbone), *170*, *191*
Coffee. *See* Caffeine
Cold exposure (hypothermia),
  emergency care, **39**
Cold hands, feet, 85, 104, 289

Cold medicines, what to look for, **94**
Cold sores, **79**, 221
Colds, 86, **93**
  airplane ear and, 68
  choosing medicines for, **94**
  ear infections and, 71
  sinusitis and, 99
  See also Flu
Colic, **251**
Colitis, ulcerative, 118, **128**
Collapsed lung, 27, 85
Collarbone, *170*
Colon, *174*
  blockage of, 117, 131
  pain referred from, *176*
  polyps, 130
  spastic, **130**
Colon cancer, 318, 320
  anemia and, 272
  tests for, 320
Coma
  in carbon monoxide
    poisoning, 205
  in encephalitis, 56
  in meningitis, 56
  in Reye's syndrome, 95
  in septic shock, 29
  See also Loss of consciousness
Compulsive exercising, in eating
  disorders, 216, 283
Compulsive-obsessive disorder,
  208
Concentration problems
  in children, **210**, 260
  with anxiety or phobias, 208
  with drug abuse, 213
  with grief, 217
  with loss of memory, wandering,
    confusion, 48
  with sleep disorders, 206
  with stress, 219
Concussion
  confusion from, 205
  dizziness from, 49
  See also Head injuries
Condoms
  female, 220
  latex allergies and, 244
  pros and cons, **220**
  safe use of, 220, 224
Confusion
  chart, **205–206**
  after blow to abdomen, 25
  after heat exposure, with fever,
    hot dry skin, 38
  with frequent headaches, dizzi-
    ness, double vision, 50
  with seizures, 41, 58
  with sudden fever, vomiting,
    sunburnlike rash, 243

See also Fever; Memory problems
Congestion
in colds or flu, 86, 93, 96, 281
returning, after using decongestant spray, 94
sinus, **98**
with headaches, 54
See also Nose problems
Congestive heart failure, **109–110**
weight gain in, 282
Conjunctivitis, 62, **63**, 145
Constipation, **116**
complementary care for, 119
during pregnancy, 241
home remedy for, **119**
premenstrual, 241
with rectal bleeding, 131
with thin stools, cramping
on left side, 121
Contact dermatitis, **149**
vaginal, 244
Contraception. *See* Birth control
Convulsions
after snakebite, 42–43
in children, 58–59, 256
See also Seizures
Coordination problems. *See* Loss of
coordination
COPD (chronic obstructive
pulmonary disease), **91**
Copperhead snake bite, **43**
Coral snake bite, **43**
Cornea, *64, 161*
Corns and calluses, **148**, 185, 199
Coronary artery disease, **104**
See also Heart attack
Cosmetics, what to watch for, 150
Cottonmouth snake bite, **42**
Coughs
chart, **85–86**
choosing medicines for, **94**
in children
barking, seal-like, 252
whooping sound, 269
with fever, 247, 248, 262, 265,
266, 267
morning, with mucus, 91
smoker's, 91
with foamy, blood-specked
mucus, 109
with high fever, mucus, 97
Counting things, over and over,
208
CPR (cardiopulmonary resuscitation)
adults, **14–15**
child one to eight years, **17**
child over eight years, **14**
infants up to one year, **16**
if you suspect choking, **18**

if you suspect head, neck, or back
injury, **36**
Crab lice, **157**
Cradle cap, 150, 249
Cramps
menstrual, 233, 234
muscle, **195**
stomach. *See* Abdominal pain
Crohn's disease, 118, 128, 132
Croup, 85, **252**
Crush fractures, *167*
Crying
in infants or children, 251, 255
with grief, 217
CTS (carpal tunnel syndrome), **188**
Cushing's syndrome, 282
Cuts
first aid, **28**
infection in, 281
on eye, 32
Cystic fibrosis, 96
Cystitis. *See* Bladder problems
Cysts
breast, 237, 238
hand (ganglion), 190
ovarian, 233

D

Dairy foods intolerance, 118, 123
Dander, animal, 84, 87
Daytime sleepiness, 286
Death, frequent thoughts of, 211
Decay, tooth, 80
Decongestants
congestion returning after
taking, 94
drug combinations to avoid
chart, **323–325**
Deep-vein thrombosis, 194
Deer tick bites, **45**
Dehydration
after diarrhea, vomiting, 120,
133, 134
after heat exhaustion, 38
after sunburn, 178
as cause of shock, 22
headache of, 53
rehydration drink recipe, 120
Delirium
after fever, severe stiff neck, 56
after snakebite, 43
after taking aspirin for viral
illness, 95
Delivery (childbirth),
emergency, **27**
Deltoid muscle, *171*

Delusions, 212
Dementia
in Alzheimer's, 48
in syphilis, 222
Dental care, 304, 305
blood infections and, 29
checkups, 82, 305
Dental plaque, 77, 80
Dentinal hypersensitivity, 81
Dentures, choking cautions
with, 19
Depression, **211**, 318
anxiety disorders and, 208
complementary care for, 209
premenstrual, 241
sexual desire and, 224
stress and, 219
Depressive reactions, 211
Dermatitis, 144, **149**
blisters from, 145
eczema, **152**, 249
swimmer's ear and, 73
vaginal, 244
Dermatologist, 309
Deviated septum, 99
Diabetes, **277**, 318
birth control and, 220
child bed-wetting as sign of, 246
during pregnancy, 277
medicines affecting blood sugar
levels, 277
muscle cramps in, 195
unconsciousness in, emergency
care, **33**
Diaper rash, **253**
Diaphragm (contraceptive),
220
Diaphragm, pain referred
from, *176*
Diarrhea, **119**
children or infants, **120**
dairy foods and, 118
hemorrhoids and, 126
persistent, 128
premenstrual, 241
rehydration after, recipe for, **120**
with abdominal cramping or
pain, 117–118
with nausea, vomiting, pain,
dehydration, 281
with rectal bleeding, 131–132
with sore mouth and tongue,
fatigue, 272
with sudden weight loss, 282
See also Nausea and vomiting
Diet
artery disease and, 107–108
best food sources of vitamins,
minerals, **298**
food guide pyramid, 297

healthy, 296–299
heart rate and, 113
high blood pressure and, 111
low-fat food chart, **297**
osteoporosis and, 196
palpitations and, 112
premenstrual syndrome and, 241
recommended dietary
    allowances, **298**
tips for creating healthy meals,
    296–299
to prevent or reverse artery
    disease, 107–108
to prevent stroke, 114
vegetables, most nutritious, **298**
Dieting
blood sugar raised by diet
    pills, 277
eating disorders and, 216
menstrual periods and, 233
Digestive system problems
abdominal pain chart, **117–118**
rectal bleeding and itching chart,
    131–132
appendicitis, **24**
constipation, **116**
Crohn's disease, 128
diarrhea, **119**
diverticulitis, **121**
food allergies, 84
food poisoning, **34**
gallstones, **122**
gas and gas pain, **123**
gastritis, **134**
heartburn, **124**
hemorrhoids, **126**
hiatal hernia, 127
inflammatory bowel disease, **128**
intestinal blockage, 117, 131
intestinal infections, 281
irritable bowel syndrome, **130**
lactose intolerance, 118
malabsorption, 283
nausea and vomiting, **133**
pancreatitis, 117
parasites, 129
peritonitis, 121
reflux (heartburn), 125
ulcerative colitis, 129
ulcers, **134**
Dilated pupils. *See* Pupils
Diphtheria vaccine, **250**, 321
Disk (spinal) problems
back pain with, 190, 192
bulging or torn disk, *166*
neck pain with, 183
Dislocations and fractures, **35**
Diverticulitis, 118, **121**
rectal bleeding in, 131
vs. constipation, 119

vs. diarrhea, 119
vs. irritable bowel syndrome, 130
Diverticulosis, 121
Dizziness
chart, **49–50**
after eating, with diarrhea, sweat-
    ing, confusion, 34
after head injury, 36
after heat exposure, with rapid
    pulse, clammy skin, 38
just before fainting, 33
premenstrual, 241
with chest pain, fainting, 105
with crushing chest pain, 37
with ear problems, 69–70
with frequent headaches, 53
with headache, odd breath, 40
with irregular heartbeat, cold
    damp skin, 22
with itching, trouble
    breathing, 22
with pasty skin, fainting, 272
with shakiness, hunger, 206
with sudden confusion, 205
with weakness, trouble seeing, 44
Doctor visits, preparing for,
    312–314
Double vision. *See* Vision problems
Douching, cautions with, 236
Dowager's hump, *167*
Drinking problem, **204**
vs. moderate drinking, 108,
    206, 296
Drooling
in seizures, 41
with diarrhea, vomiting, 34
Drowning, emergency care, **30**
Drowsiness
after cold exposure, 39
after head wound or injury, 29
after seizures, 41, 58
with confusion, headache, agita-
    tion, 205
with headache, vomiting, odd-
    smelling breath, 40
with fever, severe stiff neck, 56
Drug abuse, **213**
chart of common street drugs,
    214–215
triggering seizures, 41, 58
Drug allergies, **22, 84**
Drugs
combinations to avoid chart,
    323–325
street drugs chart, **214–215**
acetaminophen, 315
antihistamines, 22, 94
antitussives (cough suppres-
    sants), 94
aspirin, 95, 315

benzocaine, 178
benzoyl peroxide, 142
blood sugar affected by, 277
bronchodilators (inhalers), 88,
    92, 154, 155
cold medicines, choosing, 94
corticosteroids, 142, 147, 282
cortisone, 97, 147
cough medicines, 94
dangerous to diabetics, 277
decongestants, 94
diuretics, 277
ephedrine, 277
epinephrine, 23, 25, 86
estrogen, 196, 232, 235, 237
expectorants, 94
ibuprofen, 315
inhalers (bronchodilators), 88,
    92, 154, 155
laxatives, 25, 116, 126
levodopa, 57
lindane, 158
lithium, 142
methotrexate, 159
methylphenidate, 210
naproxen sodium, 315
pain relievers, choosing, **315**
permethrin, pyrethrin,
    pyrethrum shampoo, 158
phenylephrine, 277
progestin, 235
Ritalin, 210
selegiline, 57
testosterone, 225
DTaP vaccine, 250
Ductus epididymis, *175*
Ductus (vas) deferens, *175*
Duodenum, *174*
Dust and mold allergies, 84, 87, 88,
    89
Dysentery, 118, 131
Dysthymia, 213

E

Ear, *73*
Ear and hearing problems
chart, **69–70**
after being under water, 70, 73
age-related hearing loss, 69
airplane ear, **68**
background noise, constant, 74
balance problems, sudden, 49, 69
benign paroxysmal positional
    vertigo, 50
bleeding, 30
blocked or full feeling, 70
eardrum rupture, **31**, 69

earwax, **72**

emergency care, **30**

flaky skin at ear opening, 73

fluid draining, 30, 50, 69, 71

foreign object, insect, 31

foul-smelling discharge, 73

from loud noise, 74

hearing loss (sudden, temporary), 50, 69, 70, 73

in infants or young children, 50, 70, 71

infection. *See* Ear infections

injuries, emergency care, **30**

itching, 73

labyrinthitis, 50, 69

lump (painful), 70

mastoiditis, 69

Ménière's syndrome, 50, 69, 74

oily yellow scales , 149

otosclerosis, 69

presbycusis, 69

ringing, buzzing, 30, 68, 69, 70, 72

swelling behind ear, 69 , 71

swelling below ear, 264

swimmer's ear, **73**

tinnitus, **74**

vertigo, 50

with fever, 69, 70, 71

with sore throat, 100, 102

with toothache, 80

Ear infections, 69, 70, **71**

colds or flu and, 94, 96

measles and, 263

Earache. *See* Ear infections

Eating

burning in chest and throat after, sour taste, 124

gas, bloating, pain, after dairy products, 118

itchy skin rash, stomach pain after, 84

nausea, vomiting, diarrhea, cramping after, 34

See also Diet; Foods

Eating disorders, **216**, 234, 283

Ectopic pregnancy, 223, 233

Eczema, **152**, 248

Egg allergies, 84

flu shots and, 96

Ejaculation

painful, 228

premature, 224

Elbows

fractures or dislocations of, **35**

pressure point for bleeding, 13

rashes on, 159, 247, 248

tennis, 202, **203**

Electric shock, **31**

causing seizures, 41

Electrical safety, 17

Elevators, ear problems in, 68

Emergencies

ABCs of, **12**

calling 911, **21**

first-aid kits for, **21**

home medicine cabinet, **21**

recovery position for, **23**

steps to always follow, **12**

See also under specific problem or injury

Emotions

alcohol abuse, alcoholism and, **204**

anorexia and, 216

anxiety disorders, **208**

attention deficit disorder, **210**

bipolar disorder (manic depression), 212

bulimia, 216

children's (mental health resources), 271

depression, **211**

drug abuse and, **213**

eating disorders and, **216**

fears, **208**

grief, **217**

loss of interest in life, 211

loss of sexual desire, **224**

manic depression, 212

obsessive-compulsive disorder, 208

panic attacks, 208

phobias, **208**

post-traumatic stress, 208

seasonal affective disorder (SAD), 212

stress, **218**

suicidal thoughts, 212

terror, with trouble breathing, 208

time of year affecting, 212

worry, constant, 208

Emphysema, 85, **91**

Encephalitis, **55**

triggering seizures, 58

Endocrinologist, 309

Endometrial cancer, 235

Endometriosis, 139, 233

Endometrium, *175*

Enemas, 116

Enlarged prostate, 228

Epidermis of skin, *172*

Epididymitis, 227

Epiglottis, *163*

Epiglottitis, 100

Epilepsy, **58**

seizure emergency care, **41**

Epinephrine

diabetes and, 277

for emergency kits, 22, 23, 25, 86

Erection problems, 224, **226**

Esophagitis. *See* Heartburn

Esophagus, *163*

Estrogen

bone loss and, 196, 232

replacement therapy, **235**

side effects of, 237

Ethmoid sinuses, *99*

Eustachian tube, *73*

Exercise

amount needed for fitness, **294**

artery disease and, 107

benefits of, 292–295

calories burned by common activities, **293**

compulsive, 216, 283

how to keep exercising, **295**

in hot weather, 38

menstrual periods and, 234

osteoporosis and, 197

weight control and, 292–295

Exercises

for bladder control, 141

for wrists, 189

Kegel, 141

to help prevent hernia, 128

External abdominal oblique muscle, *171*

Eye, *64*

cataract surgery, *161*

Eye problems

chart, **61–62**

bleeding, 13, 32

blepharitis, 62

blood vessel broken, 62

bloodshot eye, 32, 62

bulging, 288

bump on eyelid, 67

burning feeling, 63, 67

cataracts, **60**, *161*

conjunctivitis, **63**

dry or scratchy eyes, 62, 182

emergency care, **32**

eyelashes, pus crusting on, 63

eyelids

cuts or scrapes on, 29

drooping, with trouble breathing, 34

painful red bump on, 62, 67

red and itchy, 62

eyestrain, 62

filmed-over feeling, 60

floaters in visual field, 62

foreign object, 32, 61

glaucoma, 61, **65**

inflammation (iritis, uveitis), 61

injuries, 29, **32**

itchiness, 62, 63, 67, 84

macular degeneration, 61
opaque area in eye, 60
optic neuritis, 61
pinkeye, **63**
red spot on white of eye, 62
retinal detachment, 61
rolled back, 41
scratched eyeball, 33
styes, **67**
subconjunctival hemorrhage, 62
swelling around eyes, itchiness, 63
watery eyes, 32, 61, 62, 63
    with bulging, 288
    with colds, flu, 93, 281
    with headaches, 54
    with itching, 84, 86
white area in pupil, 60, 62
with headaches, 53, 54
with sinus infection, 98
yellow-tinged eyes, 122, 123,
    274, 279
See also Vision problems
Eyebrows, oily yellow scales on or
    near, 149

F

Face
    bluish
        after coughing fit
            (children), 269
        with sudden high fever (chil-
            dren), 256
    bluish lips, 94, 97
    hair on (women), 282
    masklike, almost no blinking, 57
    numbness, with trouble seeing,
        loss of speech, 44
    pain. *See* Facial pain
    paralysis in, 44
    reddish
        from cluster headaches, 54
        with intense itching, rapid
            swelling, 23
Facial pain, *176*
    around eyes, forehead, 98
    from grinding teeth, 78, **83**
    with jaw clicking sounds, 201
Fainting, **33**
    irregular heartbeat and, 112
    with low temperature, rapid
        pulse, 29
    with pasty skin, fatigue, 272
    with severe chest pain, 104
Faintness
    with cold, damp, pale, or bluish
        skin, 22
    with panic attacks, 208

See also Dizziness
Fallopian tubes, *175*
    surgery to close, 220
Family health history, keeping track
    of, **316–317**
Family practitioner, 309
Farsightedness, 62
Fatigue
    as sign of infection, 281
    chronic fatigue syndrome, **275**
    from dehydration, 53
    in children, 247, 248, 265
    lasting longer than six
        months, 275
    leg or feet, when walking,
        104, 199
    not relieved by rest, 275
    premenstrual, 241
    with abdominal pain, yellowish
        skin, 274, 279
    with breathing problems, 86, 106
    with dizziness, 49–50
    with fever lasting weeks, bad sore
        throat, 100, 274
    with joint swelling, pain, but-
        terfly rash on face, 284
    with muscle tenderness, but no
        joint pain, 276
    with pasty skin, pale gums,
        nailbeds, 272
    with pounding headache, in
        coffee drinkers, 54
    with slow heartbeat, 112
    with sudden weight gain or loss,
        282–283
    with thyroid problems, 282
Fears, of people, places, things, 208
Febrile seizures, 256
Fecal occult blood test, 320
Feelings of dread
    with anxiety and phobias, 208
    with epileptic seizures, 58
Feet. *See* Foot problems
Female condom, 220
Female reproductive system, *175*
    inflammation of, 233, **236**
    pap smears, 320, 321
    See also Pregnancy
Femur, *170, 201*
Fever
    chart, adults and children,
        273–274
    after cut, scrape, or wound, 29
    after eating, with vomiting,
        diarrhea, 34
    after taking a new medication, 84
    after tick bite, 45
    as sign of infection, 281
    causing seizures, 41, 58, **256,**
        266, 273

high, with no sweating, after heat
    exposure, 38
lasting weeks or months, 274
rheumatic, **265**
scarlet, **266**
with a rash
    adults, 143–144
    children, 247–248
with abdominal pain, 117–118
with breathing problems, 86
with ear problems, 69, 70, 71
with headache, stiff neck, 56, 263
with painful urination, 136
with pulsing pain, tingling on
    one side of body, 160
with sore throat, 100, 102
with toothache, 80
See also Nausea and vomiting
Fever blisters, **79**
Fever seizures, 58, **256,** 266, 273
Fiber, richest food sources of, **298**
Fibrocystic breast disease, 238
    birth control drugs and, 220
Fibromyalgia, 193, **276**
Fibula, *170, 201*
Fiddleback spider bite, **43**
Fifth disease, 248, **257**
Filiform warts, **181**
Fingernails
    bluish, 37, 89
    brittle, 272
    pitted, 159
    round, scaly, itchy rash
        around, 248
Fingers
    broken or dislocated, **35**
    numbness, tingling in first
        three, 188
    sprains or strains, **44**
    stiffness, with inflamed rash
        on, 159
    trigger, 203
    warts on, 180
Fire, on clothing, how to
    smother, 26
First aid, **24–45**
    supplies for kits or home, **21**
    *See also under specific injury
        or illness*
First-degree burns, 26
Fish oil, blood sugar raised by, 277
Fixed or blank stare, 41, 58, 59
Flashbacks, 208
Flashes, hot. *See* Hot flashes
Flat warts, **181**
Flatulence, **123**
Floaters, in field of vision, 61, 62
Flossing teeth, how to, 82
Flu, 86, **95**

aspirin caution with, **95**
fever in, 274
medicines for, 94, 96
stomach, 117, **133**
vaccine, 92, 96, **321**
See also Colds
Flulike symptoms
after taking a new medication, 84
after tick bite, 45, 285
with abdominal pain, yellowish
skin, 279
with fatigue lasting more than six
months, 275
with severe stiff neck, 56, 263
Fluttering heartbeat.
See Palpitations
Flying
ear problems with, 68
jet lag, 287
Folic acid
basics of, 299
deficiency anemia, 272
richest food sources of, 298
Folliculitis, 144, 146
Food allergies, **84**
causing canker sores, 79
causing migraine headaches, 52,
55
nausea and vomiting in, 133
severe, emergency care for, **22**
Food poisoning, **34,** 117
vs. appendicitis, 24
Foods
allergies to. *See* Food allergies
causing headaches, 52, 55
drug combinations to avoid
chart, **323–325**
premenstrual cravings for, 241
with richest sources of vitamins,
minerals, **298**
Foot, pressure point to stop bleeding, 13
Foot problems
pain chart, **199**
athlete's foot, **153**
bunions, **185**
calluses, **148**
cold feet, 104
corns, **148**
discolored skin, pain at rest, 104
fractures or dislocations, **35**
hammertoes, **185**
in children, itchy rash with blisters, 258
odor that won't go away, 154
plantar fasciitis, 199
red rash on soles, fever, 243
sprains or strains, **44**
tendinitis in, 202–203
warts on soles, 181

Forearms
broken or injured, **35**
shooting pain, with tingling or
numbness, 188
See also Arms
Forehead pain
with sinus problems, 54, 98
Foreign objects
in ear, 31
in eye, 32–33, 61
in nose, 40
Foreskin tightness, 230
Forgetfulness
that gets worse over time, 48
what is "normal," **51**
with depression, 211
with extreme fatigue, fever,
joint pain, 275
with sleep problems, 206
See also Confusion; Memory
problems
Fourth-degree burns, 26
Fractures and dislocations, **35**
bleeding from, emergency
care, 13
of osteoporosis, *167,* 196
of pelvis, cautions with, 22
RICE treatment for, **198**
spinal compression (crush fracture), *167*
Frontal sinuses, *99*
Frostbite, **39**
Frozen shoulder, 186
FSH blood test, for menopause,
235
Fungal infections, **153**
drug combinations to avoid
chart, **323–325**
fungal meningitis, 56
fungal pneumonia, 97
rashes with, 144, 153–154, 248
ringworm, 248
thrush, 78, 154, 248
vs. diaper rash, 253
yeast infection, 153, 244, 248
See also Yeast infection

G

Gagging
in nosebleeds, 40
that doesn't stop, **18, 20**
Gallbladder, *123, 174*
Gallstones, 117, **122,** *123*
referred pain from, *176*
Ganglion (cyst), 190
Gangrene, 107
Gas and gas pain, **123**

after eating dairy foods, 118
in infants, **251**
vs. appendicitis, 124
with diarrhea, constipation, or
bouts of both, 130
with intense abdominal pain,
upper right side, 122
with pain in upper abdomen, 134
with weight loss, diarrhea, foul-
smelling stools, 283
See also Abdominal pain
Gastritis, 106, 118, **134**
Gastrocnemius muscle, *171*
Gastroenterologist, 309
Gastroesophageal reflux disease
(GERD), 106, **125**
drug combinations to avoid
chart, **323–325**
Generalized anxiety disorder, **208**
Genital herpes, 221
Genital warts, 181, 222
Genitals
blisters or open sores on, 221
heavy greenish-yellow or gray
discharge (women), 222
itching or burning pain, then red
bumps, 221
itchy red bumps, also in groin
area, 153
painless sores, 222
red patches on (children), 248
redness and itching
(women), 244
severe itching, dark specks on
underwear, 157
small, round, red, flat, itchy
bumps, 222
thick yellowish discharge, 222
warts, 222
watery mucus, with burning
urination, 221
See also Penis problems;
Vaginal problems
Genogram (family health history),
316–317
GERD (gastroesophageal reflux
disease), **125**
German measles, 247, **257**
maternal, newborn cataracts and,
60
vaccine, 250, 258
Gestational diabetes, 277
Giardia parasite, 119
Gingivitis (gum disease), 77, 80
Glans, *175*
Glaucoma, 61, **65,** *162*
facial pain of, *176*
headache of, 52, 53
shingles and, 160
Gluteus maximus, *171*

Gluteus medius, *171*
Goiter, 282, 283, 289
Golfer's shoulder, 202
Gonorrhea, 222
Gout, 136, **182**
Grand mal seizures, 58
Graves' disease, 289
Grief, **217**
Groin
  bulge or swelling in, 127
  itchiness in, 153
  pain, after bending or lifting, 127
  pressure point to stop bleeding, 13
Growing pains, in legs, 194
Guilty feelings, 212
Gum care tips, **82**
Gum problems
  causing bad breath, 76, 77
  gray film, 78
  receding gums, 81
  reddish, shiny gums, bleeding often, 77, 80
  See also Mouth problems

H

Haemophilus B vaccine, **250**
Hair
  follicle infection, 144
  grayish-white eggs on, 157
  shaft of, *172*
Hair loss
  after round, scaly, itchy rash, 248
  with weight gain, cold hands, low energy, 289
  with weight loss, brownish skin, 283
Halitosis. *See* Bad breath
Hallucinations, 212
  in drug abuse, 215
Hammertoes, **185**, 199
Hamstring muscles, *171*
Hand, foot, and mouth disease, 248, **258**
Hand problems
  blistered, crusty patches, 151
  blistery rash (children), 248, 258
  calluses, 148
  exercises to strengthen hands, 189
  fractures or dislocations, **35**
  ganglion cysts, 190
  knobby growths on finger joints, 182
  pain, **190**

red rash on palms, with sudden high fever, 243
shakiness, with hunger, 50, 206, 278
shooting pain, with numbness or tingling, 188
tingling or numbness, with shoulder pain, 183, 186
tingling, with sore mouth and tongue, 272
trembling, with weight loss, increased appetite, 288
tremors, 57, 204
warts, 180
Hay fever, 84
HDL levels. *See* Cholesterol
  dizziness when moving, with nausea, vomiting, 50
  lice, **157**
Head injuries
  bacterial meningitis and, 56
  bleeding, **13**
  confusion after, 205
  dizziness after, 49
  emergency care, **36**
  scalp cuts or wounds, 29
  seizures after, 58
  whiplash, 50
Headaches
  chart, **53–54**
  after blow to head, 49
  after chemical burn, 26
  after electric shock, 31
  after eye injury, 32
  after heat exposure, with clammy skin, 38
  after taking new medication, 84
  after tick bite, 45
  after whiplash injury, 50
  complementary care for, 55
  during pregnancy, 240
  in children, 247, 248, 260, 263
  morning
    with aching teeth, 83
    worse when lying down, 53
  of alcohol withdrawal, 204
  pain of, *176*
  pounding, in coffee drinkers, 54
  premenstrual, 241
  stress, 218
  sudden, severe, with paralysis, weakness, numbness, 46
  with confusion, drowsiness, sluggishness, 205
  with face, jaw pain, 94, 98
  with facial pain, clicking jaw noises, 201
  with fatigue not relieved by rest, 275

with fever, severe stiff neck, 56, 263
with pasty skin, pale gums, fatigue, 272
with shakiness, intense hunger, 206, 278
with sudden eye pain, 61, 65
with sudden high fever, rash on palms, soles, 243
with trouble seeing, odd-smelling breath, 40
Health and fitness basics
  accidents, **299**
  checkups, **312**
  dental care, 304, 305
  doctor visits, preparing for, **306**
  eight ways to feel your best, **292–305**
  exercise, 292–295
  family health history, **316**
  information sources for, C2
  nutrition, 296–299
  smoking, 299
  social support, 301
  weight, 295
Health records, how to keep track of, **316**
Healthy body weight
  chart, **296**
  maintaining your, 295
Healthy meals, tips for, 296
Hearing or seeing things that aren't there, 58
Hearing problems
  chart, **69–70**
  See also Ear and hearing problems
Heart, *168, 169, 176*
  flutters. *See* Heartbeat
  pain referred from, *176*
Heart and circulation problems
  chest pain chart, **105–106**
  artery disease, **104**
  birth control drugs and, 220
  congestive heart failure, **109**
  coronary artery disease, 104
  drug combinations to avoid chart, **323–325**
  heart attack. *See* Heart attack
  high blood pressure, **111**
  hormone replacement drugs and, 235
  Lyme disease and, 285
  mitral valve prolapse, 106
  narrowed arteries, 104
  palpitations, **112**
  peripheral vascular disease, 104
  stroke, 107, **113**
  valve problems, 106, 110
  varicose veins, **115**

Heart attack, **37**
abdominal pain of, 117
breathing problems of, 85
chest pains of, **27,** 105
congestive heart failure and, 110
dizziness of, 49
emergency care, **37**
high blood pressure and, 111
vs. heartburn, 125
Heart disease, 318
Heart palpitations, 49, 106, **112**
Heartbeat
how to check for, 12
irregular, rapid, or weak.
See Palpitations
none, CPR to restore, **14–17**
Heartburn, **124**
chest pain of, 106
complementary care for, 125
drug combinations to avoid
chart, **323–325**
during pregnancy, 125
gallstones and, 122
swallowing problems and, 101
ulcers and, 118, 134
vs. appendicitis, 24
vs. heart attack, 125
Heat exhaustion, **38**
Heat rash, 249
Heatstroke, **38**
dizziness of, 49
fever of, 273
sunburn and, 178
triggering seizures, 41
Heimlich maneuver, **18**
Helicobacter pylori bacteria, 135
Hematoma, brain, 49
Hemorrhage, brain, 49
Hemorrhoids, 115, **126,** 132
constipation and, 116
during pregnancy, 241
Hepatitis, 274, **279**
types of, **279**
vaccine for, **250,** 279, 321
Herbal teas, blood sugar raised
by, 277
Hernia, 118, **127**
heartburn and, 125
hiatal, 101, 127
in infants, 251
Herpes virus, 56, 79, 160
Hiatal hernia, 101, 127
Hib (influenza) vaccine, **250,** 321
High blood pressure, **111,** 318
antacids caution with, 125
artery disease and, 104
congestive heart failure and, 110
heartburn and, 125
palpitations and, 112
ringing in ears and, 74

stroke and, 114
with thyroid problems, 288
High-voltage wires, electric shock
from, **32**
Hips, *167*
broken or injured, emergency
care, 36
HIV infection, 221
nonlatex condoms and, 220
safe sex and, **224**
test for, 221, 224
See also AIDS
Hives, **155**
from bee or wasp stings, **25**
in allergic reactions, **23**
rash of, 143, 155, 247
Hoarseness
in children, 252
with allergies, 155
with colds, 93
with loss of voice, 86, 100
with sore throat, 100
with tonsillitis, 102
Hodgkin's disease, 177
Home pharmacy, supplies for, **21**
Home safety
for children, **17**
poisons around the home, **41**
poisonous plants, **41**
Hopelessness, 211
Hormonal drugs
drug combinations to avoid
chart, **323–325**
implants and injections (contraceptive), 223
Hormone imbalances, menstrual
periods and, 234
Hormone replacement, **235**
osteoporosis and, 196
Hot flashes
in anxiety and phobias, 208
in menopause, 232, 235
Hot weather, heat exhaustion or
stroke in, **38**
Human immunodeficiency virus.
See HIV infection
Human papilloma virus, 181
Humerus, *170*
Humidifier lung, **92**
Humidifiers and vaporizers, 99,
252
hints on, **92**
Humming only you can hear, 74
Hunchbacked posture, 193, 196
Hunger
causing headaches, 55
intense, with dizziness, 50, 206
Hydrocele, testicular, 227
Hyperactivity, child, 210
Hyperglycemia, 278

Hypertension. *See* High
blood pressure
Hyperthyroidism, 283, **288**
Hyperventilation, 106
Hypoglycemia, 50, 206, 278
Hypotension, 50
Hypothermia, **39**
after near drowning, 30
burn care and, 27
Hypothyroidism, 188, 282, **289**

I

IBD. *See* Inflammatory
bowel disease
IBS. *See* Irritable bowel syndrome
Ibuprofen, **315**
Illness, information resources,
313, 314
Immobilization, of broken
bones, **35**
Immune system, exercise benefits
to, 292
Immunizations
for adults, 321
schedule for children, **250**
Impacted teeth, 77, 80
Impetigo, 248, **259**
Implanted hormones (contracep-
tive), 223
Impotence, **226,** 282
See also Sexual health
Impulsiveness, in children, 210
Inability to escape thoughts, 208
Inability to pay attention.
See Concentration problems
Inability to relax, 208
Inability to stop talking, 214
in children, 210
Incontinence
after neck injury, 183
after seizures, 41, 58
urinary, **140**
with low back pain, 190
with prostate problems, 228–229
Indigestion. *See* Heartburn
Infants
airplane travel with, 68
bulging soft spot of skull, fever,
stiff neck, 56
choking, **18**
colic, **251**
constipation, 116
coughing loudly, barking, seal-
like, 252
CPR for, **16**
creamy yellow or white patches
in mouth, 78, 153, 248

croup, **252**

crying that won't stop, 251

dental care for, 82

diaper rash, 249, **253**, 259

diarrhea, 120

ear infection, 70, **71**

emergency care, **16, 20**

encephalitis, **56**

eye infections (newborn), 63

fever, **255, 273–274**

   temperature-taking, 255

gagging or coughs that won't stop, **20**

meningitis, **55**

red skin or small bumps, in diaper area, 253

rehydration drink for, 120

rescue breathing for, **16**

resources for parents and caregivers, 271

safeguards for, 17, 261

shrill wheezing, grunting while breathing, 252

strep throat, **267**

sudden infant death syndrome (SIDS), 253

sunscreen for, 180

thermometers, how to use on infants, 255

tugging at ear, with fever, 71

water safety with, 30

See also Newborns

Infections, **281**

   bladder, 137–138, 281

   blood (septicemia), **29**

   ear, **71**

   eye, 61, 62, 63

   fungal, **153**

   in cuts or scrapes, 29

   in wounds, 24, 29

   intestinal, 281

   lung, 29, 91

   reproductive tract (women), **236**

   respiratory, 281

   triggering seizures, 58

   urinary tract, 138

   yeast, 153, 244

Inflamed cartilage (chest), 106

Inflammatory bowel disease (IBD), 118, **128**

   kidney stones and, 136

   rectal bleeding in, 132

Influenza. *See* Flu

Information sources, for health and illness, 314

Ingrown toenails, **156**

Inhalers, for asthma, 88

Injected hormones (contraceptive), 223

Injuries

   abdominal, 22, **25**

   brain, 36, 41, 49

   eye, 29, **32**

   head, neck, and back, **36**

   life-saving skills for, **12–23**

   life-threatening, signs of, 12

   overuse, **198**

   rib, 106

   to kidney or bladder, 137

   ways to avoid, 17, 299, 301

Inner ear, *73*

Inner ear problems. *See* Ear and hearing problems

Insects

   in ear canal, 31

   See also Bites and stings

Insomnia, **286**

   complementary care for, 288

Intercourse, painful. *See under* Sexual health

Internal bleeding

   causing anemia, 272

   emergency care for, **22**

Internist, 309

Intestinal infections, **281**

Intestinal parasites, **129,** 131

Intestines, *174*

   blockage, 117, 131

   pain referred from, *176*

   See also Digestive system problems

Intrauterine device (IUD), 223, 234, 236

IPV (polio) vaccine, 250

Iris, *64, 161*

   infection (iritis), 61

Iron

   basics, 299

   food sources of, 298

Iron deficiency anemia, **272**

Irrational fears, persistent, 208–209

Irregular heartbeat.

   See Palpitations

Irregular periods.

   See Menstrual irregularities

Irritability

   in drug abuse, 213–215

   in infants or children, 251, 255

   menopausal, 232

   stress-related, 218

   with dizziness, intense hunger, 50

Irritable bladder, 140

Irritable bowel syndrome (IBS), 118, **130**

   complementary care for, 130

   kidney stones and, 136

Itching, **151**

   around swollen varicose veins, 115

   during urination (women), 244

   eyes

      after injury, 32

      of allergies, 84, 86

      of pinkeye, 62, 63

      with bump on eyelid, 62, 67

   feet, between toes, 153–154

   genital, 157, 221–222

   in ears, 73

   in nose, 40

   intense, with trouble breathing, 23, 143

   nipples, 237

   of jock itch, 153

   of lice or scabies, 157

   on eyelids, 62

   on lips or in mouth, 79

   on roof of mouth, 84

   on scalp, 157

   rectal, 126, **131–132**

   severe, at insect sting or bite, 23, 25

   skin

      extreme, constant, anywhere, 152

      See also Skin problems

   throat, 84

   vaginal, 153–155

   with puzzling tingling pain, 144, 159

   See also Rashes

IUD (intrauterine device), 223, 234, 236

J

Jaundice

   from gallstones, 122, 123

   in hepatitis, 274, 279

Jaw pain

   jaw locked shut or painful to open, 201

   upper, with stuffy nose, discharge, 94, 98

   with achy teeth upon waking, 83

   with clicking sound, 70, 78, 201

   with severe stiffness, fever, muscle spasms, 273

   with toothache, 77, 80

Jet lag, **287**

Jock itch, 153

Joint pain

   after taking a new medication, 84

   after tick bite, **45,** 144, 285

of arthritis, **182**
of bursitis, **187**
of tendinitis, **202**
severe, sudden, with red swelling
around joint, 182
with butterfly rash across nose
and cheeks, 284
with fever, 265, 281
with long-lasting fatigue, 275
Joints
arthritis, **182**
dislocation of, **35**
infection in, 281
osteoarthritis of, *165*, **182**
swollen, with sore throat,
fever, 265
Judgment problems
with drug abuse, 213
with memory loss, confusion,
wandering, 48
Jumper's knee, 200

K

Kegel exercises, 141
Kidney, *138, 174*
Kidney problems
bloody urine, 117, 136, 137
cancer, 137
chronic failure
confusion in, 206
itching and, 149
high blood pressure and, 111
infection
abdominal pain in, 117
confusion in, 206
strep throat and, 100
pain referred from, *176*
stones. *See* Kidney stones
weight gain in, 282
Kidney stones, **136,** 137, *138*
abdominal pain in, 117
urination problems with, 137
vs. appendicitis, 24
Knee, *201*
pressure point to stop
bleeding, 13
Knee problems
pain chart, **200**
dry scaly skin, itchy rash (children), 248
fractures and dislocations, **35**
Osgood-Schlatter disease, 200
patellar tendinitis, 200
sprains, **44,** 200
Kneecap, *170, 201*
Knocked-out tooth, emergency
care, **45**

L

Labyrinth, *73*
Labyrinthitis, 50, 69
Lack of energy or interest, 211
Lactose intolerance, 118
Large intestine. *See* Colon
Laryngitis, 86, 100, 101
Larynx, *163*
Latex allergies, condoms and,
244
Latissimus dorsi muscle, *171*
Laxatives, 25, 116
drug combinations to avoid
chart, **323–325**
LDL levels. *See* Cholesterol
Lead poisoning, 210, **260**
Learning disabilities, 210, 260
Legs
pain chart, **194–195**
abrupt weakness, numbness in,
on one side of body, 44
blistered, crusty patches on, 149
bones in, *170*
fractures, emergency care, **35**
low back problems and, 190
restless legs syndrome, 286
scaly dry reddish rash on, 150
scaly, reddened skin, with craterlike sores on, 149
strains and sprains, emergency
care, **44**
swelling, during pregnancy, 241
swelling, with heart
problems, 109
Lens of eye, *64, 161*
Lethargy, 213, 289
Leukemia
childhood, 247
shingles and, 177
Lice and scabies, 144, **157**
Lifting, pain during or after, 127
Ligaments
knee, *201*
pain or fatigue in, 276
sprains and strains, emergency
care, **44**
Light sensitivity
after eye injury, 32
after tick bite, 285
with blurry vision, 61
with fever, severe stiff neck, 56
with headaches, 53
with high fever, rash, 263
Light-headedness. *See* Dizziness
Lightning, being struck by, **31**
Lips
blisters on or around, 79
canker sores, **78**

cold sores, **79**
tingling or itching on, 78, 79
Liver, *174*
Liver problems
cirrhosis, 282
hepatitis, **279**
referred pain from, *176*
Lockjaw. *See* Tetanus
Longevity, increasing your,
292–305
Loose bodies (bone or cartilage),
165
Loss of appetite. *See* Appetite loss
Loss of balance
with dizziness, ear problems,
69
with sudden weakness, trouble
seeing, 44
with weakness, pale skin, 272
with weakness, tremors, 57
Loss of concentration
with depression, 211
with long-lasting fatigue, 275
with sleep disorders, 286
Loss of consciousness, **33**
after bee or wasp sting, 25
after chemical burn, 26
after cold exposure, 39
after crushing chest pain, 37
after electric shock, 31
after head injury, 36
after heat exposure, 38
after near drowning, 30
after seizures, 41, 58
CPR for an unconscious person,
14–17
emergency care, **33**
for more than a minute, 34
from choking, 18–20
if person has vomited, 34
in children, 17
in infants, 16
in severe allergic reactions, 23
in severe bleeding, 13
in shock, 22
recovery position for, 23
with weakness, numbness, 44
Loss of coordination
after cold exposure, 39
after near drowning, 30
with confusion, shakiness,
intense hunger, 206
with weakness, pasty skin, 272
with weakness, trouble seeing, 44
See also Dizziness
Loss of sexual desire, **224**
Loss of voice, 86, 100
Low back pain, *166,* **190**
complementary care for, 193,
195

with menstrual periods, 233, 234
with prostate cancer, 228
Low blood sugar. *See* Hypoglycemia
Lumbar region, *166, 191*
Lumps
in breast, **237**
in mouth or on tongue, 77, 78
in testicle, 227
Lung problems
asthma, **88,** *164*
cancer, 86
chronic bronchitis, 85, **91**
chronic obstructive pulmonary
disease (COPD), **91**
collapsed lung, 85, 105
emphysema, 85, **91**
humidifier lung, 92
infections, 29, 90
pain referred from, *176*
pneumonia, **97**
tuberculosis, 86, 274
See also Breathing problems
Lungs, *164*
Lupus, 143, **284**
Lyme disease, 45, 144, **285**
Lymph nodes
enlarged, with sores nearby, 222
painful, with flulike
symptoms, 275
swelling
in infections, 281
in neck, 183
with fever, 274
with penis problems, 230

M

Macular degeneration, 61, *162*
Malabsorption, 283
Malignant melanoma, *173,* 179
Mammograms, 320
Manic depression, 212
Mastitis, 237
Mastoiditis, 69, 71
Maxillary sinuses, *99*
Meals, creating healthy, 296–298
Measles, 86, 100, 247, **262**
baby (roseola), **265**
German, **257**
vaccine, **250**
Medications
causing glaucoma, 66
causing seizures, 41
combinations to avoid chart,
323–325
for colds or coughs, 94
pain relievers, **315**

Parkinson's disease symptoms
from, 57
safety tips, **322–325**
sudden discomfort, trouble
breathing after taking new,
22, **84**
See also Drugs
Medicine cabinet, supplies for, **21**
Meditation, 305
Melanocytes (skin), *172*
Melanoma, malignant, *173,* 179
protecting yourself from, 300
Memory problems
after blow to abdomen, 25
forgetfulness, **51**
that get worse over time, 48, 206
with alcohol abuse, 204
with drug abuse, 213
with frequent headaches, dizziness, double vision, 50, 53
with Parkinson's disease, 57
with sore mouth and tongue, 272
See also Confusion
Ménière's syndrome, 50, 69, 74
Meningitis, 53, **55,** 143, 206, 273
bacterial, in children, **56, 263**
chicken pox and, 249
ear infections and, 71
neck stiffness in, 183
triggering seizures, 58
vaccine, **250**
Menopause, **232,** 234
carpal tunnel syndrome and, 188
complementary care for, 235,236
osteoporosis and, 196
Menstrual irregularities
chart, **233–234**
absence of period, 240
breast pain in, 238
causing anemia, 272
heavy bleeding
IUDs and, 234
shock and, 22
painful urination in, 139
with eating disorders, 216, 283
with thyroid problems, 289
See also Premenstrual syndrome
Menstrual pain, 195, 233, 234
Mental confusion. *See* Confusion
Mental or psychological problems.
See under Emotions
Middle ear, *73*
airplane flying and, 68
infection, 50, 70, **71**
Migraine headaches, **52,** 53, 83
facial pain of, *176*
Milk intolerance, 118
Minerals (dietary), 299
richest sources of, 298
Miscarriage, 234

Mitral valve prolapse, 106
MMR vaccine, **250**
Mold and dust allergies, 84
Moles, *173*
ABCD test for malignant, 179
Mononucleosis, 100, 274
Mood changes
from sleep deprivation, 286, 287
in infants or children, 255
menopausal, 232
premenstrual, 241
stress-related, 218, 219
sudden, unexplained, 48,
204, 213
with depression, 211
with drug abuse, 213–215
with eating disorders, 216
with grief, 217
with long-lasting fatigue, flulike
symptoms, 275
with memory problems, 48
with weight loss, fatigue, vomiting, 283
Morning breath, 76
Morning sickness, 241
Mouth problems
chart, **77–78**
abcess, 76
bad taste, 76, 80
blisters on or around lips, 78, 79
clicking noises, 54, 70, 201
creamy yellow coating, 153
dry mouth, 34, 53, 120, 133, 182
infection, 281
itchy roof of mouth, 84
soreness, with weakness, pasty
skin, 272
sores
in children, 247, 248
with face rash, aching
joints, 258
swallowing problems, **101**
trench mouth, 78
white patches, 153, 248
white spots, with red rim, 78
Muffled hearing. *See* Ear and hearing problems
Mumps, 78, 256, **264**
vaccine, **250**
Muscle aches
of pulled muscles, 44, 106
of strains, **44**
persistent, long-lasting, without
joint pain, 276
with coughing, sneezing, congestion, sore throat, 86, 93
with fever, chills, fatigue,
headache, sore throat, 95
with fever, chills, sweating,
fatigue, 281

with fever, runny nose, swollen glands, skin rash, 262
with fever, watery diarrhea, rapid dehydration, weight loss, 131
See also Pain
Muscle cramps, **195**
Muscle spasms, with severe jaw stiffness, fever, 273
Muscle twitching, with anxiety or phobias, 208
Muscles of the body, *171*
Mushroom (wild) poisoning, 34
Murmur, heart, 168
Myopia, 61, 62, 66

N

Nails. *See* Fingernails
Naproxen sodium, **315**
Narcolepsy, 286
Nasal cavity, *163*
    See also Nose problems
Nasal decongestant sprays, 94, 99
Natural method (birth control), 224
Naturopathy, 311
Nausea and vomiting, **133**
    after blow to abdomen, 25
    after eating, with diarrhea, severe cramping, 34
    after head, neck, or back injury, 36
    after heat exposure, 38
    after spider bite or scorpion sting, 43
    blood in, 22, 282
    during pregnancy, 241
    in food poisoning, 34
    with abdominal pain, 117–118
    with breathing problems, 85–86
    with crushing or squeezing chest pain, 37
    with dizziness, 49–50
    with ear problems, 69
    with fever, 273–274
        in children, 255
    with headaches, 52, 53–54
    with hepatitis, 279
    with rectal bleeding, 131, 132
    with reddened face, intense itching, trouble breathing, 23
    with severe eye pain, 65
    with weakness on one side of body, 44
Nearsightedness, 62
Neck pain
    chart, **183–184**

from swelling neck veins, 110
from swollen lymph nodes, 281
in front, with swelling, 289
of spinal cord injury, 36
severe stiffness, with fever, 56
stress-related, 218
with headaches, 53, 54
injuries, emergency care, **36**
pressure point to stop bleeding, 13
Nervous tension
    of anxiety and phobias, 208
    premenstrual, 241
    See also Anxiety; Stress
Neuralgia, post-herpetic, 177
Neurologist, 309
Neuritis, optic, 61
Newborns
    eye infections in, 63
    maternal sexually transmitted diseases and, 221, 222
    See also Infants
Nicotine
    drug combinations to avoid chart, **323**
    See also Smoking and illness
Night sweats
    with HIV or AIDS, 221, 274
    with menopause, 232
    with tuberculosis, 274
Nightmares, 208
911 calls, what to say, **21**
Nipples, pain or change in, 237
Nits (lice), 157
Noise
    constant background (hearing), 74
    damage to hearing, 74
    not heard by others, 69, 70, 74
    sensitivity to, with headaches, 53
Nose problems
    blisters, 177
    bloody (nosebleed), 40
    broken, 40
    deviated septum, 99
    emergency care, **40**
    foreign object, 40
    foul smell, 40, 98
    oily yellow scales, 149
    postnasal drip, 76, 98, 99
    rashes, 143, 145
    runny or stuffy
        with colds, flu, 93, 95, 281
        with conjunctivitis, pinkeye, 63
        with earache, 71
        with green, yellow discharge, 98
        with migraine or cluster headache, 54

with rashes, 247, 248, 262, 265
    with sneezing, itchy eyes, 84
small growths, 98
sores, 284
Nosebleeds, emergency care, **40**
Numbness
    abrupt, on one side of body, 44
    after cold exposure, 39
    after fractures or dislocations, 35
    after head, neck, or back injury, 49, 183
    in fingers, 188
    in hands, 106
    in legs or buttocks, low back pain, 190
    with shakiness, intense hunger, 206
    with spinal problems, 183, 186, 190, 192
    with thyroid problems, 289
Nummular dermatitis, 149
Nut allergies, 84
Nutrition
    recommended dietary allowances, **298**
    tips for healthy, 296–299
    vegetables, most nutritious, **298**
    vitamins and minerals, richest food sources of, **298**
    See also Diet

O

Obesity
    Heimlich maneuver and, 18
    See also Overweight
Obsessive-compulsive disorder, 208
Obstetrician/Gynecologist (OB/GYN), 309
Obstructive sleep apnea, 286
Odors
    mouth, 76, 77–78
    odd-smelling breath, 40
    unique, in seizures, 58
Ophthalmologist, 309
Optic nerve, *64, 161*
Optic neuritis, 61
Oral cancer, 77
Orchialgia, 227
Organs of the body, *174*
    referred pain from, *176*
Orgasm, 224
Orthopedist, 309
Osgood-Schlatter disease, 200
Osteoarthritis, *165*, 182
Osteoporosis, *167*, 193, **196**

calcium food sources to
  prevent, **298**
Otitis externa, **73**
Otitis media, **71**
Otalryngologist, 309
Otosclerosis, 69, 74
Ovarian cancer, 233
Ovarian cyst, 233
Ovaries, *175*
Over-the-counter medicines
  cold or cough, 94
  drug combinations to avoid
    chart, **323–325**
  pain relievers, **315**
Overeating
  during stress, 217, 218
  of eating disorders, 216, 282
  See also Overweight
Oversleeping, 211
Overuse injuries, **198**
  bursitis and, **187**
  carpal tunnel syndrome and, 188
  hand pain from, 190
  leg pain from, 194
  tendinitis and, 199
Overweight
  artery disease and, 104
  gallstones and, 123
  healthy body weight chart, **296**
  heartburn and, 125
  Heimlich maneuver and, 18
  See also Weight gain; Weight loss

P

Pain
  pain charts
    abdominal, **117–118**
    ankle, **199**
    back, **192–193**
    breast, **237–238**
    chest, **105–106**
    foot, **199**
    headaches, **53–54**
    knee, **200**
    leg, **194–195**
    neck, **183–184**
    shoulder, **186**
  *See also under specific part of body
    or problem*
  facial. *See* Facial pain
  gas, **123**
  joint. *See* Joint pain
  low back, **190**
  menstrual, 195, 233, 234, 241
  muscle cramps, **195**
  referred, from internal
    organs, *176*

Pain relievers
  choosing, **315**
  drug combinations to avoid
    chart, **323–325**
  overuse of, ulcers and, 135
  Reye's syndrome and, **95**
Painful intercourse. *See under*
  Sexual health
Painful urination. *See*
  Urinary problems
Palpitations, 49, 106, **112**
  caffeine and, 110
Pancreas, *174*
  referred pain from, *176*
Pancreatitis, 117
Panic
  attack, 106, 208
  feeling, of an impending heart
    attack, 37
  in allergic reactions, 85
  in asthma attacks, 88
  shortness of breath with, 42
Panic disorder, 106, **208**
Pap smears, 320
Paralysis
  facial nerve, 71, 285
  in neck injury, 183
  sudden, with droopy eyelids,
    blurry vision, 34
  sudden, on one side of body, 44
Paranasal sinuses, *99*
Paranoid thinking
  depression and, 212
  with drug abuse, 214–215
Parasites, 119, **129**, 131, 222
Parkinson's disease, **57**
  muscle cramps and, 195
  swallowing problems with, 101
  urinary incontinence and, 140
Parvovirus, 257
Patella (kneecap), *170, 201*
  See also Knee problems
Patellar tendinitis, 200
Peanut allergy, 84
Pectoralis major muscle, *171*
Pedialyte, 120
Pediatrician, 309
Pelvic inflammatory disease (PID),
  223, **236**
Pelvis (pelvic girdle), *170*
  fracture, 22
Penicillin allergy, 22, 84
Penis, *175*
Penis problems, **230**
  bend in penis, 230
  cancer, 230
  erection problems, 224, **226**, 230
  itching or burning pain, then red
    bumps, 221
  pain, with trouble urinating, 137

painless sores, 222
pimplelike sore, 230
round, itchy, flat bumps, 222
soreness, inflammation of
  tip, 230
thick yellowish discharge, 222
tight foreskin, 230
watery mucus, 221
with being uncircumcised, 230
Pep pills, blood sugar raised by, 277
Peptic ulcers, **134**
Perforated eardrum, 69, 71, 72
  emergency care, **30**
Perforated ulcer, 117
Periodontitis, 77
Periods, irregular. *See*
  Menstrual irregularities
Peripheral vascular disease, 104,
  194, 199
Peripheral vision loss, 61, 65
Peritonitis, 121
Pernicious anemia, 272
Personality changes, 48, 53, 284
Peyronie's disease, 230
Pertussis (whooping cough),
  86, **269**
  vaccine, **250**
Pessimism, 211, 219
Petit mal seizures, 58
Peyronie's disease, 230
Pharynx, 163
Pharyngitis. *See* Sore throat
Phimosis, 230
Phlebitis, 194
Phobias, **208**
Physicians, 308, 309
PID. *See* Pelvic inflammatory
  disease
Piles. *See* Hemorrhoids
The Pill (contraceptive), 220
Pimples, 142, 145
Pinkeye, **63**
Pinworm, 131
Pituitary gland disorders, 137
Plantar fasciitis, 199
Plantar warts, **181**, 199
Plants, poisonous, **41**
Plaque (artery), 104, 113, *169*
Plaque (dental), 76, 77, 80
Pleurisy, 27, 86, 105
PMS. *See* Premenstrual syndrome
Pneumonia, **97**
  bacterial meningitis and, 56
  flu and, 96
  pleurisy and, 105
  vaccine, 92, 321
Poison oak or ivy, 144, **151**
Poisoning
  blood, 29
  carbon monoxide, 40, 205

emergency care, **40**
food, **34**
from household substances, **41**
from plants, **41**
lead, **260**
poison control centers, using, 41
seizures from, 58
Poisonous snakebites, **42**
Poisonous spider bites, **43**
Polio vaccine, **250**
Pollen allergies, 84
Polyps, colon, 130
Porous bones. *See* Osteoporosis
Post-traumatic stress disorder, 208
Post-herpetic neuralgia, 177
Postnasal drip, 76, 98, 99
Posture, stooped or hunched, 193, 196
Pounding heart. *See* Palpitations
Power lines, electric shock from, **32**
Pregnancy, **238**
back pain in, 192
breast pain in, 237
carpal tunnel syndrome and, 188
comfort measures during, 240–241
danger signs in, **240**
diabetes (gestational) in, 277
ectopic, 233
flu shots and, 96
Heimlich maneuver during, 18
hemorrhoids and, 126
high blood pressure and, 111
laxative caution with, 116
miscarriage, 234, 257
seizures and, 58, 59
trouble getting pregnant, PID and, 236
yeast infection and, 153
Premature ejaculation, 224
Premenstrual syndrome (PMS), **241**
complementary care for, 242
Presbyopia, 62
Pressure points, to stop bleeding, 13
Priapism, 230
Proctitis, 131
Prostate gland, *175*
Prostate problems, **228**
cancer, 228, 230
complementary care for, 231
enlarged prostate, 228, 229, 230, 231
PSA test for, 231, 321
symptoms chart, **229**
urinary problems with, 137, 140
Prostatitis, 230, 231
Protruded disk, neck pain in, 183

PSA (prostate-specific antigen) test, 231, 321
Psoriasis, 144, **159**
rectal bleeding in, 132
swimmer's ear and, 73
Psychiatrist, 309
Psychological problems. *See under* Emotions
Pulled muscle (strain), **44,** 106
Pulmonary valve, 168
Pulse
how to check for, **12**
in infants, **16**
irregular, with crushing chest pain, **37**
none, CPR to restore, **14–17**
weak, with cold, damp, bluish skin, **22**
Puncture wounds, emergency care, **28**
Pupils, *64, 161*
different sizes, 32
white area visible in, 60, 62
widened, with cold, clammy skin, irregular pulse, 22
Purpura, allergic, 247
Pus
draining from ear, 30–31, 71
draining from eye, 63
from bump on eyelid, 67
in cuts, scrapes, or wounds, 29

Q

Quadriceps muscle, *171*
Quadriceps tendon, *201*

R

Rabies, 24
Racing heartbeat. *See* Palpitations
Radius, *170*
Rashes
charts
in adults, **143–144**
in children, **247–249**
after bee or wasp sting, 25
after eating, 84
after tick bite
bull's-eye shaped, 45, 285
pink, starts near wrists, ankles, 45
blistered, crusty, or scaly skin in round patches, 149
bumpy red or purplish, with stiff neck, 56

butterfly-shaped, across cheeks, nose, 284
itchy red bumps with pale centers, 155
oily yellow scales on or near face, 149
painless purple spots, on ankles, elbows, shins, buttocks, 247
painless small gray or white bumps inside mouth, 262
raised patches of itchy pink skin, white scales, 159
red bumps and blisters that weep, crust over, 149
red, painful, blistery, on one side of body, 160
resembling sunburn, on palms, soles, 243
scaly, reddened skin, craterlike sores, on lower legs, 149
Rattlesnake bite, **42**
RDA (recommended dietary allowance) chart, **298**
Rebound congestion, from nasal sprays, 94
Receding gums, 81
Recommended dietary allowance (RDA) chart, **298**
Recovery from illness, ways to speed, 314
Recovery position, emergency, **23**
cautions with head, neck, or back injuries, 36–37
Rectal bleeding and itching chart, **131–132**
after blow to abdomen, 25
bright red bleeding, 131
itching and bright red blood in stool, 132
stools with red blood, or blood on toilet paper, 126
with vomiting or coughing blood, abdominal tenderness, 22
with watery diarrhea or pus, fever, rapid weight loss, 131
See also Bowel movements
Rectal exams, 320, 321
Rectum, *175*
Rectus abdominis muscle, *171*
Referred pain, from internal organs, *176*
Reflux, gastroesophageal, **125**
Rehabilitation, ways to speed, 314
Rehydration drink recipe, 38, **120**
Relaxation, **303**
exercises, 305
inability to achieve, 208
techniques, 305
See also Health and fitness basics

INDEX

Repeated actions, in obsessive-compulsive disorder, 208
Repetitive motion injuries. *See* Overuse injuries
Reproductive systems, *175*
Rescue breathing
for adults, **14–15**
for infants and children, **16–17**
Respiratory infections, 281
See also Breathing problems
Restless legs syndrome, 286–287
Restlessness
in infants, 50, 71, 254
with drug abuse, 213, 214
Retina, *64, 161*
macular degeneration of, 61
Retinal detachment, 61, 162
Reye's syndrome, **95,** 256
Rheumatic fever, 100, **265,** 267
Rheumatoid arthritis, 182
Rheumatologist, 309
Rhinitis, allergic, 84
Rhythm method
(birth control), 224
Ribs, *170*
injuries, 27, 106
RICE treatment, 35, **198**
Ringing in ears, 30, 68, 69, 70, 72
tinnitus, **74**
Ringworm, 144, 248
Rocky Mountain spotted fever, **45,** 143
Rosacea, **145**
Roseola, 248, **265**
Rotator cuff injury, 186
Rubella (German measles), 247, **257**
maternal, 60
vaccine, 60, **250,** 258, 263
Rumbling sounds from abdomen, 118
Running injuries, 198, 200
shin splints, 194
Runny nose. *See under* Nose problems
Ruptured eardrum, 69, 71, 72
emergency care, **30**

S

Sacrum (base of spine), *170, 191*
SAD (seasonal affective disorder), 212
Sadness, persistent, 211
Safe sex, **224**
condoms and, 220
Safety measures
infants or children, **17, 261**

to stay healthy, 299, 301
Saliva
sticky, with dry mouth, 53, 120, 133
Salivary gland disorders, 78
mumps, **264**
Scabies and lice, 144, **157**
Scalp problems
cuts, scrapes, or wounds, 29
oily yellow scales, 149
round, scaly, itchy rash, with later bald spots, 248
small grayish-white oval eggs, 157
yellow, scaly rash (infants), 149, 249
Scapula (shoulder blade), *170*
Scarlet fever, 247, **266,** 274
Sciatic nerve, *166*
Scorpion stings, **43**
Scrapes
emergency care, **28**
infections in, 281
Scrotum, pain or swelling in, 227
Seafood allergies, 84
Seasonal affective disorder (SAD), 212
Seborrheic dermatitis, 149
in children, 249
Second-degree burns, 26
Secondary glaucoma, 65–66
Seeing or hearing things that aren't there, 58
Seeing problems. *See* Vision problems
Seizures, **58**
after chemical burn, 26
after heat exposure, **38**
after snakebite, **43**
emergency care for, **41**
fever, **256,** 273
when to call for help, **41**
with fever, trouble seeing, odd-smelling breath, 40
with frequent headaches, double vision, 50
with high fever, severe stiff neck, 56
Self-destructive behavior, 217
Self-exams, **319**
breast, **239,** 319
skin cancer, 319
testicular, 319
weight, 319
See also Tests
Sensitive teeth, **81**
Sensitivity to light. *See* Light sensitivity
Septic shock, 29
Septicemia, **29**

Severe bleeding. *See* Bleeding
Sexual health
anal intercourse, 131
birth control health risks, 220–224
loss of sexual desire, **224**
premenstrual, 241
painful intercourse
with infections, 138, 221, 233, 244
with menopause, 232
with penis or erection problems, 228, 230
safe sex, **224**
See also AIDS
Sexually transmitted diseases (STDs)
chart, **221–222**
AIDS, 221
cold sores, **79**
hepatitis, **279**
intrauterine devices and, 223
painful urination in, 137, 138
pelvic inflammatory disease, **236**
rectal bleeding in, 131
yeast infections, 153, 244
Shaking. *See* Trembling
Shampoos, for head lice, 157–158
Shingles, 144, **160**
chest pain of, 106
Shins
pain in, with or after exercise, 194
purple rash on, 247
Shivering
with drowsiness, clumsiness, after cold exposure, 30, **39,** 205
See also Trembling
Shock
anaphylactic (from allergy), **22**
electric, **31**
emergency care, **22**
septic, 29
severe bleeding and, **13**
Shock from allergy, **22,** 85, 143, 205
Shortness of breath
breathing problems chart, **85–86**
emergency care, **42**
in anxiety and phobias, 208
See also Breathing problems
Shoulder blade, *170*
Shoulder pain
chart, **186**
with headaches, 54
Sickle-cell anemia, 230, 257
Side vision, loss of, 61, 65
SIDS (sudden infant death syndrome), **253**
Sigmoidoscopy, 320
Sinus headaches, 52, 54

Sinus infection. *See* Sinusitis
Sinuses, 98, *99, 163*
Sinusitis, **98**
  airplane ear and, 68
  bacterial meningitis and, 56
  bad breath of, 76
  colds or flu and, 94, 96
  headaches of, 52, 54
  toothache and, 80
Sitting up quickly, dizziness
  from, 50
Skeletal system, *170*
Skin cancer, *173,* **179**
  itching and, 149
  protecting yourself from, **300**
  sunburn and, 178
Skin problems
  charts
    rashes in adults, **143–144**
    rashes in children, **247–249**
  acne, **142**
  athlete's foot, 153
  blisters, **145**
  bluish or pale skin
    with crushing chest pain, 37
    with trouble breathing, 22
  boils, **146**
  bruises, **147**
  calluses, **148**
  cancer. *See* Skin cancer
  carbuncles, 146
  constant, extreme itchiness any-
    where, 154
  corns, **148**
  crusty, scaly round patches, 152
  darkened color, with weight loss,
    hair loss, 283
  dermatitis, **149**
  discoloring, 104
  eczema, **152**
  frostbite, **39**
  fungal infections, **153**
  hives, **155**
  hot, reddened skin, with itching,
    trouble breathing, 23
  ingrown toenails, **156**
  itching (mild), without rash, 149
  jock itch, 153
  knobby lumps on elbows, finger
    joints, 182
  lice, **157**
  oily yellow scales on or near
    face, 149
  painful tingling, extreme sensi-
    tivity, on one side, 160
  paleness, with pale gums,
    nailbeds, 272
  pink or red rash, after chemical
    contact, 149

poison oak or ivy, **151**
psoriasis, **159**
purple rash, spots, 56, 143, 247,
  273
red blotches, in hot weather, 249
red bumps and blisters that weep,
  crust over, 149
rosacea, 145
round, oozing red spots, 149
scaly, reddened skin, with craterlike sores, 149
shingles, **160**
sunburn, **178**
skin products and, **150**
thick, itchy, dry red patches, 149
warts, **180**
yellow skin, 122, 123, 204, 216,
  274, 279, 282
Skin products, choosing, 150
Skin self-exam, **178**
Skull, *170*
Skull fractures
  bacterial meningitis and, 56
  See also Head injuries
Slapped cheek disease (fifth disease), 248, **257**
Sleep problems, **286**
  adenoids and, 103
  apnea, 103, 206, 287
  constant urge to move legs while
    trying to sleep, 287
  depression and, 211
  falling asleep suddenly (day-
    time), 211
  insomnia, 287
  jet lag, 287
  narcolepsy, 287
  restless legs syndrome, 287
  stiff neck from sleeping wrong
    way, 184
  stress-related, 217, 218
  too little or too much sleep, 55
  tooth grinding and, 78, **83**
  with chronic fatigue or pain, 193,
    275, 276, 282,
  with menopause, 232, 235
Sleepiness. *See* Drowsiness
Sleeping pills, drug combinations
  to avoid chart, **323–325**
Slings, for fractures or
  dislocations, **35**
Slurred speech. *See*
  Speech problems
Small intestine, *174*
  blockage of, 117, 131
  referred pain from, *176*
Smell
  unique, in seizures, 58
Smoker's cough, 86, 90

Smoking and illness, **299**
  birth control pills and, 220, 325
  quitting smoking, 299
Snakebites, **42**
Sneezing
  with allergies, 84
  with colds or flu, 93, 95
  with conjunctivitis, 63
  with respiratory infections, 281
Snoring, 286, 287
Snorting, while asleep, 286
Social support, to stay healthy,
  301, 303
Social withdrawal
  stress-related, 219
  with depression, 211, 212
  with eating disorders, 216
Sore throat, **100**
  after tick bite, (lyme disease), 285
  strep throat, 100, **267**
  with colds, 93
  with cough, fever, red bumps,
    (measles), 262
  with ear infection, 71
  with flu, 86, 95, 274
  with long-lasting fatigue, joint
    pain, 275
  with lost voice, 86
  with low fever, swollen glands,
    fatigue, 100, 274
  with pinkeye, 63
  with purple spotted rash, 247
  with red or white spots on
    tonsils, 102
  with respiratory infections, 281
  with scarlet fever, 247, 274
Spasms. *See* Muscle spasms
Specialists, 309
Speech problems
  after cold exposure, 205
  after head injury, 36, 205
  after snakebite, 43
  in epileptic seizures, 58
  sudden, with weakness on one
    side of body, 44
  with memory loss, wandering,
    confusion, 48
Spermicides, 223
Sphenoid sinuses, *99, 163*
Sphincter muscle tear, 131, 132
Spider bites, **43**
Spider veins. *See* Varicose veins
Spinal column, *166, 167, 170, 191*
Spinal compression fractures, *167*
Spinal cord, *166,* 183
Spinal curvature, of
  osteoporosis, *167*
Spinal injuries
  emergency care, **36**
  neck pain of, 183

INDEX

Spinal stenosis, 192
Spinal tumor, 192
Spine, *166, 167, 170, 191*
Spleen, *174*
Splints, for fractures or dislocations, **35–36**
Spondylitis, ankylosing, 192
Spondylosis, cervical, 183
Sprains, **44**
    back, 191, 193
    knee, 200
    leg, 194
    RICE treatment for, 198
Squamous cell carcinoma, 179
Squamous cells of skin, *172*
Standing up quickly, dizziness in, 50
Stare, blank or fixed, 41, 57, 58, 260
Stasis dermatitis, 150
STDs. *See* Sexually transmitted diseases
Sterility
    from STDs, 221
    mumps and, 264
Sterilization (contraceptive), 220
Sternum, *170*
Steroid inhalers, 88, 154, 155
Stiffness
    from sleeping wrong way, 184
    morning, in arthritis, 182
    of fingers or toes, with scaly rash, 159
    of neck (severe), with flulike symptoms, 56, 263
    with headaches, 53, 56, 263
    See also Pain
Stings and bites. *See* Bites and stings
Stomach, *174*
    abdominal pain chart, **117–118**
    anemia, from bleeding in, 272
    cancer, 272
    drug combinations to avoid chart, **323–325**
    food allergies, **84**
    gastritis, **134**
    heartburn, **124**
    hiatal hernia, 127
    nausea and vomiting, **133**
    pain referred from, *176*
    stomach flu, 117, 133
    stress-related problems, 218, 219
    ulcers, 117, **134**
    See also Abdominal pain; Digestive system problems
Stools, blood in. *See* Blood in stools
Stooped or hunched posture, 193, 196
Strains, **44**

back, 191, 193
    leg, 194
    neck, 184
Strangulated hernia, 127, 131
Street drugs
    chart of common, **214–215**
    blood poisoning and, 29
Strep throat, 100, **267**
    bad breath and, 76
    colds and, 94
    in children, **267**
    tonsillitis and, 103
Stress, **218**
    how to reduce, 219, 292, 303, 305
    in low back pain, 191, 193
    rating your level of, **302–303**
Stress disorder, post-traumatic, 208
Stress incontinence, 140
Stroke, **44**, 49, 53, **113**
    artery disease and, 104
    confusion in, 205
    dizziness in, 49
    emergency care, **44**
    eye and vision problems with, 61
    high blood pressure and, 111
    urinary incontinence in, 140
Stuffy nose. *See under* Nose problems
Stumbling. *See* Loss of coordination
Styes, 62, **67**
Subdural hematoma, 49
Subdural hemorrhage, 49
Sudden infant death syndrome (SIDS), **253**
Suicidal thoughts, 211–212
Sunburn, **178**
Sunglasses, choosing, 60
Sunlight
    cataracts and, 60
    hives from, 155
    sensitivity to, 284
    skin cancer and, 178–180
    wrinkles and, 178
Sunscreen, 178, 180
    sun protection factor (SPF) and, **180**
    quiz to rate your knowledge of, 300
Swallowing problems, **101**
    after spider bite or scorpion sting, 43
    with pain in front of neck, 289
    with sore throat, 100
    with stiff jaw, muscle spasms, 273
    with trouble breathing, nausea, vomiting, diarrhea, 34
    See also Choking
Sweat glands in skin, *172*

Sweating
    heavy
        after spider bite, 43
        with clammy skin, headache, dizziness, 38
        in feverish children, 255
        just before fainting, 33
        night
            in HIV or AIDS, 221, 274
            with menopause. *See* Hot flashes
            with tuberculosis, 274
        with food poisoning, 34
        with infections, 281
        with kidney stones, 117
        with shakiness, hunger, 206, 278
        with sudden, crushing chest pain, 37
        with thyroid problems, 283, 288
Swelling
    after skin burns, 26
    after snakebite, 42
    after spider bite or scorpion sting, 43
    deep swelling in eyelids, lips, tongue, or genitals, 155
    during pregnancy, 115, 240, 241
    in fractures or dislocations, 35
    in front of neck (goiter), 282, 283, 289
    in infection, 281
    in lymph nodes. *See* Lymph nodes
    in sprains or strains, 44
    in testicles, scrotum, 227
    in varicose veins, 115, 195
    rapid, of face, tongue, with trouble breathing, 23
Swimmer's ear, 70, **73**
Syndromes
    carpal tunnel, **188**
    chronic fatigue, 219, **275**
    Cushing's, 282
    irritable bowel, 118, 129, **130,** 136
    Ménière's, 50, 69, 74
    premenstrual, **241**
    restless legs, 286
    Reye's, **95,** 256
    toxic shock, 49, 143, 206, **243,** 273
Synovial fluid, 165
Syphilis, 222

T

Tailbone, *170*
Talking excessively, 210, 214

Tampons, 243, 244
Tarsals, *170*
Taste
  bad, in mouth, 76, 77, 78, 80
  unusual, in seizures, 58
TB. *See* Tuberculosis
Td vaccine, **250**, 321
Teary eyes. *See* Eye problems
Teas, herbal, 277
Teeth. *See* Tooth problems
Teething, **268**
  caring for first teeth, **268**
Temperature, how to take, **255**
Temporomandibular disorder
  (TMD), 54, 70, 78, **201**
  toothache and, 80
Temporomandibular joint (TMJ),
  170, 202
Tendinitis, 186, 199, 200, **202**
  RICE treatment for, 198
Tendon pain, with no joint
  pain, 276
Tennis elbow, 202, **203**
Tension
  from stress, 218
  headaches, **52**, 54
  nervous (anxiety), 208
Terror, feelings of, with rapid
  heartbeat, 208
Testes, *175*
Testicle problems, **227**
  self-exam for, 319
  with sharp back pains, trouble
    urinating, 136
  with swollen neck glands below
    ear, low fever, 264
Testicular cancer, 227
Testicular torsion, 227
Tests (diagnostic)
  blood pressure, 319
  cholesterol, 319
  fecal occult blood, 320
  menopause, 235
  Pap, 320
  PSA, 321
  to stay healthy, 319–321
  See also Self-exams
Tetanus (lockjaw), 273
  vaccine, **250**, 321
Tetanus and diphtheria (TD)
  vaccine, **250**, 321
Thermometers, how to choose, 255
Thinking difficulty
  with drug abuse, 213–215
  with chronic fatigue, joint
    pain, 275
  with low energy, weight gain for
    no reason, 289
  with memory loss, confusion,
    wandering, 48

Third-degree burns, 26
Thirst (extreme)
  with cold, damp skin,
    faintness, 22
  with need to urinate often,
    277, 283
  with sticky saliva, dry mouth,
    headache, 53, 133, 134
Thoracic region of spine, *191*
Throat problems
  adenoids enlarged, 103
  burning, sour taste, 124
  burning pain, with foul-smelling
    white debris, 102
  creamy yellow or white coating,
    78, 153, 248
  feeling of lump, trouble getting
    food down, 101
  itching, with runny eyes, sneez-
    ing, 84
  red all over, or red streaks, 100
  red tonsils, or tonsils with white
    or yellow spots, 102
  sore throat, **100**
  sores, with swollen joints,
    butterfly-shaped rash, 284
  strep throat, 100, **267**
  swallowing difficulty, **101**
  throat swelling shut, with trouble
    breathing, 22
  tonsillitis, **102**
  with high fever, fuzzy tongue,
    bright red rash, 266–267
Thrombophlebitis, 194
Thrush, 78, 88, 153, 248
Thyroid problems, **288**
  carpal tunnel syndrome and, 188
  hyperthyroidism, 283, 288
  hypothyroidism, 188, 282,
    289
  muscle cramps with, 195
  thyroiditis, 183, 289
  weight gain or loss in, 282, 283
Thyroiditis, 183, **289**
TIA. *See* Transient ischemic attack
Tibia, *170, 201*
Tibialis anterior muscle, *171*
Tick bites
  first aid, **45**
  Lyme disease and, 45, 144, **285**
  Rocky Mountain spotted fever
    and, 45, 143
Tinea cruris (jock itch), 153
Tinea pedis (athlete's foot), 153
Tingling
  after electric shock, 31
  in fingers, with shooting wrist
    pain, 188
  in legs or buttocks, with low back
    pain, 190

  in skin, with blistery rash, 160
  of seizures, 41
  on lips or in mouth, 78, 79
  with back pain, 190, 192
  with neck pain, 183, 186
  See also Numbness
Tinnitus, 70, **74**
TMD. *See* Temporomandibular
  disorder
TMJ (temporomandibular joint),
  170, 202
Tobacco hazards. *See* Eight Ways to
  Feel Your Best
Toddlers
  safety cautions for, **261**
  water cautions with, 30, 261
  See also Infants
Toenails, ingrown, **156**
Toes
  athlete's foot, 153
  bent in clawlike position, 185
  big toe pain, swelling, 185, 187
  bluish, 194
  broken or injured, **35**
  bunions, **185**
  corns or calluses, **148**
  hammertoes, **185**
  itching, scaling, redness
    between, 153
  joint pain in, 182, 185
  lump on side of big toe, 185
  stiffness, with scaly rash, 159
Tongue, *163*
Tongue problems
  canker sores, 78
  fuzzy, with fever, red rash, 266
  lump, 77
  peeling, 267
  rapid swelling, with trouble
    breathing, 23
  soreness, with pale skin,
    fatigue, 272
  tingling just before a sore
    appears, 78
  white or gray sores, with red
    rims, 78
Tonic-clonic seizures, 58
Tonsillectomy, 102
Tonsillitis, **102**
Tonsils, *102, 163*
  bright red, 100, 102
  white coating on, 103, 267
  white coating on, with fuzzy
    tongue (children), 274
Tooth problems
  chart, **77–78**
  abscess, 77, **80**
  decay, 80
  enamel damage, from constant
    vomiting, 216

grinding, 80, **83**, 201
knocked-out tooth, emergency
care, **45**
pressure, especially upper jaw, 98
sensitivity, 81
taking care of your teeth, **82,
304–305**
toothache, 76, 77, **80**
upon waking, 83
Toothpaste, choosing, 82
Torsion, testicular, 227
Tourniquets, for snakebite, 43
Toxic shock syndrome, 49, 143,
206, **243**, 273
Trachea (windpipe), *163*
Tranquilizers, drug combinations
to avoid chart, **323–325**
Transient ischemic attack (TIA),
61, 205
See also Stroke
Trapezius muscle, *171*
Trembling
after cold exposure, 39
hands or head, with weakness,
depression, 57
hands, with increased appetite,
weight loss, 288
in alcohol or drug abuse, 204,
214, 215
with intense hunger, dizziness,
50, 206, 278
Tremors
after snakebite, 43
of head or hands, 57
Trench mouth, 78
Triceps muscle, *171*
Trichomoniasis, 222
Tricuspid (atrial) valve, 168
Trigger finger, 203
Triple vision, 60
Tubal ligation, 220
Tuberculosis (TB), 86, 274
pleurisy and, 105
Twitching muscles
in anxiety and phobias, 208
of muscle cramps, 195
with seizures, 41
Twitching skin, after snakebite, 43

U

Ulcerative colitis, 118, **128**, 132
Ulcers, 106, 118, 133, **134**
anemia and, 272
perforated, 117
Ulna bone, *170*
Ultraviolet (UV) rays, 60, 178, 180,
300

Umbilical cord cutting, in emer-
gency childbirth, **28**
Unconsciousness. *See* Loss of con-
sciousness
Uncoordinated movements. *See*
Loss of coordination
Uneven heartbeat
See Palpitations
Upper Respiratory, 163
Upset stomach. *See* Abdominal
pain; Nausea and vomiting
Ureter, *138, 174, 175*
Urethra, *174, 175*
enlarged prostate and, 228
infections in, 138
Urge incontinence, 140
Uric acid, gout and, 182
Urinary bladder, *174, 175*
Urinary problems
chart, **137**
bladder infections, 137, 138, 281
bladder, pain referred from, *176*
blood in urine, 25, 117, 137,
233, 281
burning with urination, 138,
222, 244
complementary care for, 140
dark, cloudy, or murky urine,
117, 136, 138, 274, 279, 282,
284
dark yellow urine, after diarrhea,
vomiting, 120, 133, 134
during pregnancy, 241
frequent urinating, 110, 136,
233, 277, 281
incontinence, **140**
interstitial cystitis, 137
Kegel exercises for, 141
kidney failure, 137
kidney stones, 117, **136,** *138*
leaking urine, 140
painful urination, **138,** 281
smelly urine, 117, 138
urge to urinate you can't
control, 140
weak stream, 228
with prostate problems, 228
with sudden weight gain or loss,
282, 283
Urinary tract infections, 138, 281
causing incontinence, 140
during pregnancy, 241
kidney stones and, 136
Urologist, 309
Uterine fibroids, 234
Uterus, *175*
UVA or UVB rays. *See*
Ultraviolet (UV) rays
Uveitis, 61

V

Vaccinations
for adults, 321
schedule for children, **250**
Vagina, *175*
Vaginal problems, **244**
dryness, in menopause, 232, 235
fishy odor, with watery grayish or
yellow discharge, 244
foul-smelling discharge, aching
abdomen, 236
heavy greenish-yellow
discharge, 222
thick, white, cheesy discharge,
153, 244
thick yellowish discharge, burning urination, 222
unusual bleeding, after blow to
abdomen, 25
urination problems with, 137
vaginosis, bacterial, 244
watery mucus, burning with
urination, 221
with diabetes, 283
with IUDs, 236
with menstrual irregularities,
233
yeast infections, 153, 244
yellow or green and foul-smelling
discharge, 222, 244
Vaporizers. *See* Humidifiers
and vaporizers
Varicella zoster virus (Var)
vaccine, **250**
Varicocele, testicular, 227
Varicose veins, **115**
during pregnancy, 241
in scrotum, 227
leg pain in, 195
See also Hemorrhoids
Vasectomy, 220
Vegetables, top ten most
nutritious, 298
Veins
blue or purple, with swelling,
itching, 115
deep-vein thrombosis, 194
in anus, inflamed or swollen, 126
in leg, hard, cordlike swelling
of vein, with pain, burning,
194
in leg, swelling, warmth, redness
throughout, bluish toes, 194
in neck, swollen, painful, 110
in scrotum, swollen, 227
phlebitis or thrombosis, 194
spider, 115
Ventricle, left, *168*

Ventricle, right, *168*
Vertebrae, *166, 167*
Vertebral column (spine), *170*
Vertigo, in inner ear problems, 50
Violent or aggressive feelings, behavior, 208, 214–215
Viral infections, 281
Vision problems
  chart, **61–62**
  after eye injury, 32
  after tick bite, 45, 285
  blurred vision
    fogged-over feeling, 60, 62
    in near or farsightedness, 62
    with intense thirst, frequent urination, 277
    with severe eye pain, 61, 65
    with trouble breathing, muscle paralysis, 34
  cataracts, **60**, 62, 161, *162*
  dark, empty area in center of vision, 61, *162*
  dim or distorted vision, 61, 161, *162*
  double vision
    in one eye only, 60
    with frequent headaches, 50, 53
  eyestrain, 62
  flashes of light, 54, 61
  floaters across field of vision, 61, 62
  glaucoma, 53, 61, **65,** *162*
  halos around lights, 61, 65
  headaches, 56
  iritis, 61
  light sensitivity, 32, 53, 56, 60
  macular degeneration, 61, *162*
  peripheral vision loss, 61, 65, *162*
  retinal detachment, 61, *162*
  "second sight," 60
  straight lines looking wavy, 61
  sudden blindness, often in one eye only, 44
  temporary change in near vision, 60
  triple vision, 60
  uveitis, 61
  with epileptic seizures, 58
  with headaches, 52, 53–54
  with shakiness, hunger, 206
  with sudden weakness on one side of body, 44
  See also Eye problems
Vitamins, 298, **299**
  richest food sources of, 298
  vitamin B12 deficiency anemia, 272

vitamin C, 94, 298, 299
vitamin E, 108
Vivid dreams, 286
Vocal cords, *163*
Voice, loss of, 86, 100
Vomiting, 117–118, **133,** 281
  See also Nausea and vomiting
Vulva, redness, itching on, 244

W

Waking too early, 211
Walking pneumonia, 97
Wandering, with memory loss, confusion, 48
Warning signs, of impending seizure, 58
Warts, **181 ,** 199, 222
Washing hands, over and over, 208
Wasp stings, **25**
  allergic reaction to, **22,** 25
  emergency care, **23**
  removing the stinger, 25
Water moccasin snake bite, **42**
Water safety, for infants or children, 17
Watery eyes. *See* Eye problems
Weakness
  abrupt, on one side of body, 44
  after neck injury, 183
  in arms and legs, with neck pain, 183, 186
  in one or both legs, with low back pain, 190
  with pain, chronic cough, 86
  with light-headedness, just before fainting, 33
Weight
  healthy body weight chart, **296**
  how to maintain a healthy, 295
Weight gain
  sudden gain or loss chart, **282–283**
  from fluid retention, 110
  in depression, 211
  premenstrual, 241
Weight loss
  sudden gain or loss chart, **282–283**
  abdominal pain and, 118, 131
  despite increased appetite, 288
  rapid, with diarrhea, fever, 118, 131
Wheals, of hives, 155
Wheezing
  even after light activity, or lying down, 109

from smoking, 86
high-pitched, with choking, 18, 20
with asthma, 42, 85, 88
with bronchitis, 42, 85, 90, 91
See also Breathing problems
When you are sick, steps to follow, **312–315**
Whiplash, 50, 184
Whiteheads, 142
Whooping cough, 86, 256, **269**
  vaccine, **250**
Withdrawal symptoms
  from alcohol, 204
  from caffeine, 54
Women's health resources, **245**
Worry, severe, persistent, 208
Wounds
  bleeding, with object still stuck in, 13
  blood poisoning from, 29
  emergency care, **29**
  from animal bites, 24
  infection in, 29, 281
  internal bleeding and, 22
  puncture, 29
  severe bleeding, emergency care, **13**
  tetanus and, 273
  See also Bleeding
Wrinkles, premature, 178
Wrist bones, *170*
Wrist problems
  arthritis and, 182
  broken or injured, 35
  carpal tunnel syndrome and, **188**
  exercises for, **189**
  pain, 188, **190**
  pressure point to stop bleeding, 13
  tendinitis, 203

Y

Yawning
  to open up ears, 68
  with light-headedness, just before fainting, 33
Yeast infection, **153,** 244, 248
Yellow skin or eyes, 122, 123, 204, 216, 274, 279, 282

The Self-Care Advisor

Editor
John Poppy

Art Director
Robin Terra

Executive Editor
Eric Olsen

Senior Editors
Anne Milner, Annie Stine

Copy Editors
Ellen Rush, *chief*
Will Rose, Cynthia Rubin

Associate Art Director
Margery Cantor

Designers
Crystal Guertin, Shannon Laskey

Writers
Barbara Boughton, Ingfei Chen,
Jeanie Puleston Fleming,
Deborah Franklin, Katherine
Griffin, Sarah Henry, Peter Jaret,
Katherine Kam, Susan LaCroix,
Lisa Margonelli, Constance
Matthiessen, Clark Norton,
Mary Purpura, Laurie Udesky,
Rob Waters

Researchers
Felicity John, Masaye Waugh,
Kimberly Wong

Indexer
Karen Hollister

Production Manager
Pat E. Jensen

Consulting Editor
Susan West

HEALTH MAGAZINE

Editor-in-Chief
Barbara Paulsen

Executive Editor
Bruce K. Kelly

Managing Editor
Constance Hale

Manufacturing Director
Linda K. Smith

TIME INC HEALTH

Chief Operating Officer
Martha A. Lorini

TIME LIFE INC.

Chairman & CEO
Jim Nelson

President & COO
Steven L. Janas

TIME-LIFE
TRADE PUBLISHING

Vice President & Publisher
Neil Levin

**Senior Director of Acquisitions
& Editorial Resources**
Jennifer Pearce

**Director of New
Product Development**
Carolyn Clark

Director of Marketing
Inger Forland

**Director of New
Product Development**
Teresa Graham

Director of Trade Sales
Dana Hobson

Director of Custom Publishing
John Lalor

Director of Special Markets
Robert Lombardi

Director of Design
Kate L. McConnell

THE SELF-CARE ADVISOR

Project Manager
Robert Somerville

Technical Specialist
Monika Lynde

Production Manager
Jim King

Quality Assurance
Stacy L. Eddy

Pre-Press Services
Time-Life Imaging Center

Color illustrations for The Body Illustrated by **Enid V. Hatton.**

Color photograph and modifications, page 162: Kevin Candland.

Black-and-white illustrations: Neil Hardy: pages 64, 73, 201, 202. Jeffrey Smith: 13, 14, 15, 16, 18, 19, 20, 23, 32, 36, 99, 123, 138, 189, 191, 239.

Color photographs, page 173: Moles A, B, and D: Custom Medical Stock Photo. Mole C: Biophoto Associates/Photo Researchers, Inc.

Cover photographs: left to right, Peter Correz/Stone, Laurence Monneret/Stone, Scott T. Baxter/PhotoDisc.

Acknowledgments

This book would not be as helpful and accurate as it is without the assistance of health professionals in every part of the United States—men and women who answered hundreds of questions, offered guidance and resources, and repeatedly displayed their commitment to improving information about health care. We owe them our sincerest thanks.

Lifesaving Skills & First Aid
Sheldon Clark, M.D.
R. Scott Jacobs, M.D.
Eric A. Weiss, M.D.

Head & Nervous System
Seymour Diamond, M.D.
Robert G. Feldman, M.D.
R. Michael Gallagher, D.O.
Howard Gruetzner, M.Ed.
W. Michael Scheld, M.D.
Mark Spitz, M.D.
Cathi Thomas, R.N., M.S.

Eyes
Ronald M. Burde, M.D.
Monica L. Monica, M.D., Ph.D.

Ears
Richard Goode, M.D.
Michael Seidman, M.D.

Mouth
Bruce Bagley, M.D.
Donald Collins, D.D.S., M.P.H.
Jon Richter, D.M.D., Ph.D.
Thomas Weida, M.D.

Nose, Throat, Lungs & Chest
Stephen Astor, M.D.
Robert Breiman, M.D.
James Cook, M.D.
Donald Donovan, M.D.
Dominick Iacuzio, Ph.D.
Clayton Kersting, M.D.
Barry Make, M.D.
Harold Nelson, M.D.
Carol Reid, M.D.
Nathan Schultz, M.D.

Heart & Circulation
Ralph S. Paffenbarger, Jr.,
   M.D., Dr.P.H.
Rodman D. Starke, M.D.
Katharine Weiser, M.D.

Stomach, Abdomen & Digestive System
Quan-Yang Duh, M.D.
Johannes Koch, M.D.
Peter McNally, D.O.
Stephen Pardys, M.D.
Theodore R. Schrock, M.D.
Marvin Schuster, M.D.

Skin, Scalp & Nails
Deborah Allen, M.D.
William Epstein, M.D.
Glenn B. Gastwirth, D.P.M.
Richard Glogau, M.D.
Michael Heffernan, M.D.
Robert Jackson, M.D.
Mark Lebwohl, M.D.
Jerome Z. Litt, M.D.
Alan R. Shalita, M.D.
David Taplin
Stephen Tyring, M.D., Ph.D.

Muscles, Bones & Joints
Daniel Benson, M.D.
Stanley Bigos, M.D.
Doyt Conn, M.D.
Scott Dye, M.D.
James Garrick, M.D.
David Kell, M.D.
Nancy Liu, M.D.
John Rugh, Ph.D.
Cody Wasner, M.D.

Behavior & Emotions
Robert Bailey, M.D.
Herbert Freudenberger, Ph.D.
Nancy Kennedy, Dr.P.H.
Vivian Hanson Meehan, R.N.,
   B.A., D.Sc.
Robert Sapolsky, Ph.D.
Rick Seymour, M.A.
Joe Takamine, M.D.
Scott Thomas, Ph.D.

Sexual, Men's & Women's Health
Stanley Althof, Ph.D.
Sondra Lynne Carter, M.D.
Stuart Howards, M.D.
Tom F. Lue, M.D.
Joseph E. Oesterling, M.D.
Michael Spence, M.D., M.P.H.
Paul Stumpf, M.D.

Children's Health
David Batts
Armando Correa, M.D.
Robert Prentice, M.D.
S. Norman Sherry, M.D.
Donald Shifrin, M.D.

General Problems
Grover Bagby, Jr., M.D.
Kathleen Bliese, M.D.
Alan Blum, M.D.
Robert Katz, M.D.
Rick Kellerman, M.D.
Clete Kushida, M.D., Ph.D.
Emmanuel Mignot, M.D., Ph.D.

Staying Healthy
Pamela Stitzlein Davies, R.N., M.S.
Bruce Gollub, M.D.
Stirling Puck, M.D.
Robert Rakel, M.D.
Rachel Naomi Remen, M.D.
John Stoeckle, M.D.
David Stutz, M.D.
Mary Wade
Ssu Weng, M.D.

Medicines: Playing It Safe
Hemlata Chopra, Pharm.D.
Frederic J. Zucchero, M.A., R.Ph.

If I'd known I was going to live this long,
I'd have taken better care of myself.